BASIC AND CLINICAL SCIENCE COURSE™

Ophthalmic Pathology and Intraocular Tumors

Section 4

2015–2016

(Last major revision 2011–2012)

AMERICAN ACADEMY® OF OPHTHALMOLOGY
The Eye M.D. Association

The American Academy of Ophthalmology is accredited by the Accreditation Council for Continuing Medical Education to provide continuing medical education for physicians.

The American Academy of Ophthalmology designates this enduring material for a maximum of 10 *AMA PRA Category 1 Credits*™. Physicians should claim only the credit commensurate with the extent of their participation in the activity.

Originally released June 2011; reviewed for currency September 2, 2014; CME expiration date: June 1, 2016. *AMA PRA Category 1 Credits*™ may be claimed only once during this period.

BCSC® volumes are designed to increase the physician's ophthalmic knowledge through study and review. Users of this activity are encouraged to read the text and then answer the study questions provided at the back of the book.

To claim *AMA PRA Category 1 Credits*™ upon completion of this activity, learners must demonstrate appropriate knowledge and participation in the activity by taking the posttest for Section 4 and achieving a score of 80% or higher. For further details, please see the instructions for requesting CME credit at the back of the book.

Cover image: From BCSC Section 12, *Retina and Vitreous*. Ultra-wide-field fundus photograph from a patient with von Hippel–Lindau disease. *Courtesy of Colin A. McCannel, MD.*

MIX
Paper from responsible sources
FSC www.fsc.org FSC® C103061

Basic and Clinical Science Course

Louis B. Cantor, MD, Indianapolis, Indiana, *Senior Secretary for Clinical Education*
Christopher J. Rapuano, MD, Philadelphia, Pennsylvania, *Secretary for Ophthalmic Knowledge*
George A. Cioffi, MD, New York, New York, *BCSC Course Chair*

Section 4

Faculty

Robert H. Rosa, Jr, MD, *Chair,* Temple, Texas
Ronald Buggage, MD, New York, New York
George J. Harocopos, MD, St Louis, Missouri
Theresa Retue Kramer, MD, Tucson, Arizona
Tatyana Milman, MD, New York, New York
Nasreen Syed, MD, Iowa City, Iowa
Matthew W. Wilson, MD, Memphis, Tennessee
Jacob Pe'er, MD, *Consultant,* Jerusalem, Israel
Robert G. Fante, MD, Denver, Colorado
Practicing Ophthalmologists Advisory Committee for Education
Ron W. Pelton, MD, PhD, Colorado Springs, Colorado
Practicing Ophthalmologists Advisory Committee for Education

The Academy wishes to acknowledge the American Association of Ophthalmic Pathology for recommending faculty members to the BCSC Section 4 committee.

Financial Disclosures

Academy staff members who contributed to the development of this product state that within the past 12 months, they have had no financial interest in or other relationship with any entity discussed in this course that produces, markets, resells, or distributes ophthalmic health care goods or services consumed by or used in patients, or with any competing commercial product or service.

The authors state the following financial relationships:

Dr Buggage: Novartis Pharmaceuticals, employee, equity ownership/stock options

Dr Rosa: Genentech, grant recipient; National Eye Institute, grant recipient

The other authors state that they have no significant financial interest or other relationship with the manufacturer of any commercial product discussed in the chapters that they contributed to this course or with the manufacturer of any competing commercial product.

Recent Past Faculty

Patricia Chévez-Barrios, MD
Sander Dubovy, MD
Debra J. Shetlar, MD

In addition, the Academy gratefully acknowledges the contributions of numerous past faculty and advisory committee members who have played an important role in the development of previous editions of the Basic and Clinical Science Course.

American Academy of Ophthalmology Staff

Richard A. Zorab, *Vice President, Ophthalmic Knowledge*
Christine A. Arturo, *Publishing Services Manager*
Stephanie Tanaka, *Publications Manager*
D. Jean Ray, *Production Manager*
Ann McGuire, *Medical Editor*
Crissa M. Williams, *Administrative Coordinator*

American Academy® of Ophthalmology
The Eye M.D. Association

655 Beach Street
Box 7424
San Francisco, CA 94120-7424

Contents

General Introduction

The Basic and Clinical Science Course (BCSC) is designed to meet the needs of residents and practitioners for a comprehensive yet concise curriculum of the field of ophthalmology. The BCSC has developed from its original brief outline format, which relied heavily on outside readings, to a more convenient and educationally useful self-contained text. The Academy updates and revises the course annually, with the goals of integrating the basic science and clinical practice of ophthalmology and of keeping ophthalmologists current with new developments in the various subspecialties.

The BCSC incorporates the effort and expertise of more than 80 ophthalmologists, organized into 13 Section faculties, working with Academy editorial staff. In addition, the course continues to benefit from many lasting contributions made by the faculties of previous editions. Members of the Academy's Practicing Ophthalmologists Advisory Committee for Education serve on each faculty and, as a group, review every volume before and after major revisions.

Organization of the Course

The Basic and Clinical Science Course comprises 13 volumes, incorporating fundamental ophthalmic knowledge, subspecialty areas, and special topics:

1 Update on General Medicine
2 Fundamentals and Principles of Ophthalmology
3 Clinical Optics
4 Ophthalmic Pathology and Intraocular Tumors
5 Neuro-Ophthalmology
6 Pediatric Ophthalmology and Strabismus
7 Orbit, Eyelids, and Lacrimal System
8 External Disease and Cornea
9 Intraocular Inflammation and Uveitis
10 Glaucoma
11 Lens and Cataract
12 Retina and Vitreous
13 Refractive Surgery

In addition, a comprehensive Master Index allows the reader to easily locate subjects throughout the entire series.

References

Readers who wish to explore specific topics in greater detail may consult the references cited within each chapter and listed in the Basic Texts section at the back of the book.

These references are intended to be selective rather than exhaustive, chosen by the BCSC faculty as being important, current, and readily available to residents and practitioners.

Study Questions and CME Credit

Each volume of the BCSC is designed as an independent study activity for ophthalmology residents and practitioners. The learning objectives for this volume are given on page 1. The text, illustrations, and references provide the information necessary to achieve the objectives; the study questions allow readers to test their understanding of the material and their mastery of the objectives. Physicians who wish to claim CME credit for this educational activity may do so by following the instructions given at the end of the book.

Conclusion

The Basic and Clinical Science Course has expanded greatly over the years, with the addition of much new text and numerous illustrations. Recent editions have sought to place a greater emphasis on clinical applicability while maintaining a solid foundation in basic science. As with any educational program, it reflects the experience of its authors. As its faculties change and as medicine progresses, new viewpoints are always emerging on controversial subjects and techniques. Not all alternate approaches can be included in this series; as with any educational endeavor, the learner should seek additional sources, including such carefully balanced opinions as the Academy's Preferred Practice Patterns.

The BCSC faculty and staff are continually striving to improve the educational usefulness of the course; you, the reader, can contribute to this ongoing process. If you have any suggestions or questions about the series, please do not hesitate to contact the faculty or the editors.

The authors, editors, and reviewers hope that your study of the BCSC will be of lasting value and that each Section will serve as a practical resource for quality patient care.

Objectives

Upon completion of BCSC Section 4, *Ophthalmic Pathology and Intraocular Tumors,* the reader should be able to

- describe a structured approach to understanding major ocular conditions based on a hierarchical framework of topography, disease process, general diagnosis, and differential diagnosis
- summarize the steps in handling ocular specimens for pathologic study, including obtaining, dissecting, processing, and staining tissues
- explain the basic principles of special procedures used in ophthalmic pathology, including immunohistochemistry, flow cytometry, molecular pathology, and diagnostic electron microscopy
- communicate effectively with the pathologist regarding types of specimens, processing, and techniques appropriate to the clinical situation
- summarize the histopathology of common ocular conditions
- correlate clinical and pathological findings
- list the steps in wound healing in ocular tissues
- summarize current information about the most common primary tumors of the eye
- identify those ophthalmic lesions that indicate systemic disease and are potentially life threatening
- provide useful genetic information to families affected by retinoblastoma
- summarize current treatment modalities for ocular tumors in terms of patient prognosis and ocular function

PART I

Ophthalmic Pathology

CHAPTER 1

Introduction to Part I

The purpose of BCSC Section 4, *Ophthalmic Pathology and Intraocular Tumors,* is to provide a general overview of the fields of ophthalmic pathology and ocular oncology. Although there is some overlap between the 2 fields, it is useful to approach specific disease processes from the standpoint of 2 separate disciplines. This book contains numerous illustrations of entities commonly encountered in an ophthalmic pathology laboratory and in the practice of ocular oncology. In addition, important but less common entities are included for teaching purposes. For more comprehensive reviews of ophthalmic pathology and ocular oncology, the reader is referred to the excellent textbooks listed in Basic Texts at the end of this volume.

Part I of this text provides a framework for the study of ophthalmic pathology, with the following hierarchical organizational paradigm (explained in detail in the next section): topography, disease process, general diagnosis, differential diagnosis. Chapter 2 briefly covers basic principles and specific aspects of wound repair as it applies to ophthalmic tissues, which exhibit distinct responses to trauma, including end-stage processes such as phthisis bulbi. Chapter 3 discusses specimen handling, including orientation and dissection, and emphasizes the critical communication between the ophthalmologist and the pathologist. Although most ophthalmic pathology specimens are routinely processed and slides are stained with hematoxylin and eosin (H&E), special procedures are used in selected cases. Chapter 4 details several of these procedures, including immunohistochemical staining, flow cytometry, polymerase chain reaction (PCR), and electron microscopy. Also discussed are indications in some instances for special techniques in obtaining the specimen, such as fine-needle aspiration biopsy, and special ways of preparing slides for examination, such as frozen sections. Chapters 5 through 15 apply the organizational paradigm to specific anatomical locations.

Organization

Chapters 5 through 15 are each devoted to a particular ocular structure. Within the chapter, the text is organized from general to specific, according to the following hierarchical framework:

- topography
- disease process
- general diagnosis
- differential diagnosis

Topography

The microscopic evaluation of a specimen, whether on a glass slide or depicted in a photograph, should begin with a description of any normal tissue. For instance, the topography of the cornea is characterized by nonkeratinized stratified squamous epithelium, the Bowman layer, stroma, the Descemet membrane, and endothelium. By recognizing a particular structure, such as the Bowman layer or the Descemet membrane, in a biopsy specimen, an examiner might be able to identify the topography in question as cornea. It may not be possible, however, to identify the specific tissue source from the topography present on a glass slide or in a photograph. For example, a specimen showing the topographic features of keratinized stratified squamous epithelium overlying dermis with dermal appendages may be classified as skin; however, unless specific eyelid structures such as a tarsal plate are identified, that skin is not necessarily from the eyelid. See BCSC Section 2, *Fundamentals and Principles of Ophthalmology,* for a review of ophthalmic anatomy.

Disease Process

After identifying a tissue source, the pathologist should attempt to categorize the general disease process. These processes include

- congenital anomaly
- inflammation
- degeneration and dystrophy
- neoplasia

Congenital anomaly

Congenital anomalies usually involve abnormalities in size, location, organization, or amount of tissue. An example of congenitally enlarged tissue is congenital hypertrophy of the retinal pigment epithelium (CHRPE) (see Chapter 11, Fig 11-5; and Chapter 17, Fig 17-10). Many congenital abnormalities may be classified as choristomas or hamartomas.

A *choristoma* consists of normal, mature tissue at an abnormal location. It occurs when 1 or 2 embryonic germ layers form mature tissue that is abnormal for a given topographic location. An example of a choristoma is a *dermoid:* skin that is otherwise normal and mature present at the abnormal location of the limbus. A tumor made up of tissue derived from all 3 embryonic germ layers is called a *teratoma* (Fig 1-1).

In contrast, the term *hamartoma* describes an exaggerated hypertrophy and hyperplasia (abnormal amount) of mature tissue at a normal location. An example of a hamartoma is a *cavernous hemangioma,* an encapsulated mass of mature venous channels in the orbit.

Inflammation

The next disease process in the schema, inflammation, is classified in several ways. It may be acute or chronic in onset and focal or diffuse in location. Chronic inflammation is subdivided further as either granulomatous or nongranulomatous. For example, a bacterial corneal ulcer is generally an acute, focal, nongranulomatous inflammation, whereas sympathetic ophthalmia is a chronic, diffuse, granulomatous inflammation.

Polymorphonuclear leukocytes (PMNs), eosinophils, and basophils all circulate in the blood and may be present in tissue in early phases of the inflammatory process (Figs 1-2,

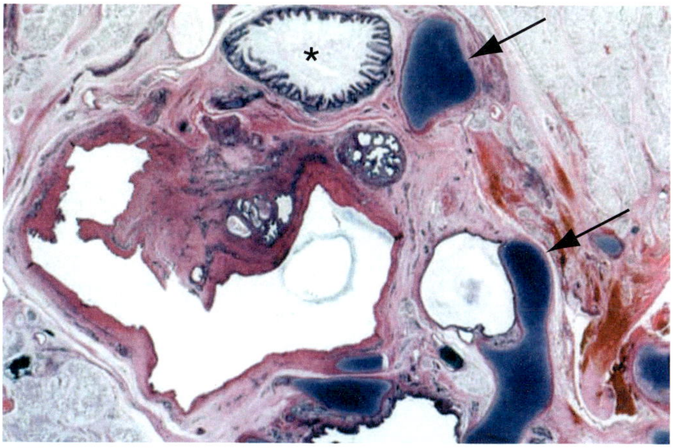

Figure 1-1 Orbital teratoma with tissue from 3 germ layers. Note gastrointestinal mucosa *(asterisk)* and cartilage *(arrows)* in the tumor. *(Courtesy of Hans E. Grossniklaus, MD.)*

1-3, 1-4). The types of leukocytes present at the site of inflammation vary according to the inflammatory response. PMNs, also known as *neutrophils,* typify acute inflammatory cells and can be recognized by a multisegmented nucleus and intracytoplasmic granules. They may be present in a variety of acute inflammatory processes; for example, they are associated with bacterial infection and found in the walls of blood vessels in some forms of vasculitis. *Eosinophils* have bilobed nuclei and prominent intracytoplasmic eosinophilic granules. They are commonly found in allergic reactions, although they may also be present in chronic inflammatory processes such as sympathetic ophthalmia. *Basophils* contain basophilic intracytoplasmic granules. *Mast cells* are the tissue-bound equivalent of the bloodborne basophils.

Inflammatory cells that are relatively characteristic of chronic inflammatory processes include monocytes (Fig 1-5) and lymphocytes (Fig 1-6). *Monocytes* may migrate from the intravascular space into tissue, in which case they are classified as *histiocytes,* or *macrophages.* Histiocytes have eccentric nuclei and abundant eosinophilic cytoplasm. In some instances, histiocytes may take on the appearance of epithelial cells, with abundant eosinophilic cytoplasm and sharp cell borders, becoming known in the process as *epithelioid histiocytes.* Epithelioid histiocytes may form a ball-like aggregate known as a *granuloma,* the sine qua non for granulomatous inflammation. These granulomas may contain only histologically intact cells ("hard" tubercles, Fig 1-7), or they may exhibit necrotic centers ("caseating" granulomas, Fig 1-8). Epithelioid histiocytes may merge to form a syncytium with multiple nuclei known as a *multinucleated giant cell.* Giant cells formed from histiocytes come in several varieties, including

- Langhans cells, characterized by a horseshoe arrangement of the nuclei (Fig 1-9)
- Touton giant cells, which have an annulus of nuclei surrounded by a lipid-filled clear zone (Fig 1-10)
- foreign body giant cells, with haphazardly arranged nuclei (Fig 1-11)

Lymphocytes are small cells with round, hyperchromatic nuclei and scant cytoplasm. Circulating lymphocytes infiltrate tissue in all types of chronic inflammatory processes.

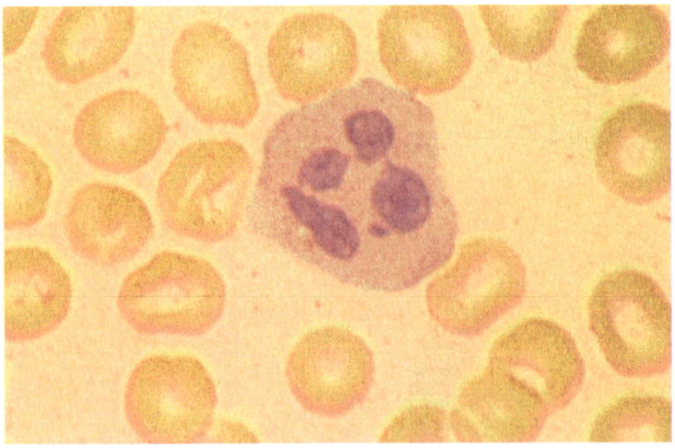

Figure 1-2 Polymorphonuclear leukocyte with multilobulated nucleus. *(Courtesy of Hans E. Grossniklaus, MD.)*

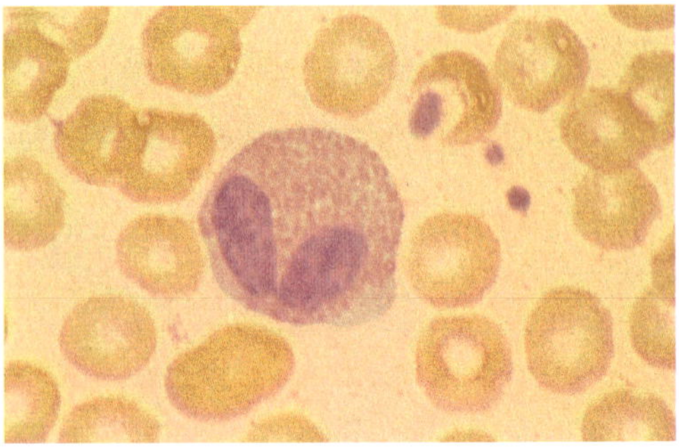

Figure 1-3 Eosinophil with bilobed nucleus and intracytoplasmic eosinophilic granules. *(Courtesy of Hans E. Grossniklaus, MD.)*

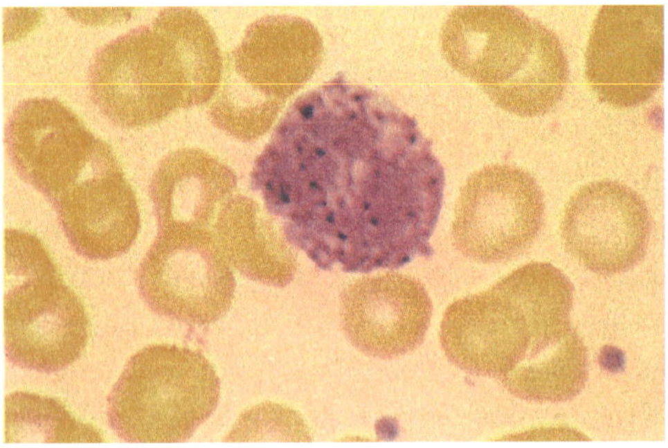

Figure 1-4 Basophil with intracytoplasmic basophilic granules. *(Courtesy of Hans E. Grossniklaus, MD.)*

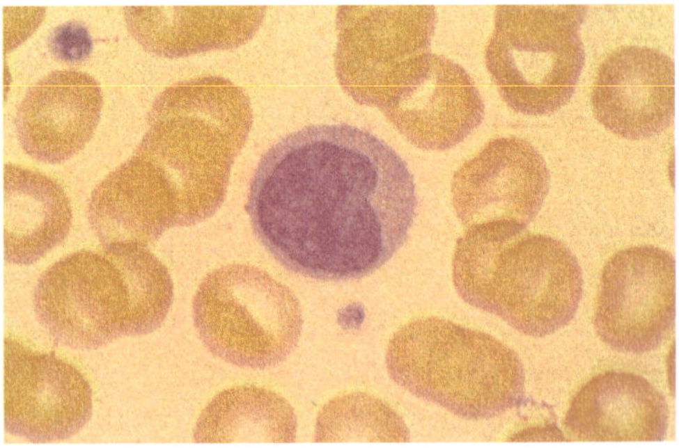

Figure 1-5 Monocyte with indented nucleus. *(Courtesy of Hans E. Grossniklaus, MD.)*

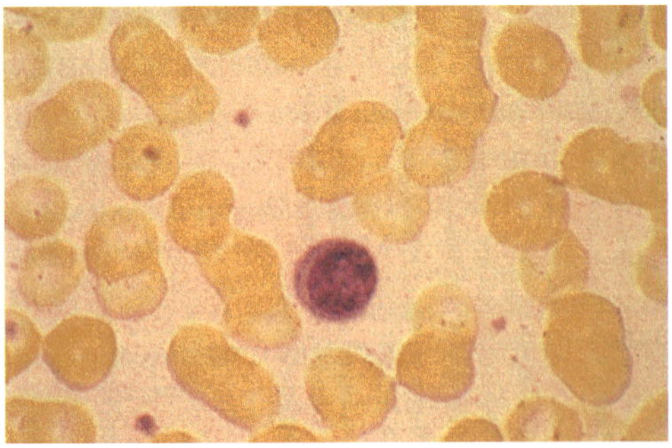

Figure 1-6 Lymphocyte with small, hyperchromatic nucleus and scant cytoplasm. *(Courtesy of Hans E. Grossniklaus, MD.)*

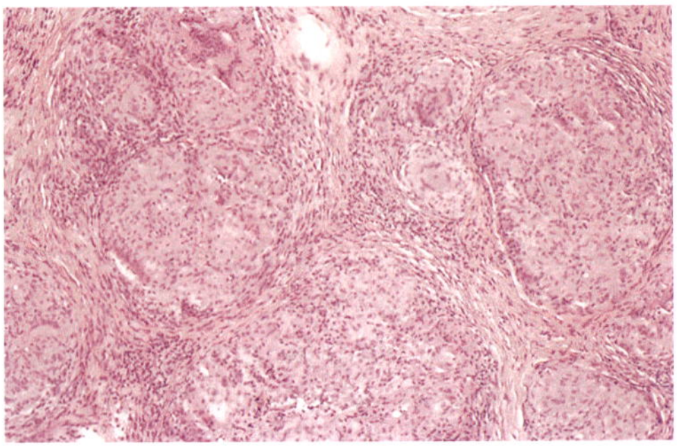

Figure 1-7 Noncaseating granulomas, or "hard" tubercles, are formed by aggregates of epithelioid histiocytes. *(Courtesy of Hans E. Grossniklaus, MD.)*

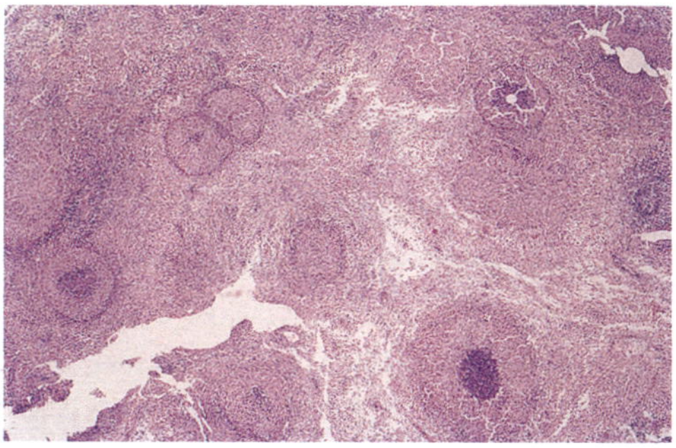

Figure 1-8 Granulomas with necrotic centers are classified as caseating granulomas. *(Courtesy of Hans E. Grossniklaus, MD.)*

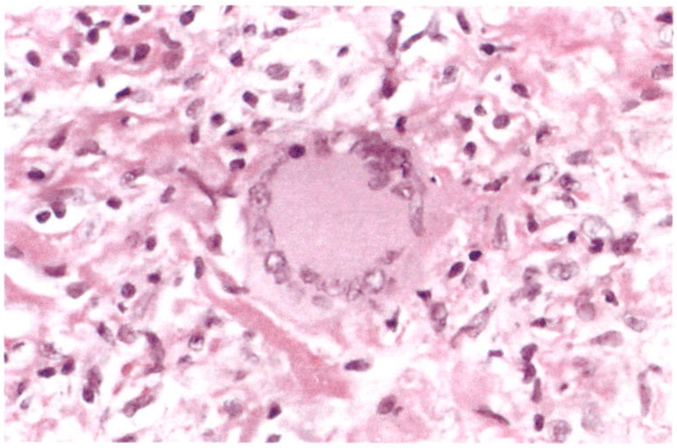

Figure 1-9 Langhans giant cell.

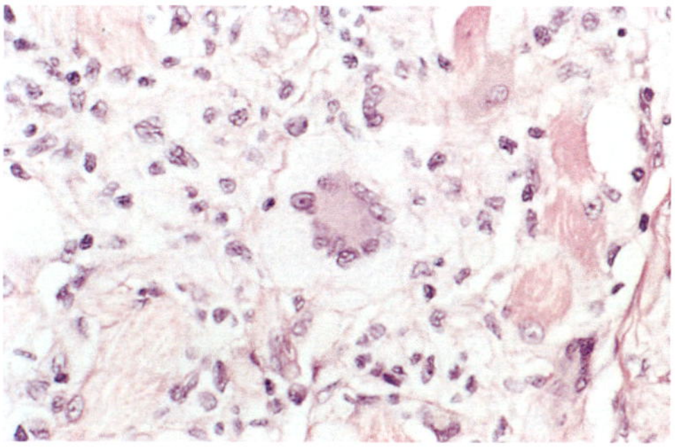

Figure 1-10 Touton giant cell.

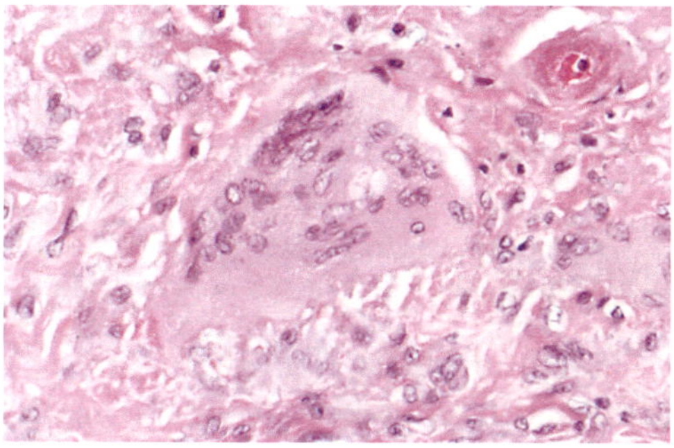

Figure 1-11 Foreign body giant cell.

These cells terminally differentiate in the thymus *(T cells)* or bursa equivalent *(B cells),* although it is not possible to distinguish between B and T lymphocytes with routine histologic stains. B cells may produce immunoglobulin and differentiate into *plasma cells,* with eccentric "cartwheel," or "clockface," nuclei and a perinuclear halo corresponding to the Golgi apparatus. These cells may become completely distended with immunoglobulin and form *Russell bodies,* which may be extracellular. BCSC Section 9, *Intraocular Inflammation and Uveitis,* discusses the cells involved in the inflammatory process in depth in Part I, Immunology.

Degeneration and dystrophy

The term *degeneration* refers to a wide variety of deleterious tissue changes that occur over time. Degenerative processes are not usually associated with a proliferation of cells; rather, there is often an accumulation of acellular material or a loss of tissue mass. Extracellular deposits may result from cellular overproduction of normal material or metabolically abnormal material. These processes, which have a variety of pathologic appearances, may occur in response to an injury or an inflammatory process. As used in this book, "degeneration" is an artificial category used to encompass a wide variety of disease processes. Various categories of diseases, such as those due to vascular causes, normal aging or involutional causes, and trauma, could be considered separately. However, in order to efficiently convey the hierarchical scheme used in this book, these causes are lumped under the rubric of "degeneration." *Dystrophies* are defined as bilateral, symmetric, inherited conditions that appear to have little or no relationship to environmental or systemic factors.

Degeneration of tissue may be seen in conjunction with other general disease processes. Examples include calcification of the lens (degeneration) in association with a congenital cataract (congenital anomaly); corneal amyloid (degeneration) in association with trachoma (inflammation); and orbital amyloid (degeneration) in association with a lymphoma (neoplasm). The ophthalmic manifestations of diabetes mellitus can be classified as degenerative changes associated with a metabolic disease.

Neoplasia

A *neoplasm* is a stereotypic, monotonous new growth of a particular tissue phenotype. Neoplasms can occur in either benign or malignant forms. Examples found in particular tissues include

- adenoma (benign) versus adenocarcinoma (malignant) in glandular epithelium
- topography + *oma* (benign) versus topography + *sarcoma* (malignant) in soft tissue
- hyperplasia/infiltrate (benign) versus leukemia/lymphoma (malignant) in hematopoietic tissue

Some neoplastic proliferations are called *borderline,* in that they are difficult to classify histologically as benign or malignant. Although most of the neoplasms illustrated and discussed in this text are classified as benign or malignant, the reader should be aware that tissue evaluation in a particular disease can give only a static portrait of a dynamic process. Thus, it may be impossible to determine whether the process will ultimately be benign or malignant, and in some instances "indeterminate" or "borderline" is a legitimate interpretation. Table 1-1 summarizes the origin, general classification of benign versus malignant, and growth pattern of neoplasms originating in various tissues.

The growth patterns described in Table 1-1 are shown in Figure 1-12. General histologic signs of malignancy include nuclear and cellular pleomorphism, necrosis, hemorrhage, and mitotic activity.

Table 1-1 Classification of Neoplasia

Tissue Origin	Benign	Malignant	Growth Pattern
Epithelium	Hyperplasia/adenoma	Carcinoma Adenocarcinoma	Cords Tubules
Soft tissue	Topography + *oma*	Topography + *sarcoma*	Coherent sheets
Hematopoietic tissue	Hyperplasia/infiltrate	Leukemia Lymphoma	Loosely arranged

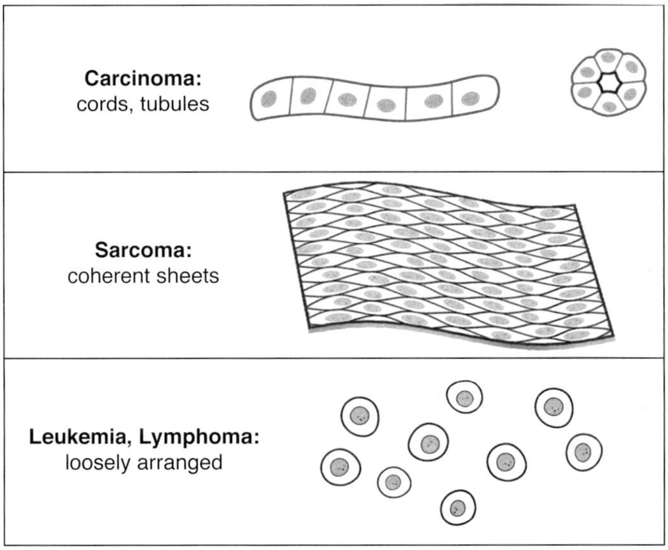

Figure 1-12 General classification and growth patterns of malignant tumors. *(Illustration by Christine Gralapp.)*

General Diagnosis

After considering the topography and disease process, the examiner formulates the general diagnosis. Recognizing a tissue *index feature* is a critical step in arriving at the general diagnosis. Index features are morphologic identifiers that help to define the disease process more specifically. Examples include the presence of pigment in a pigmented neoplasm, necrosis in a necrotizing granulomatous inflammation, and accumulation of smudgy extracellular material in a smudgy eosinophilic corneal degeneration. The index feature should differentiate the particular specimen from others demonstrating the same general disease process. For instance, retinoblastoma and melanoma are both intraocular malignant neoplasms; the former is a retinal malignancy, and the latter is a uveal tract malignancy. Other index features for distinguishing between these lesions could be “small, round, blue cell tumor” for the retinoblastoma and “melanocytic proliferation” for the melanoma. Although the most basic index features can be recognized without great difficulty, it takes experience and practice to identify subtle index features.

Differential Diagnosis

After the examiner has distinguished a key index feature and formulated a general diagnosis, developing a differential diagnosis is the next step. The differential diagnosis is a limited list of specific conditions resulting from pathologic processes that were identified in the general diagnosis. For instance, the differential diagnosis based on the features of noncaseating granulomatous inflammation of the conjunctiva includes sarcoidosis, foreign body, fungus, and mycobacterium. The differential diagnosis of melanocytic proliferation of the conjunctiva includes nevus, primary acquired melanosis, and melanoma.

Readers are encouraged to practice working through the hierarchical framework by verbalizing each step in sequence while examining a pathologic specimen. Chapters 5 through 15 of this book provide tissue-specific examples of the differential diagnoses for each of the 4 disease process categories. The expanded organizational paradigm is shown in Table 1-2.

Table 1-2 Organizational Paradigm for Ophthalmic Pathology

Topography
Conjunctiva
Cornea
Anterior chamber/trabecular meshwork
Sclera
Lens
Vitreous
Retina
Uveal tract
Eyelids
Orbit
Optic nerve
Disease process
Congenital anomaly
Choristoma versus hamartoma
Inflammation
Acute versus chronic
Focal versus diffuse
Granulomatous versus nongranulomatous
Degeneration (includes dystrophy)
Neoplasia
Benign versus malignant
Epithelial versus soft tissue versus hematopoietic
General diagnosis
Index feature
Differential diagnosis
Limited list

CHAPTER 2

Wound Repair

General Aspects of Wound Repair

Wound healing, though a common physiologic process, requires a complicated sequence of tissue events. The purpose of wound healing is to restore the anatomical and functional integrity of an organ or tissue as quickly and perfectly as possible. Repair may take a year, and the result of wound healing is a scar with variable consequences (Fig 2-1). A series of reactions follows a wound, including an acute inflammatory phase, regeneration/repair, and contraction:

- The *acute inflammatory phase* may last from minutes to hours. Blood clots quickly in adjacent vessels in response to tissue activators. Neutrophils and fluid enter the extracellular space. Macrophages remove debris from the damaged tissues, new vessels form, and fibroblasts begin to produce collagen.
- *Regeneration* is the replacement of lost cells; this process occurs only in tissues composed of labile cells (eg, epithelium), which undergo mitosis throughout life. *Repair* is the restructuring of tissues by granulation tissue that matures into a fibrous scar.
- Finally, *contraction* causes the reparative tissues to shrink so that the scar is smaller than the surrounding uninjured tissues.

Healing in Specific Ocular Tissues

The processes summarized in the following sections are also discussed in other volumes of the BCSC; consult the *Master Index.* Also see the appropriate chapters in this volume for a specific topography.

Cornea

A corneal *abrasion,* a painful but rapidly healing defect, is limited to the surface corneal epithelium, although the Bowman layer and superficial stroma may also be involved. Within an hour of injury the parabasilar epithelial cells begin to slide and migrate across the denuded area until they touch other migrating cells; then *contact inhibition* stops further migration. Simultaneously, the surrounding basal cells undergo mitosis to supply additional cells to cover the defect. Although a large corneal abrasion is usually covered by migrating epithelial cells within 24–48 hours, complete healing, which includes restoration of the full thickness of epithelium (4–6 layers) and re-formation of the anchoring

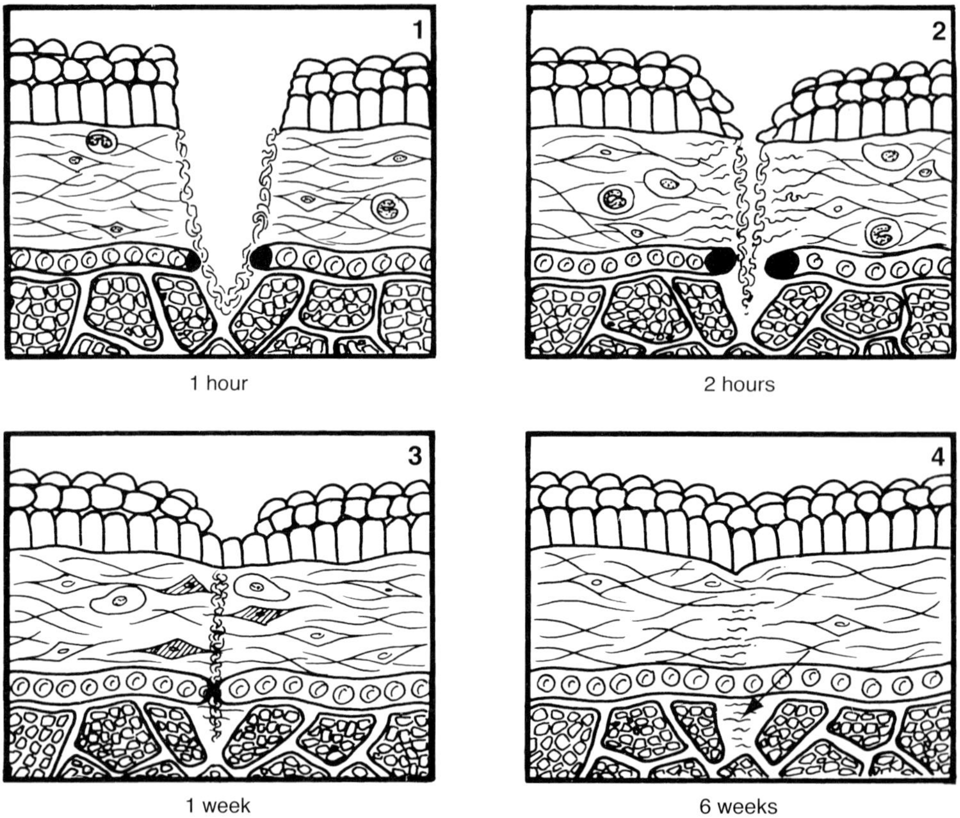

Figure 2-1 Sequence of general wound healing with an epithelial surface. **1,** The wound is created. Blood clots in the vessels; neutrophils migrate to the wound; the wounded edges begin to disintegrate. **2,** The wound edges are reapposed with the various tissue planes in good alignment. The epithelium is lost over the wound but starts to migrate. The subcutaneous fibroblasts enlarge and become activated. Fibronectin is deposited at the wound edges. The blood vessels begin to produce buds. **3,** The epithelium seals the surface. Fibroblasts and blood vessels enter the wound and lay down new collagen. Much of the debris is removed by macrophages. **4,** As the scar matures, the fibroblasts subside. Newly formed blood vessels recanalize. New collagen strengthens the wound, which contracts. Note that the striated muscle cells (permanent cells) at bottom are replaced by scar *(arrow).*

fibrils, takes 4–6 weeks. The epithelial cells are labile; that is, some are continuously active mitotically and thus are able to completely replace the lost cells. If a thin layer of anterior cornea is lost with the abrasion, the shallow crater will be filled by epithelium, forming a facet.

Corneal stromal healing is avascular. Unlike with other tissues, healing in the corneal stroma occurs by means of fibrosis rather than by fibrovascular proliferation. This avascular aspect of corneal wound healing is critical to the success of penetrating keratoplasty as well as photorefractive keratectomy (PRK), laser in situ keratomileusis (LASIK), laser epithelial keratomileusis (LASEK), and other corneal refractive surgical procedures.

Following a central corneal wound, neutrophils are carried to the site by the tears (Fig 2-2), and the edges of the wound swell. Healing factors derived from vessels are not present. The matrix glycosaminoglycans, which in the cornea are keratan sulfate and chondroitin sulfate, disintegrate at the edge of the wound. The fibroblasts of the stroma become activated, eventually migrating across the wound, laying down collagen and fibronectin. The direction of the fibroblasts and collagen is not parallel to stromal lamellae. Hence, cells are directed anteriorly and posteriorly across a wound that is always visible microscopically as an irregularity in the stroma and clinically as an opacity. If the wound edges are separated, the gap is not completely filled by proliferating fibroblasts, and a partially filled crater results.

Both the epithelium and the endothelium are critical to good central wound healing. If the epithelium does not cover the wound within days, the subjacent stromal healing is limited and the wound is weak. Growth factors from the epithelium stimulate and sustain

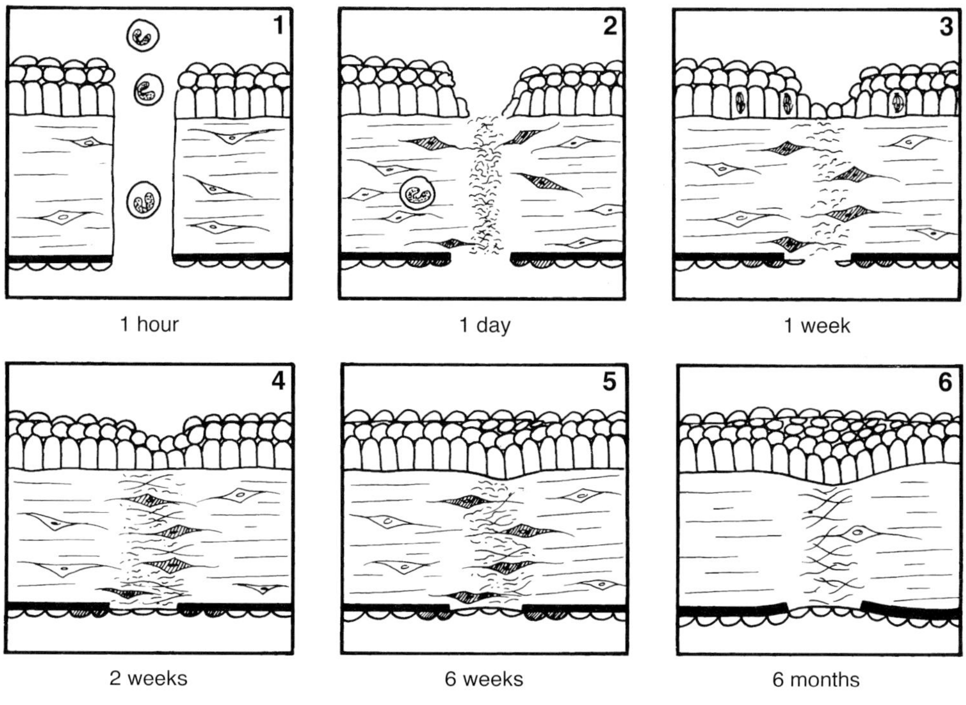

Figure 2-2 Clear corneal wound. **1,** The tear film carries neutrophils with lysozymes to the wound within an hour. **2,** With closure of the incision, the wound edge shows early disintegration and edema. The glycosaminoglycans at the edge are degraded. The nearby fibroblasts are activated. **3,** At 1 week, migrating epithelium and endothelium partially seal the wound; fibroblasts begin to migrate and supply collagen. **4,** Fibroblast activity and collagen and matrix deposition continue. The endothelium, sealing the inner wound, lays down new Descemet membrane. **5,** Epithelial regeneration is complete. Fibroblasts fill the wound with type I collagen and repair slows. **6,** The final wound contracts. The collagen fibers are not parallel with the surrounding lamellae. The number of fibroblasts decreases.

healing. The endothelial cells adjacent to the wound slide across the posterior cornea; a few cells are replaced through mitotic activity. Endothelium lays down a new thin layer of the Descemet membrane. If the internal margin of the wound is not covered by Descemet membrane, stromal fibroblasts may continue to proliferate into the anterior chamber as fibrous ingrowth, or the posterior wound may remain permanently open. The initial fibrillar collagen is replaced by stronger collagen in the late months of healing. The Bowman layer does not regenerate when incised or destroyed. In an ulcer, the surface is covered by epithelium, but little of the lost stroma is replaced by fibrous tissue. Modification of the healing process by use of topical antimetabolites, such as 5-fluorouracil and mitomycin C, may be desirable in certain clinical situations (see BCSC Section 10, *Glaucoma,* Chapter 8).

Sclera

The sclera differs from the cornea in that the collagen fibers are randomly distributed rather than laid down in orderly lamellae, and the glycosaminoglycan is dermatan sulfate. Sclera is relatively avascular and hypocellular. When stimulated by wounding, the episclera migrates down the scleral wound, supplying vessels, fibroblasts, and activated macrophages. The final wound contracts, creating a pinched-in appearance. If the adjacent uvea is damaged, uveal fibrovascular tissue may enter the scleral wound, resulting in a scar with a dense adhesion between uvea and sclera. Indolent episcleral fibrosis produces a dense coat around an extrascleral foreign body such as an encircling scleral buckling element or a glaucoma drainage device.

Limbus

The limbus is a complex region of corneal, scleral, and episcleral tissues. Wounds of the limbus cause swelling in the cornea and shrinking of the sclera. Healing involves episcleral ingrowth and clear corneal fibroblastic migration. Collector channels in the sclera do not contribute to the healing. Alterations in surgical technique between clear corneal and limbal incisions may produce different healing responses. Differences include

- the potential for vascular ingrowth from episcleral vessels into a limbal wound and the absence of vascularity of a clear corneal wound
- surface remodeling of epithelium over a clear corneal wound that does not occur over a limbal wound

Uvea

Under ordinary circumstances, wounds of the iris do not stimulate a healing response in either the stroma or the epithelium. Though richly endowed with blood vessels and fibroblasts, the iridic stroma does not produce granulation tissue to close a defect. The pigmented epithelium may be stimulated to migrate in some circumstances, such as excessive inflammation, but its migration is usually limited to the subjacent surface of the lens capsule, where subsequent adhesion of epithelial cells occurs. When fibrovascular tissue forms, it usually does so on the anterior surface of the iris as an exuberant and aberrant membrane (eg, rubeosis iridis) that may cross iridectomy or pupillary openings. The fibrovascular tissue may arise from the iris, the chamber angle, or the cornea.

Stroma and melanocytes of the ciliary body and choroid do not regenerate after injury. Debris is removed, and a thin fibrous scar develops that appears white and atrophic clinically.

Dunn SP. Iris repair: putting the pieces back together. *Focal Points: Clinical Modules for Ophthalmologists.* San Francisco: American Academy of Ophthalmology; 2002, module 11.

Lens

Small rents in the lens capsule are sealed by nearby lenticular epithelial cells. When posterior synechiae make the lenticular epithelium anoxic or hypoxic, a metaplastic response occurs, producing fibrous plaques intermixed with basement membrane.

Retina

The retina is made of terminally differentiated cells that typically do not regenerate when injured. Glial cells (Müller cells and fibrous astrocytes) proliferate in response to retinal trauma. Surgical techniques to close openings in the peripheral retina are successful when the neurosensory retina and retinal pigment epithelium (RPE) are destroyed (eg, cryotherapy, photocoagulation) and the surrounding tissues form an adhesive, atrophic scar.

Retinal scars are produced by glia rather than fibroblasts. After inflammatory cells have cleared away the debris, the tissues most damaged by the therapeutic modality remain as a thin, atrophic area in the center of the scar. Increasing numbers of residual viable cells encircle the zone of greatest destruction. Adhesion between the residual neurosensory retina and Bruch membrane develops according to the size of the original wound and the type of injury. The internal limiting membrane and the Bruch membrane provide the architectural planes for glial scarring. Adhesions from the internal limiting membrane to the Bruch membrane may incorporate a rare residual glial cell, and variable numbers of retinal cells and RPE may be present between the membranes. If the wound has damaged the Bruch membrane, choroidal fibroblasts and vessels may participate in the formation of the final scar. The end result is a metaplastic collagenous plaque in the sub–neurosensory retina and sub-RPE areas. The RPE usually proliferates rather exuberantly in such scars, giving rise to the dense black clumps seen clinically in scars of the fundus.

Vitreous

The vitreous has few cells and no blood vessels. Nonetheless, in conditions that cause vitreal inflammation, mediators stimulate the formation of membranes composed of new vessels and the proliferation of glial and fibrous tissue. With contraction of these membranes, the retina becomes distorted and detached.

Eyelid, Orbit, and Lacrimal Tissues

The rich blood supply of the skin of the eyelids supports rapid healing. On about the third day after injury to the skin, myofibroblasts derived from vascular pericytes migrate around the wound and actively contract, resulting in a volumetric decrease in the size of the wound. The eyelid and orbit are compartmentalized by intertwining fascial membranes enclosing muscular, tendinous, fatty, lacrimal, and ocular tissues that are distorted by scarring. Exuberant contracting distorts muscle action, producing dysfunctional scars. The striated muscles of the orbicularis oculi and extraocular muscles are made of terminally differentiated cells that do not regenerate, but the viable cells may hypertrophy.

Histologic Sequelae of Ocular Trauma

Rupture of the Descemet membrane may occur after minor trauma (eg, in keratoconus; Fig 2-3) or major trauma (eg, after forceps injury; Fig 2-4).

The anterior chamber angle structures, especially the trabecular beams, are vulnerable to distortion of the anterior globe. *Cyclodialysis* results from disinsertion of the longitudinal muscle of the ciliary body from the scleral spur (Fig 2-5). This condition can lead to hypotony because the aqueous of the anterior chamber now has free access to the suprachoroidal space; and because the blood supply to the ciliary body is diminished, the production of aqueous is decreased.

Traumatic recession of the anterior chamber angle is due to a tear in the ciliary body between the longitudinal and circular muscles with posterior displacement of the iris root (Fig 2-6). Concurrent damage to the trabecular meshwork may lead to glaucoma.

The uveal tract is attached to the sclera at 3 points: the scleral spur, the internal ostia of the vortex veins, and the peripapillary tissue. This anatomical arrangement is the basis of the evisceration technique and explains the vulnerability of the eye to expulsive choroi-

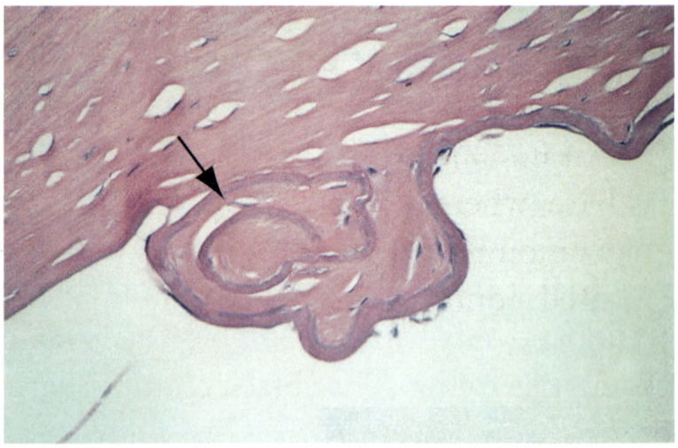

Figure 2-3 A break in the Descemet membrane in keratoconus shows anterior curling of Descemet membrane toward the corneal stroma *(arrow)*. *(Courtesy of Hans E. Grossniklaus, MD.)*

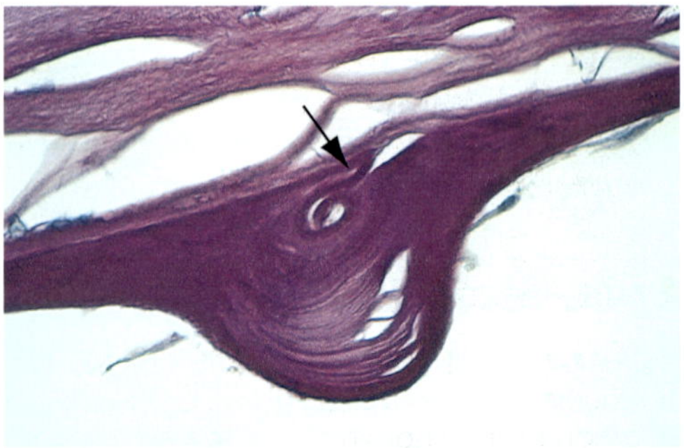

Figure 2-4 A break in the Descemet membrane as a result of forceps injury shows anterior curling of the original membrane *(arrow)* and production of a secondary thickened membrane. *(Courtesy of Hans E. Grossniklaus, MD.)*

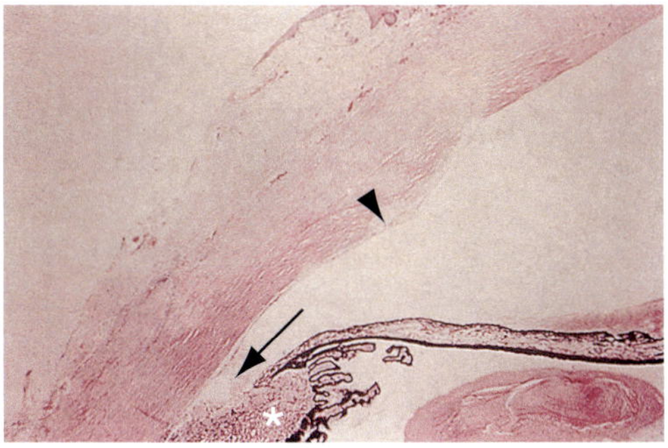

Figure 2-5 Cyclodialysis *(arrow)* shows disinsertion of ciliary body muscle *(asterisk)* from the scleral spur *(arrowhead)*. *(Courtesy of Hans E. Grossniklaus, MD.)*

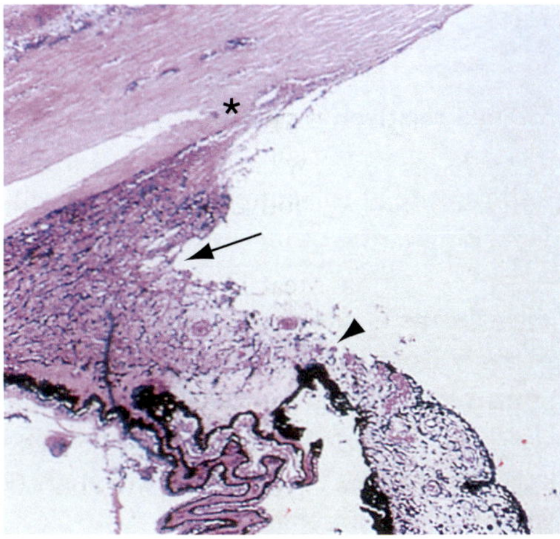

Figure 2-6 Angle recession shows a rupture in the ciliary body in the plane between the external longitudinal muscle fibers and the internal circular and oblique fibers *(arrow)*; the iris root is displaced posteriorly *(arrowhead)*. Note the scleral spur *(asterisk)*.

dal hemorrhage. The borders of the dome-shaped choroidal hemorrhage are defined by the position of the vortex veins and the scleral spur (Fig 2-7).

An *iridodialysis* is a rupture of the iris at the thinnest portion of the diaphragm, the iris base, where it inserts into the supportive tissue of the ciliary body (Fig 2-8). Only a small amount of supporting tissue surrounds the iris sphincter. If the sphincter muscle is ruptured, contraction of the remaining muscle will create a notch at the pupillary border.

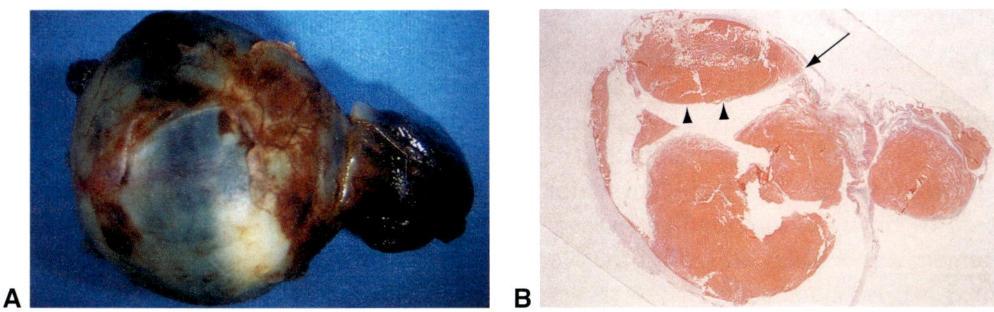

Figure 2-7 **A,** This eye developed an expulsive hemorrhage after a corneal perforation. **B,** The intraocular choroidal hemorrhage is dome shaped *(arrowheads)*, delineated anteriorly by the insertion of the choroid at the scleral spur *(arrow)*. *(Courtesy of Hans E. Grossniklaus, MD.)*

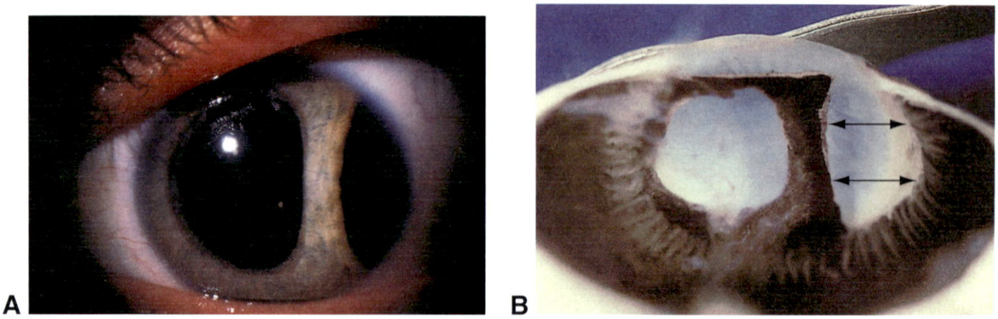

Figure 2-8 **A,** Clinical photograph showing iridodialysis with a tear in the base of the iris. **B,** Gross photograph showing posterior view of iridodialysis *(arrows)*. *(Part A courtesy of Hans E. Grossniklaus, MD.)*

The iris diaphragm may be lost completely through a relatively small limbal rupture associated with 360° iridodialysis.

A *Vossius ring* appears when compression and rupture of iris pigment epithelial cells against the anterior surface of the lens occur, depositing a ring of melanin pigment concentric to the pupil.

A *cataract* may form immediately if the lens capsule is ruptured. The lens capsule is thinnest at the posterior pole, a point farthest away from the lens epithelial cells. The epithelium of the lens may be stimulated by trauma to form an anterior lenticular fibrous plaque. The lens zonular fibers are points of relative weakness; if they are ruptured, displacement of the lens can be partial (subluxation) or complete (luxation). Focal areas of zonular rupture may allow formed vitreous to enter the anterior chamber.

Commotio retinae (Berlin edema) often complicates blunt trauma to the eye. Most prominent in the macula, commotio retinae can affect any portion of the retina. Originally, the retinal opacification seen clinically was thought to result from retinal edema (extracellular accumulation of fluid), but experimental evidence shows that a disruption in the architecture of the photoreceptor elements causes the loss of retinal transparency.

Retinal dialysis is most likely to develop in the inferotemporal or superonasal quadrant. The retina is anchored anteriorly to the nonpigmented epithelium of the pars plana. This union is reinforced by the attachment of the vitreous base, which straddles the ora serrata. Deformation of the eye can result in a circumferential retinal tear at the point of attachment of the ora or immediately posterior to the point of attachment of the vitreous base. Vitreoretinal traction may cause tears in a retina weakened by necrosis.

Intraocular *fibrocellular proliferation* may occur after a penetrating injury. Such proliferation may lead to vitreous/subretinal/choroidal hemorrhage; traction retinal detachment; proliferative vitreoretinopathy (PVR), including anterior PVR (Fig 2-9); hypotony; and ultimately phthisis bulbi. Formation of proliferative intraocular membranes may affect the timing of vitreoretinal surgery. The timing of the drainage of a ciliochoroidal hemorrhage is based on lysis of the blood clot (10–14 days). Hemosiderin forms at approximately 72 hours after hemorrhage. Sequelae of intraocular hemorrhage include siderosis bulbi, cholesterosis, and hemoglobin spherulosis.

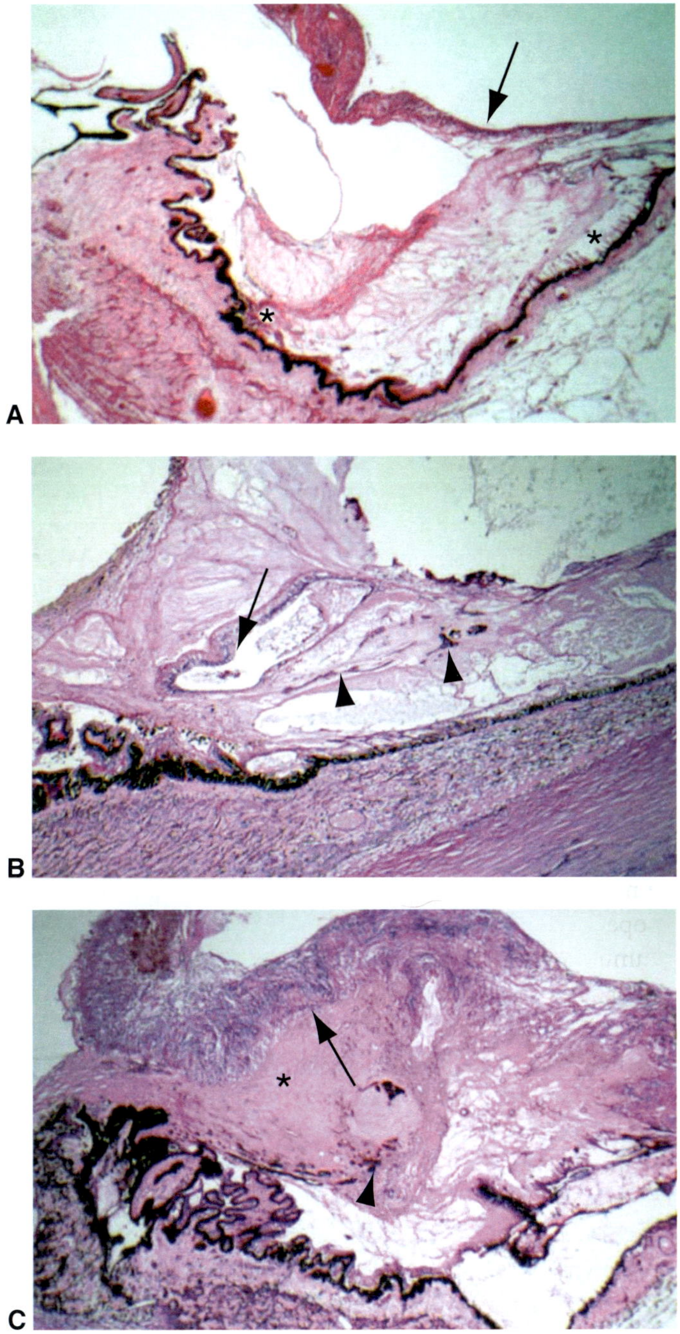

Figure 2-9 Anterior proliferative vitreoretinopathy (PVR). **A,** Traction of the vitreous base on the peripheral retina *(arrow)* and ciliary body epithelium *(asterisks)*. **B,** Incorporation of peripheral retinal *(arrow)* and ciliary body tissue *(arrowheads)* into the vitreous base. **C,** Condensed vitreous base *(asterisk)*, adherent retina *(arrow)*, and RPE hyperplasia *(arrowhead)*. *(Courtesy of Hans E. Grossniklaus, MD.)*

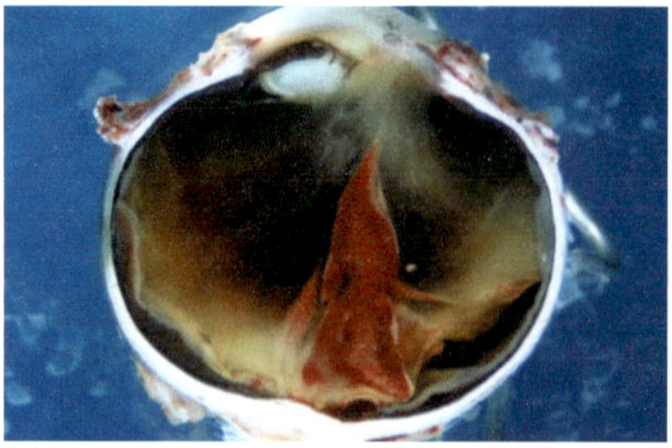

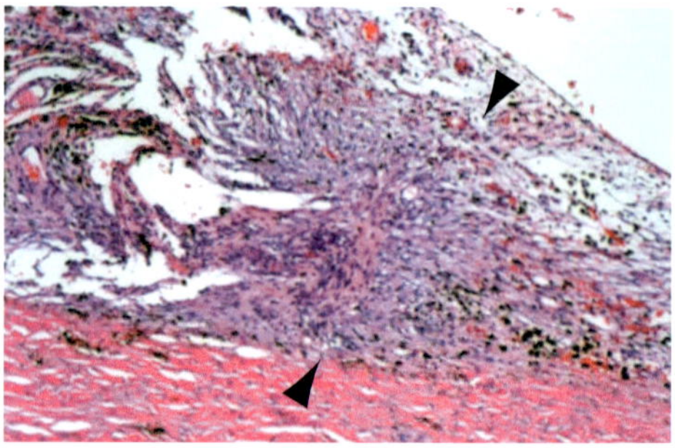

Figure 2-10 Focal posttraumatic choroidal granulomatous inflammation. **A,** Enucleated eye with a projectile causing a perforating limbal injury that extends to the posterior choroid. **B,** Microscopic examination shows a focus of choroidal granulomatous inflammation *(between arrowheads)*. *(Courtesy of Hans E. Grossniklaus, MD.)*

Rupture of the Bruch membrane or *choroidal rupture* may occur after direct or indirect injury to the globe. Choroidal neovascularization, granulation tissue proliferation, and scar formation may occur in an area of choroidal rupture. A subset of direct choroidal ruptures, those usually occurring after a projectile injury, may result in *focal posttraumatic choroidal granulomatous inflammation* (Fig 2-10). This may be related to foreign material introduced into the choroid. A chorioretinal rupture and necrosis is known as *sclopetaria.*

Phthisis bulbi is defined as atrophy, shrinkage, and disorganization of the eye and intraocular contents. Not all eyes rendered sightless by trauma become phthisical. If the nutritional status of the eye and near-normal intraocular pressure (IOP) are maintained during the repair process, the globe will remain clinically stable. However, blind eyes are at high risk of repeated trauma with cumulative destructive effects. Slow, progressive functional decompensation may also prevail. Many blind eyes pass through several stages of atrophy and disorganization into the end stage of phthisis bulbi:

- *Atrophia bulbi without shrinkage.* Initially, the size and shape of the eye are maintained. The atrophic eye often has elevated IOP. The following structures are most sensitive to loss of nutrition: the lens, which becomes cataractous; the retina, which atrophies and becomes separated from the RPE by serous fluid accumulation; and the aqueous outflow tract, where anterior and posterior synechiae develop.
- *Atrophia bulbi with shrinkage.* The eye becomes soft because of ciliary body dysfunction and progressive diminution of IOP. The globe becomes smaller and assumes a squared-off configuration as a result of the influence of the 4 rectus muscles. The anterior chamber collapses. Associated corneal endothelial cell damage results initially in corneal edema followed by opacification from degenerative pannus, stromal scarring, and vascularization. Most of the remaining internal structures of the eye will be atrophic but recognizable histologically.
- *Phthisis bulbi* (Fig 2-11). The size of the globe shrinks from a normal average diameter of 24–26 mm to an average diameter of 16–19 mm. Most of the ocular contents become disorganized. In areas of preserved uvea, the RPE proliferates and drusen may be seen. Extensive calcification of the Bowman layer, lens, retina, and drusen usually occurs. Osseous metaplasia of the RPE with bone formation may be a prominent feature. The sclera becomes massively thickened, particularly posteriorly.

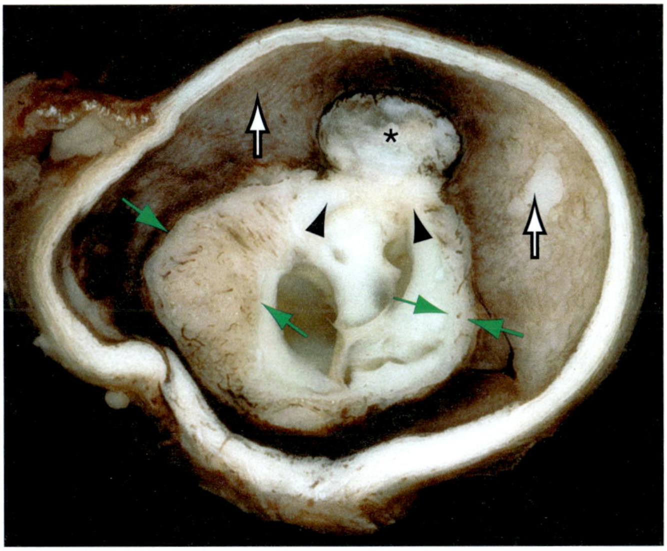

A

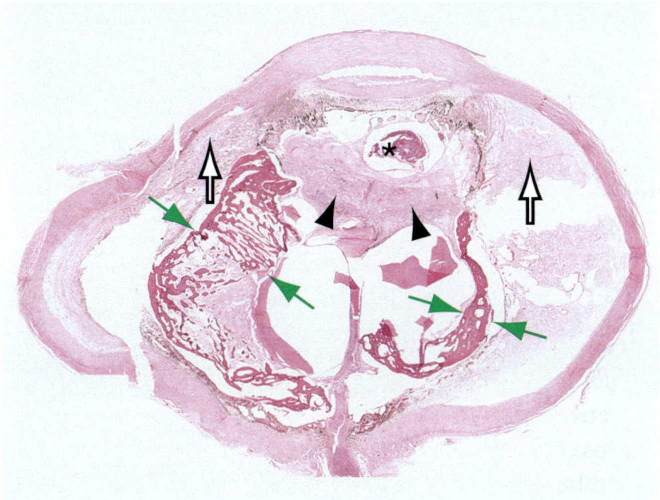

B

Figure 2-11 Phthisis bulbi. **A,** Gross photograph showing globe with irregular contour, cataractous lens with calcification *(asterisk)*, cyclitic membrane with adherent retina *(arrowheads)*, organized ciliochoroidal effusion *(open arrows)*, and bone formation *(between green arrows)*. **B,** Photomicrograph demonstrating histopathologic correlation with gross photograph in **A.** *(Courtesy of Robert H. Rosa, Jr, MD.)*

CHAPTER 3

Specimen Handling

Communication

Communication with the pathologist before, during, and after surgical procedures is an essential aspect of quality patient care. Standards for the technical handling of specimens and reporting of results have been developed and are available on the website of the College of American Pathologists (www.cap.org). The final histologic diagnosis reflects successful collaborative work between clinician and pathologist. The ophthalmologist should provide a relevant and reasonably detailed clinical history when the specimen is submitted to the laboratory. This history facilitates clinicopathologic correlation and enables the pathologist to provide the most accurate interpretation of the specimen.

Where there is an ongoing relationship between a pathologist and an ophthalmologist, communication usually can be accomplished through the pathology request form and the pathology report. However, if a malignancy is suspected or if the biopsy will be used to establish a critical diagnosis, direct and personal communication between the ophthalmic surgeon and the pathologist can be essential. This preoperative consultation allows the surgeon and pathologist to discuss the best way to submit a specimen. For example, the pathologist may wish to have fresh tissue for immunohistochemical stains and molecular diagnostic studies, glutaraldehyde-fixed tissue for electron microscopy, and formalin-fixed tissue for routine paraffin embedding. If the tissue is simply submitted in formalin, the opportunity for a definitive diagnosis may be lost. Communication between clinician and pathologist is especially important in ophthalmic pathology, where specimens are often very small and require very careful handling. In some cases, careful selection of the surgical facility is necessary to ensure proper specimen handling. Biopsies may be incisional, in which only a portion of the tumor is sampled, or excisional, in which the entire lesion is removed. See BCSC Section 7, *Orbit, Eyelids, and Lacrimal System,* for further discussion.

Any time a previous biopsy has been performed at the site of the present pathology, the sections of the previous biopsy should be requested and reviewed with the pathologist who will interpret the second biopsy. The surgical plan may be altered substantially if the initial biopsy was thought to represent, for example, a basal cell carcinoma when in fact the disease was a sebaceous carcinoma. In addition, the pathologist will be able to interpret intraoperative frozen sections more accurately when the case has been reviewed in advance.

If substantial disagreement arises between the clinical diagnosis and the histologic diagnosis, the ophthalmologist should contact the pathologist directly and promptly to resolve the discrepancy. Mislabeling of pathology specimens or reports through a simple typing error, for example, can have serious consequences. Merely correcting the patient age on the pathology request form may change the interpretation of melanotic lesions of the conjunctiva. Benign melanotic lesions in children may have a histologic appearance similar to that of malignant melanotic lesions in adults. Whether the patient is age 4 or age 44 makes a tremendous difference in interpretation.

Orientation

Globes may be oriented according to the location of the extraocular muscles and of the long posterior ciliary arteries and nerves, which are located in the horizontal meridian. The medial, inferior, lateral, and superior rectus muscles insert progressively farther from the limbus. Locating the insertion of the inferior oblique muscle is very helpful in distinguishing between a right and a left eye (Fig 3-1). The inferior oblique inserts temporally over the macula, with its fibers running inferiorly. Once the laterality of the eye is determined, the globe may be transilluminated and dissected.

Transillumination

Eyes are transilluminated with bright light prior to gross dissection. This helps to identify intraocular lesions such as a tumor that blocks the transilluminated light and casts

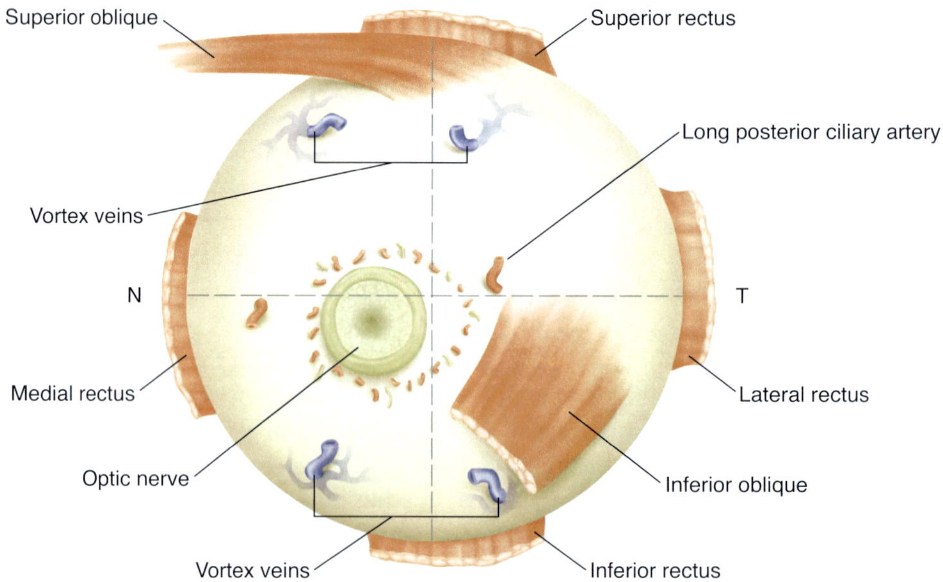

Figure 3-1 Posterior view of right globe. *N* = nasal, *T* = temporal. *(Modified by C.H. Wooley from an illustration by Thomas A. Weingeist, PhD, MD.)*

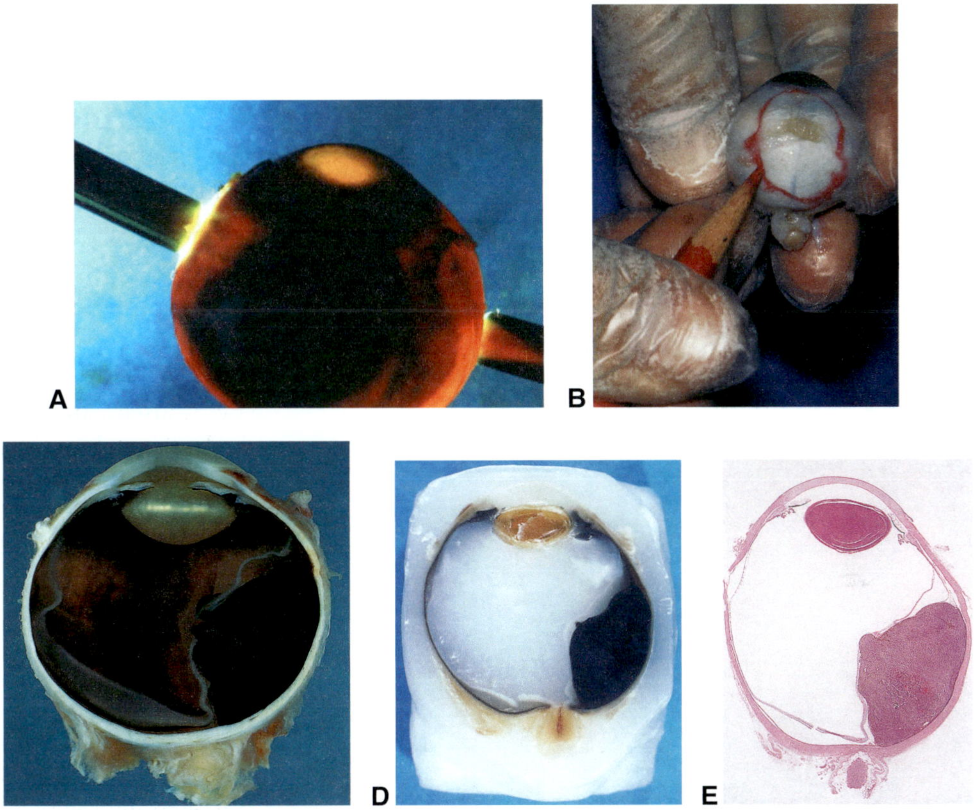

Figure 3-2 Preparation of an intraocular tumor specimen. **A,** Transillumination shows blockage to light secondary to an intraocular tumor. **B,** The area of blockage to light is marked with a marking pencil. **C,** The opened eye shows the intraocular tumor that was demonstrated by transillumination. **D,** The paraffin-embedded eye shows the intraocular tumor. **E,** The H&E-stained section shows that the maximum extent of the tumor demonstrated by transillumination is in the center of the section, which includes the pupil and optic nerve. *(Courtesy of Hans E. Grossniklaus, MD.)*

a shadow (Fig 3-2A). The shadow can be outlined with a marking pencil on the sclera (Fig 3-2B). This outline can then be used to guide the gross dissection of the globe so that the center of the section will include the maximum extent of the area of interest (Figs 3-2C to 3-2E).

Gross Dissection

A globe is opened so as to display as much of the pathologic change as possible on a single slide. The majority of eyes are cut so that the pupil and optic nerve are present in the same section, the *PO section.* The meridian, or clock-hour, of the section is determined by the unique features of the case, such as the presence of an intraocular tumor or a history of previous surgery or trauma. In routine cases, with no prior surgery or intraocular neoplasm, most eyes are opened in the horizontal meridian, which includes the macula in the same section as the pupil and optic nerve (Fig 3-3). Globes with a surgical or nonsurgical

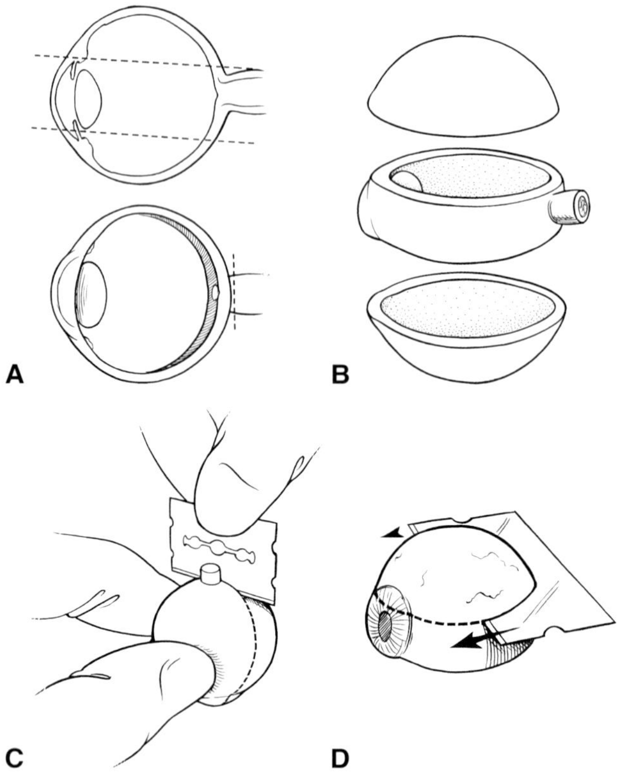

Figure 3-3 **A,** The goal of sectioning is to obtain a pupil–optic nerve (PO) section that contains the maximum area of interest. **B,** Two caps, or *calottes,* are removed to obtain a PO section. **C,** The first cut is generally performed from posterior to anterior. **D,** The second cut will yield the PO section. *(Illustration by Christine Gralapp.)*

wound should be opened so the wound will be perpendicular to, and included in, the PO section, which often means opening the globe vertically. Globes with intraocular tumors are opened in a way (horizontal, vertical, or oblique) that places the center of the tumor as outlined by transillumination in the PO section.

The globe can also be opened coronally with separation of the anterior and posterior compartments. The tumor can be visualized directly with this technique, and a section including the maximum extent of the tumor may then be obtained.

Processing and Staining

Fixatives

The most commonly used fixative is 10% neutral buffered formalin. Formalin is a 40% solution of formaldehyde in water that stabilizes protein, lipid, and carbohydrates and prevents postmortem enzymatic destruction of the tissue (autolysis). In specific instances, other fixatives may be preferred, such as glutaraldehyde for electron microscopy, ethyl alcohol for cytologic preparations, and Michel medium for immunofluorescence studies. Table 3-1 lists examples of some commonly used fixatives.

Formalin diffuses rather quickly through tissue. Because most of the functional tissue of the eye is within 2–3 mm of the surface, it is not necessary or desirable to open the eye. Opening the eye before fixation may damage or distort sites of pathology, making histologic interpretation difficult or impossible. The adult eye measures approximately 24 mm in diameter, and formalin diffuses at a rate of approximately 1 mm/hr; therefore, globes should be fixed at least 12 hours prior to processing. It is generally desirable to suspend an eye in formalin in a volume of approximately 10:1 for at least 24 hours prior to processing to ensure adequate fixation. Different institutions may use different protocols, and preoperative consultation is critical.

Tissue Processing

The infiltration and embedding process removes most of the water from the tissue and replaces the water with paraffin. Organic solvents used in this process will dissolve lipid and may dissolve some synthetic materials. Routine processing usually dissolves intraocular lenses made of polymethylmethacrylate (PMMA), polypropylene, and silicone, although the PMMA may fall out during sectioning. Silk, nylon, and other synthetic sutures do not dissolve during routine processing. Specimens are routinely processed through increasing concentrations of alcohol followed by xylene or another clearing agent prior to infiltration with paraffin. Alcohol dehydrates water, and xylene replaces alcohol prior to paraffin infiltration. The paraffin mechanically stabilizes the tissue, making possible the cutting of sections.

The processing of even a "routine" specimen usually takes a day. Thus, it is unreasonable for a surgeon to expect an interpretation of a specimen sent for permanent sections to be available on the same day as the biopsy. Techniques for the rapid processing of special surgical pathology material are generally reserved for biopsy specimens that require emergent handling. Because the quality of histologic preparation after rapid processing is usually inferior to that of standard processed tissue, it should not be requested routinely. Surgeons should communicate directly with their pathologists about the availability and shortcomings of these techniques.

Table 3-1 Common Fixatives Used in Ophthalmic Pathology

Fixative	Color	Examples of Use
Formalin	Clear	Routine fixation of all tissues
Bouin solution	Yellow	Small biopsies
B5	Clear	Lymphoproliferative tissue (eg, lymph node)
Glutaraldehyde	Clear	Electron microscopy
Ethanol/methanol	Clear	Crystals (eg, urate crystals of gout)
Michel fixative	Light pink	Immunofluorescence
Zenker acetic fixative	Orange	Muscle differentiation

Tissue Staining

Tissue sections are usually cut at 4–6 µm. A tissue adhesive is sometimes used to secure the thin paraffin section to a glass slide. The cut section is colorless except for areas of indigenous pigmentation, and various tissue dyes—principally hematoxylin and eosin (H&E) and periodic acid–Schiff (PAS)—are used to color the tissue for identification (Fig 3-4). Other histochemical stains used in ophthalmic pathology are alcian blue or colloidal iron for acid mucopolysaccharides, Congo red for amyloid, Gram stain for bacteria, Masson trichrome for collagen, Gomori methenamine silver stain for fungi, and oil red O for lipid. A small amount of resin is placed over the stained section and covered with a thin glass coverslip to protect and preserve it. Table 3-2 lists some common stains and gives examples of their use in ophthalmic pathology.

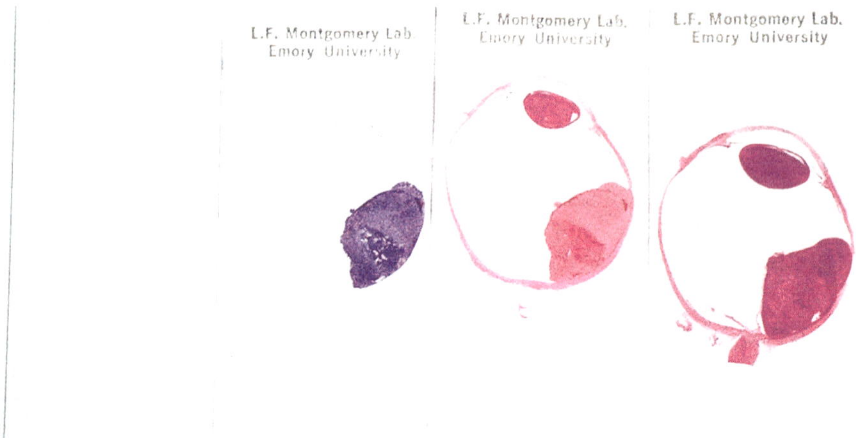

Figure 3-4 The section of a melanoma at the far left is colorless except for mild indigenous pigmentation in the tissue. Moving to the right, note the slides stained with hematoxylin only, eosin only, and both hematoxylin and eosin. *(Courtesy of Hans E. Grossniklaus, MD.)*

Table 3-2 Common Stains Used in Ophthalmic Pathology

Stain	Material Stained: Color	Example
Hematoxylin and eosin (H&E)	Nucleus: blue Cytoplasm: red	General tissue stain (Fig 3-2E)
Periodic acid–Schiff (PAS)	Glycogen and proteoglycans: magenta	Descemet membrane (Fig 6-17E)
Alcian blue	Acid mucopolysaccharide: blue	Cavernous optic atrophy (Fig 15-10B)
Alizarin red	Calcium: red	Band keratopathy
Colloidal iron	Acid mucopolysaccharide: blue	Macular dystrophy (Fig 6-21C)
Congo red	Amyloid: orange, red-green dichroism	Lattice dystrophy (Fig 6-23C, D)
Ziehl-Neelsen	Acid-fast organisms: red	Atypical mycobacterium
Gomori methenamine silver (GMS)	Fungal elements: black	*Fusarium* (Fig 6-7B)
Crystal violet	Amyloid: purple, violet	Lattice dystrophy
Gram stain (tissue Brown & Brenn [B&B] or Brown & Hopps [B&H] stain)	Bacteria positive: blue Bacteria negative: red	Bacterial infection
Masson trichrome	Collagen: blue Muscle: red	Granular dystrophy (Fig 6-22C) Red deposits
Perls Prussian blue	Iron: blue	Fleischer ring
Thioflavin T (ThT)	Amyloid: fluorescent yellow	Lattice dystrophy
Verhoeff–van Gieson (elastic stain)	Elastic fibers: black	Temporal artery elastic layer (Fig 15-6B)
von Kossa	Calcium phosphate salts: black	Band keratopathy (Fig 6-12C)

CHAPTER 4

Special Procedures

New technologies have contributed to improvements in the diagnosis of infectious agents and tumors as well as to the classification of tumors, especially the non-Hodgkin lymphomas (NHLs), childhood tumors, and sarcomas. Use of a more extensive test menu of paraffin-active monoclonal antibodies for immunohistochemistry; molecular cytogenetic studies, including standard cytogenetics; multicolor fluorescence in situ hybridization (FISH); polymerase chain reaction (PCR) and its many variations; and locus-specific FISH; as well as developments in high-resolution techniques, including microarray gene expression profiling, proteomics, and array comparative genomic hybridization (CGH), allow a more accurate diagnosis and more precise definition of biomarkers of value in risk stratification and prognosis. The ophthalmic surgeon is responsible for appropriately obtaining and submitting tissue for evaluation and consulting with the ophthalmic pathologist. See Table 4-1 for a checklist of important considerations when submitting tissue for pathologic consultation.

Immunohistochemistry

Pathologists making a diagnosis take advantage of the property that a given cell can express specific antigens. The immunohistochemical stains commonly used in ophthalmic pathology work because a primary antibody binds to a specific antigen in or on a cell, and because that antibody is linked to a chromogen, usually through a secondary antibody (Fig 4-1). The color product of the chromogens generally used in ophthalmic pathology is brown or red in tissue sections, depending on the chromogen selected for use (Fig 4-2). Red chromogen is especially helpful in working with ocular pigmented tissues and melanomas, because it differs from the brown melanin pigment (see Fig 4-7).

The precise cell or cells that display the specific antigen can be identified using these methods. Many antibodies are used routinely for diagnosis, treatment, and prognosis:

- cytokeratins for lesions composed of epithelial cells (adenoma, carcinoma)
- desmin, myoglobin, or actin for lesions with smooth muscle or skeletal muscle features (leiomyoma, rhabdomyosarcoma)
- S-100 protein for lesions of neuroectodermal origin (schwannoma, neurofibroma, melanoma)
- HMB-45 and Melan A for melanocytic lesions (nevus, melanoma)

Table 4-1 Checklist for Requesting an Ophthalmic Pathologic Consultation

Routine Specimens (cornea, conjunctiva, eyelid lesions)
1. Fill out requisition form
   a. Sex and age of patient
   b. Location of lesion (laterality and exact location)
   c. Previous biopsies of the site and diagnosis
   d. Pertinent clinical history
   e. Clinical differential diagnosis
   f. Ophthalmologist phone and fax numbers
2. Specimen submitted in adequately sealed container with
   a. Ample amount of 10% formalin (at least 5 times the size of the biopsy)
   b. Label with patient's name and location of biopsy
3. Drawing/map of site of biopsy for orientation of margins (eyelid lesions for margins, en bloc resections of conjunctiva, sclera, and ciliary body/iris tumors)

Frozen Sections
1. If possible, previous communication with ophthalmic pathologist
2. Fill out specific frozen section requisition form, specifying the reason for submitting tissue, such as
   a. Margins
   b. Diagnosis
   c. Adequacy of sampling
   d. Obtaining tissue for molecular diagnosis (retinoblastoma, rhabdomyosarcoma, metastatic neuroblastoma, etc) or flow cytometry
3. Map/diagram of lesion indicating margins and orientation
4. Labeling of tissue (ink, sutures) to orient according to the diagram (for margins)

Fine-Needle Aspiration Biopsy and Cytology
1. Previous communication with ophthalmic pathologist to discuss
   a. Logistics of the biopsy
      i. Possible adequacy check during the biopsy (intraocular tumors)
      ii. Fixative to be used
      iii. Fresh tissue for possible molecular diagnosis
   b. Specific cytology form to be filled out

Flow Cytometry
1. Previous communication with ophthalmic pathologist to discuss
   a. Fresh tissue is critical.
   b. Adequate sample is essential.
   c. Geographic proximity to the laboratory

Molecular Techniques and Electron Microscopy
1. Previous communication with ophthalmic pathologist to discuss
   a. Differential diagnosis
   b. Fixative (fresh vs alcohol vs glutaraldehyde vs other)
   c. Logistics of the biopsy
      i. Time and date (availability of specialized personnel)
      ii. Geographic proximity to laboratory

- chromogranin and synaptophysin for neuroendocrine lesions (metastatic carcinoid [see Fig 4-2], small cell carcinoma)
- leukocyte common antigen for lesions of hematopoietic origin (leukemia, lymphoma)
- CD antigens for subtyping white blood cells
- Her2Neu and c-Kit for prognosis and treatment (metastatic breast carcinoma, mastocytosis)

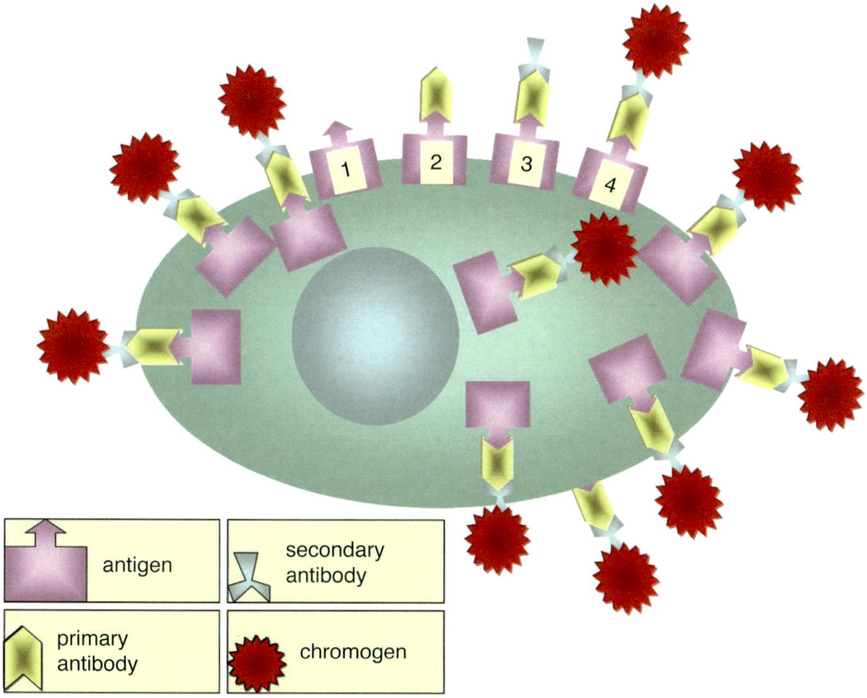

Figure 4-1 Schematic representation of the general immunohistochemistry method. *1,* The cellular antigen is recognized by the specific primary antibody, *2.* A secondary antibody, *3,* directed against the primary antibody, reacts with the enzymatic complex to create the chromogen, *4.* The final product allows the visualization of the cell containing the antigen. *(Courtesy of Patricia Chévez-Barrios, MD.)*

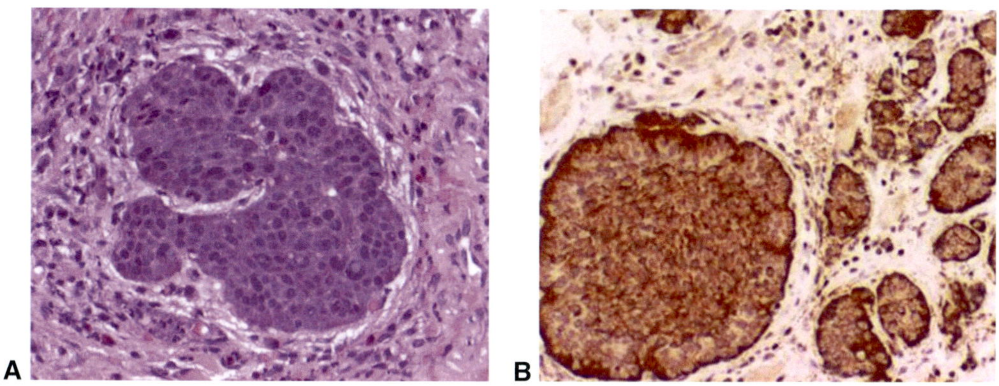

Figure 4-2 A metastatic carcinoid to the orbit seen by H&E **(A)** shows bland epithelial characteristics. **B,** Chromogranin antibody highlights the neuroendocrine nature of the cells. *(Courtesy of Patricia Chévez-Barrios, MD.)*

These antibodies vary in their specificity and sensitivity. Specificities and sensitivities of new antibodies are continually being evaluated (for examples, see the online immunohistology query system at www.immunoquery.com). Automated equipment and antigen retrieval techniques are currently used to increase sensitivity and decrease turnaround time.

Flow Cytometry, Molecular Pathology, and Diagnostic Electron Microscopy

Flow Cytometry

Flow cytometry is used to analyze the physical and chemical properties of particles or cells moving in single file in a fluid stream (Fig 4-3, *a*). An example of flow cytometry is immunophenotyping of leukocytes. The cells need to be fresh (unfixed). Fluorochrome-labeled specific antibodies bind to the surface of lymphoid cells, and a suspension of labeled cells is sequentially illuminated by a light source (usually argon laser) for approximately 10^{-6} second (Fig 4-3, *b*). As the excited fluorochrome returns to its resting energy level, a specific wavelength of light is emitted (Fig 4-3, *c*), which is sorted by wavelength stream (Fig 4-3, *d*) and received by a photodetector (Fig 4-3, *e*). This signal is then converted to

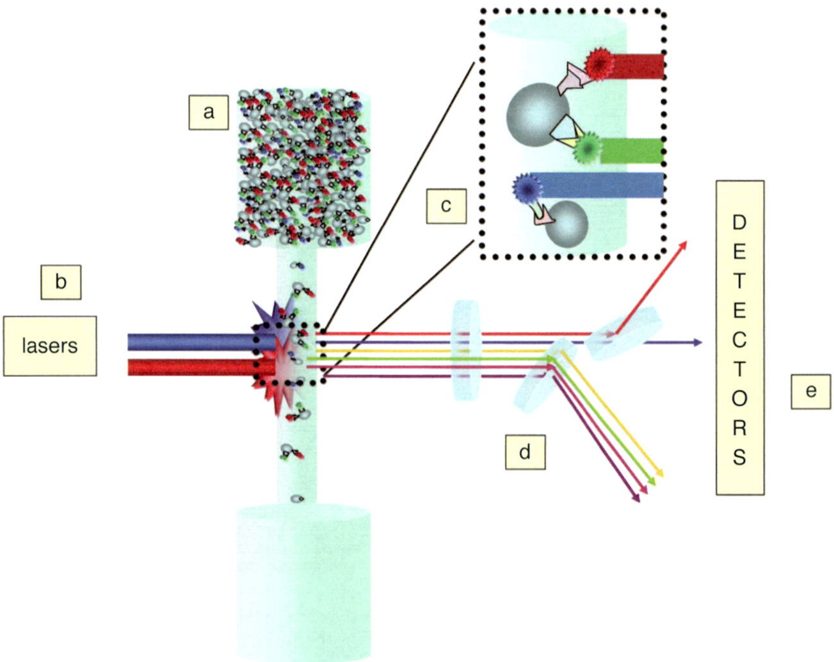

Figure 4-3 Flow cytometry analyzes particles or cells moving in single file in a fluid stream *(a)*. Fluorochrome-labeled specific antibodies bind to the surface of cells, and a suspension of labeled cells is sequentially illuminated by a laser *(b)*. As the excited fluorochrome returns to its resting energy level, a specific wavelength of light is emitted *(c)*, which is sorted by wavelength *(d)* and received by a photodetector *(e)*. This signal is then converted to electronic impulses, which are in turn analyzed by computer software. *(Courtesy of Patricia Chévez-Barrios, MD.)*

electronic impulses, which are in turn analyzed by computer software. The results may be imaged by a multicolored dot-plot histogram (Fig 4-4). The most common use of flow cytometry in clinical practice is for immunophenotyping hematopoietic proliferations. This procedure may be performed on vitreous, aqueous, or ocular adnexal tissue.

In addition, multiple antibodies and cellular size can be analyzed, and the relative percentages of cells may be displayed. For example, CD4 (helper T cells), CD8 (suppressor T cells), both $CD4^+$ and $CD8^+$, or either $CD4^+$ or $CD8^+$ may be displayed for a given lymphocytic infiltrate. The advantage of this method is that it actually shows the percentages of particular cells in a specimen. Disadvantages are the failure to show the location and distribution of these cells in tissue and the possibility of sampling errors. Depending on the number of cells in the sample and on clinical information, the flow cytometrist chooses the panel of antibodies to be tested. Flow cytometric data should therefore be used as an adjunct to morphologic H&E and sometimes immunohistochemistry interpretation. Flow cytometric analysis is particularly useful for the evaluation of lymphoid proliferations.

Molecular Pathology

Molecular biology techniques are used increasingly in diagnostic ophthalmic pathology and extensively in experimental pathology (Table 4-2). More recently, their use has expanded to include prognostication of disease and determination of treatment. Molecular pathology is used to identify tumor-promoting or tumor-inhibiting genes (CGH, PCR, array CGH), such as the retinoblastoma gene; and viral DNA or RNA strands, such as those seen in herpesviruses and Epstein-Barr virus (PCR, in situ hybridization [ISH]). The evolution of molecular pathology techniques has made it possible not only to recognize the presence or absence of a strand of nucleic acid but also to localize specific DNA

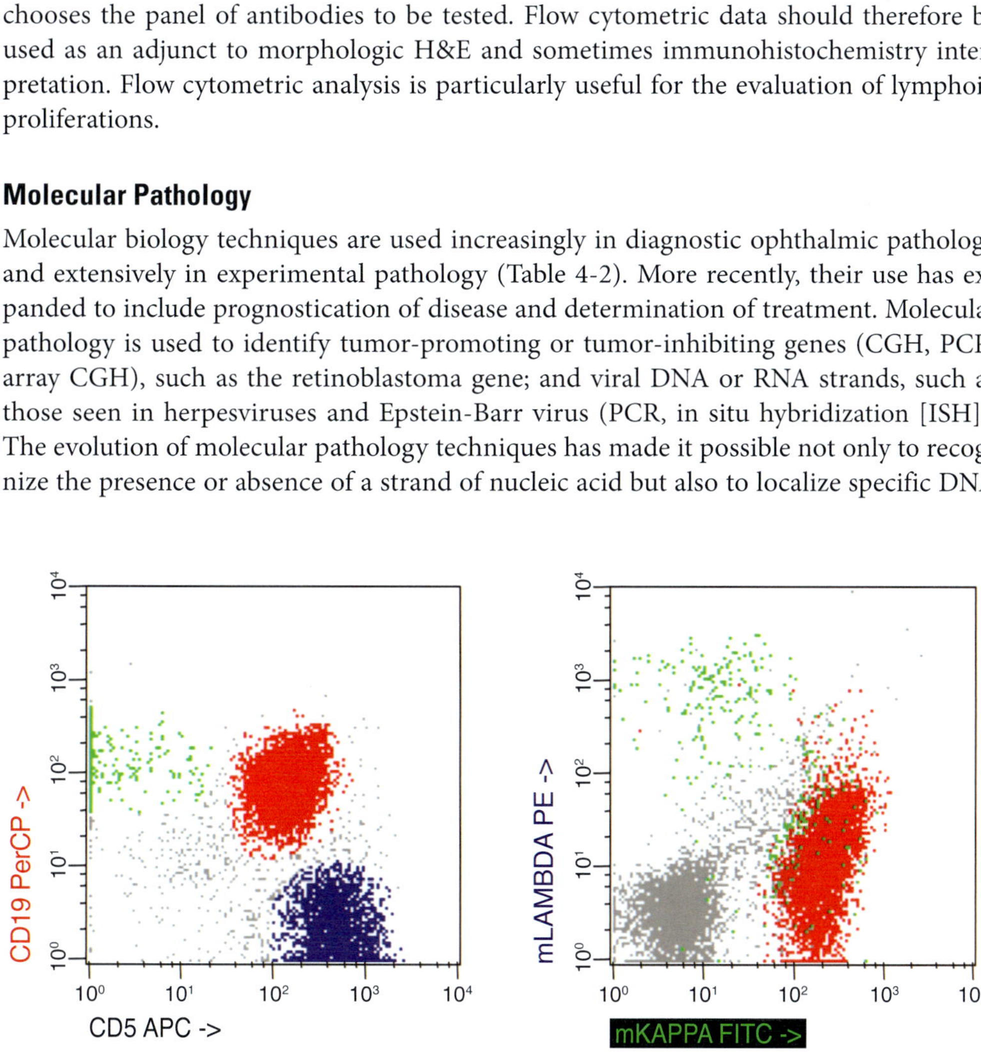

Figure 4-4 Flow cytometry scatter graphs showing a clonal population of $CD19^+$ kappa restricted lymphocytes. Note that most of the $CD19^+$ *(red in left graph)* cells fail to express lambda light chains; however, the cells do exhibit strong kappa expression *(red in right graph)*. *(Courtesy of Patricia Chévez-Barrios, MD.)*

Table 4-2 Summary of Molecular Techniques Used in Diagnostic Pathology

Technique	Method	Advantages	Disadvantages
SNP oligonucleotide microarray analysis (SOMA)	Type of DNA microarray used to detect single nucleotide polymorphisms (SNPs), the most frequent type of variation in the genome, within a population. Uses array that contains immobilized nucleic acid sequences and 1 or more labeled allele-specific oligonucleotide (ASO) probes	1. SNPs are highly conserved between species and within a population and serve as a genotypic marker for research. 2. Able to detect copy number neutral loss of heterozygosity to uniparental disomy 3. Has huge potential in cancer diagnostics	Unable to detect mosaicism, balanced chromosomal translocations, inversions, and whole-genome ploidy changes
Multiplex ligation-dependent probe amplification (MLPA)	Amplification of multiple targets using only a single primer pair within a single PCR mixture to produce amplicons of varying sizes that are specific to different DNA sequences	Additional information may be gained from a single test run.	Targets must be different enough to form distinct bands when visualized by gel electrophoresis.
Fluorescence in situ hybridization (FISH)	Chromosome region-specific, fluorescently labeled DNA probes (cloned pieces of genomic DNA) able to detect their complementary DNA sequences	Microfluidic chip allows automation and clinical use.	Known type and location of expected aberrations
Polymerase chain reaction (PCR)	Amplification of a single strand of DNA (nucleic acid) based on thermal cycles of repeated heating and cooling of the reaction for DNA melting and enzymatic replication of the DNA. Clinically used for early detection of cancer, hereditary diseases, and infectious diseases	Quality snap-frozen tissue (optimal) and archival paraffin-embedded tissue	1. Variable success rate of DNA extraction 2. Contamination with other nucleic acid material

Table 4-2 *(continued)*

Technique	Method	Advantages	Disadvantages
Reverse transcriptase-polymerase chain reaction (RT-PCR)	Amplifies DNA from RNA. Clinically used to determine the expression of a gene	Quality snap-frozen tissue (optimal) and archival paraffin-embedded tissue	1. Variable success rate of RNA extraction 2. Contamination with other nucleic acid material
Real-time quantitative PCR (RT-PCR)	Measurement of PCR-product accumulation during the exponential phase of the PCR reaction using a dual-labeled fluorogenic probe	Direct detection of PCR-product formation by measuring the increase in fluorescent emission continuously during the PCR reaction	Variable success rate of RNA extraction
Comparative genomic hybridization (CGH)	Molecular cytogenetic method for analysis of copy number changes (gains/losses) in the DNA content of an individual, often in tumor cells. Uses epifluorescence and quantitative, regional differences in the fluorescence ratio of gains/losses vs control DNA to identify abnormal regions in the genome at a resolution of 20–80 base pairs	1. Detects and maps alterations in copy number of DNA sequences 2. Analyzes all chromosomes in a single experiment and no dividing cells required	Inability to detect mosaicism, balanced chromosomal translocations, inversions, and whole-genome ploidy changes
Microarray-based CGH (array CGH)	Differentially labeled test and reference DNAs, hybridized to cloned fragments, genomic DNA or cDNA, which are spotted on a glass slide (the array). The DNA copy number aberrations measured by detecting intensity differences in the hybridization patterns	High resolution	1. Inability to detect aberrations not resulting in copy number changes 2. Limited in its ability to detect mosaicism

sequences within specific cells (FISH, ISH). Two major techniques have markedly advanced our knowledge of developmental biology and tumorigenesis: PCR (and its variations) and microarray (and its subtypes).

Polymerase chain reaction

A common molecular biology technique is the *polymerase chain reaction (PCR),* which amplifies a single strand of nucleic acid across several orders of magnitude, generating thousands to millions of copies of a particular DNA sequence (Fig 4-5). The PCR method

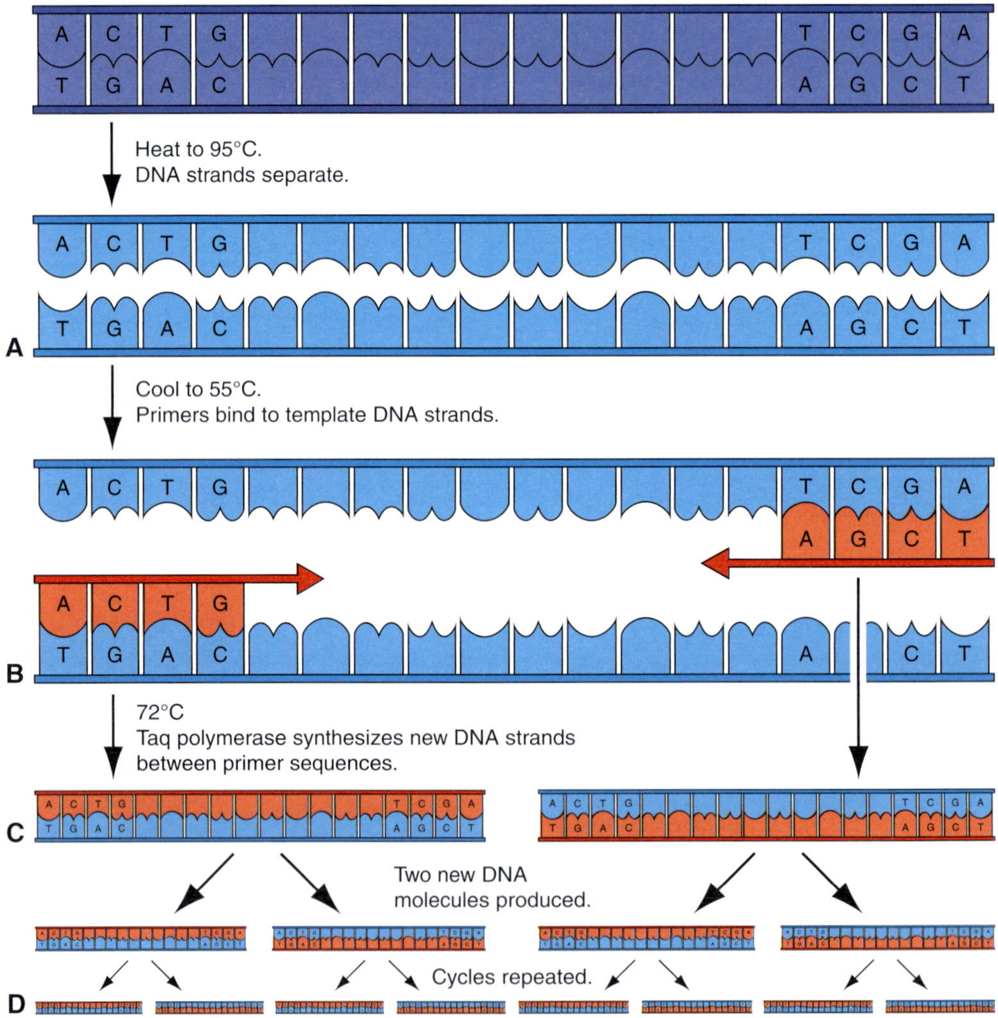

Figure 4-5 A, A polymerase chain reaction (PCR) starts with a denaturing step where DNA samples are heated to 95°C to separate the target DNA into single strands. **B,** Next, the temperature is lowered to 55°C to allow the primers to anneal to their complementary sequences. The primers are designed to bracket the DNA region to be amplified. **C,** The temperature is raised to 72°C to allow Taq polymerase to attach at each priming site and extend or synthesize a new DNA strand between primer sequences producing 2 new DNA molecules. **D,** Step C is repeated multiple times to generate thousands of copies. *(Courtesy of Theresa Kramer, MD.)*

relies on thermal cycles of repeated heating and cooling of the DNA sample for DNA melting and enzymatic replication. *Primers,* which are short DNA fragments containing sequences complementary to the target region, DNA polymerase, and nucleotides are the components required in order for selective and repeated amplification to occur. The selectivity of PCR is due to the use of primers that are complementary to the DNA region targeted for amplification.

The techniques of PCR have advanced considerably in recent years, and there are now approximately 20 variations on PCR, including real-time and quantitative real-time PCR. The variations center around quantification; increased definition of the sequence amplified (allele, single nucleotide, generation of long sequences with overlap technology, intersequences, flanking sequences and genomic inserts, methylation-specific sequences, conserved sequences, simultaneous multiple gene amplification); isothermal amplification methods for use in living cells (PAN-AC); and increased resolution of the sequence (multiplex ligation-dependent probe amplification, MLPA). MLPA permits multiple targets to be amplified simultaneously with only a single primer pair and is becoming important in prognostication of tumors. The clinical relevance of detecting a PCR product depends on numerous variables, including the primers selected, the laboratory controls, and the demographic considerations. Thus, for the clinician making a clinicopathologic diagnosis, PCR should be used mainly to derive supplementary information. See also Part III, Genetics, in BCSC Section 2, *Fundamentals and Principles of Ophthalmology.*

Microarray

Microarrays are used to survey the expression of thousands of genes in a single assay, the output of which is called a *gene expression profile.* Using microarray technology, scientists and clinicians can attempt to understand fundamental aspects of growth and development, as well as to explore the molecular mechanisms underlying normal and dysfunctional biological processes and elucidate the genetic causes of many human diseases. DNA microarray, microRNA microarray (MMChips), protein microarray, tissue microarray (Fig 4-6), cellular (or transfection) microarray, antibody microarray, and carbohydrate (glycoarray) microarray are some of the different types of microarrays available.

Although there are a variety of DNA microarray platforms, the basic process underlying all of them is straightforward: A glass slide or chip is spotted or "arrayed" with oligonucleotides or DNA fragments that represent specific gene coding regions (called *probes*). Fluorescently or chemiluminescently labeled purified cDNA or cRNA (called *target*) is hybridized to the "arrayed" slide/chip. After the chip is washed, the raw data are obtained by laser scanning, entered into a database (some public, others mined), and analyzed by statistical methods.

An example of one of these microarray platforms is the DualChip low-density microarray. These DNA microarrays were developed as a flexible tool capable of reliably quantifying the expression of a limited number of genes of clinical relevance, but DualChip technology has also been applied to tumor diagnosis and tumor-acquired drug resistance. Validation of the results of microarray experiments is a critical step in the analysis of gene expression. Quantitative real-time PCR is the method of choice for validation of gene expression profiling.

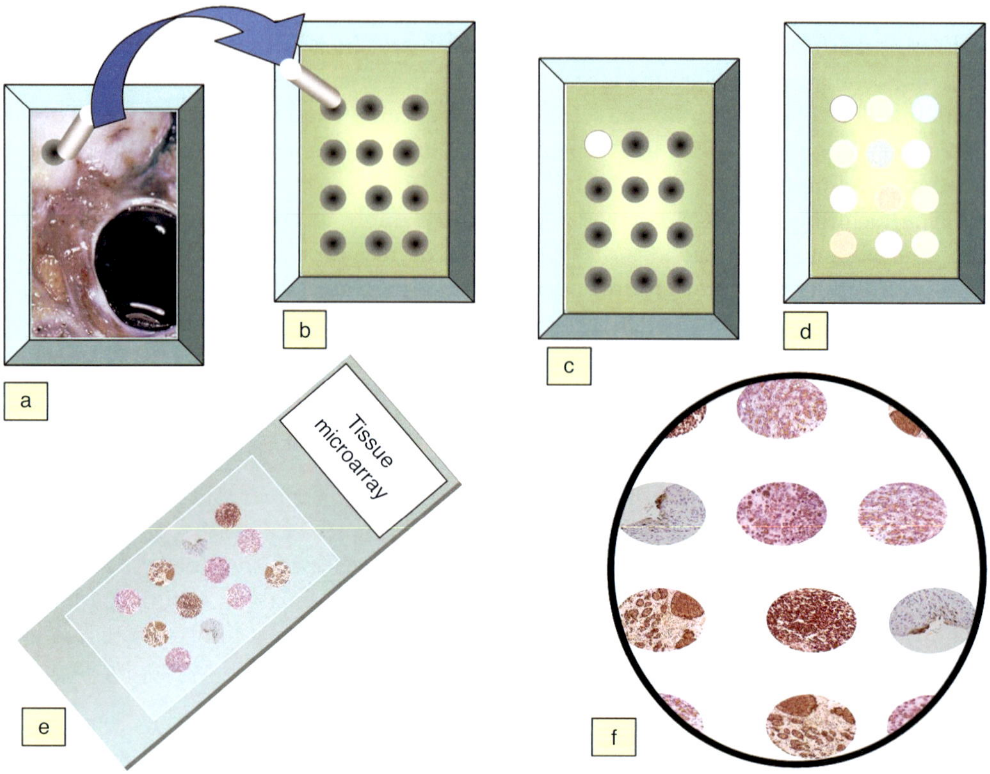

Figure 4-6 Tissue microarrays are constructed with small core biopsies of different tumors/tissues. A core is obtained from the donor paraffin block of the tumor *(a)*. A recipient paraffin block is prepared, creating empty cores *(b)*. The cores are incorporated into the slots *(c)* until all are occupied *(d)*. Glass slides are prepared and stained with a selected antibody *(e)*. Microscopic examination reveals the different staining patterns of each core *(f)*. *(Courtesy of Patricia Chévez-Barrios, MD.)*

Clinical use of PCR and microarray

Routine clinical use of PCR and microarray is limited to the diagnosis of leukemias, lymphomas, soft-tissue tumors, and tumors with nondiagnostic histopathology results. Commercial microarray and PCR platforms now exist that can be used for assigning biopsy-sized tumor samples to 1 of 2 distinct molecular classes, based on gene expression analysis that distinguishes low-grade tumors from high-grade tumors. The selection of commercially available microarray and PCR kits is growing rapidly.

Leukemias, lymphomas, and soft-tissue tumors represent a heterogeneous group of lesions whose classification continues to evolve as a result of advances in cytogenetic and molecular techniques. In the 1990s, traditional diagnostic approaches were supplemented by the successful application of these newer techniques (see Table 4-2) to formalin-fixed, paraffin-embedded tissue, making it possible to subject a broader range of clinical material to molecular analysis. Thus, molecular genetics has already become an integral part of the workup of tumors, such as pediatric orbital tumors (rhabdomyosarcomas, neuroblastomas, peripheral neuroectodermal tumors [PNET]), that demonstrate characteristic translocations. Based on the results, treatment can be directed and prognostic features associated with certain mutations and translocations.

Hicks J, Mierau GW. The spectrum of pediatric tumors in infancy, childhood, and adolescence: a comprehensive review with emphasis on special techniques in diagnosis. *Ultrastruct Pathol.* 2005;29(3-4):175–202.

Oostlander AE, Meijer GA, Ylstra B. Microarray-based comparative genomic hybridization and its applications in human genetics. *Clin Genet.* 2004;66(6):488–495.

Diagnostic Electron Microscopy

Diagnostic electron microscopy (DEM) is used primarily to indicate the cell of origin of a tumor of questionable differentiation rather than to distinguish between benign and malignant processes. Although immunopathologic studies are less expensive and performed more rapidly than DEM, in some cases, DEM complements immunopathologic studies. The surgeon should consult with the pathologist before surgery to determine whether DEM might play a role in the study of a particular tissue specimen.

Special Techniques

Fine-Needle Aspiration Biopsy

Fine-needle aspiration biopsy (FNAB) has been used instead of excisional biopsy by nonophthalmic surgeons and pathologists. It is especially useful if the physician performing the biopsy can grasp the lesion (usually between the thumb and forefinger) and make several passes with the needle to obtain representative areas. The use of FNAB (with the results interpreted by a well-trained cytologist or ophthalmic pathologist) is becoming more common in ophthalmology.

Intraocular FNAB may be useful in distinguishing between primary uveal tumors and metastases, and biopsy specimens can undergo genetic analysis using a microsatellite assay in order to identify monosomy 3 in uveal melanoma, which would indicate a poor prognosis. Intraocular FNAB has also been utilized in the diagnosis of primary intraocular lymphoma, and the biopsy specimens can undergo flow cytometric analysis, immunocytologic analysis, cytokine analysis, or molecular biological analysis (using PCR on both fixed and nonfixed material). Special fixatives are used for cytology specimens.

The procedure is performed under direct visualization through a dilated pupil. Iris tumors may be accessible for FNAB during slit-lamp biomicroscopy. However, FNAB alone cannot reliably predict the prognosis of a uveal melanoma because the sample with intraocular FNAB is limited. Intraocular FNAB may also enable tumor cells to escape the eye; this possibility is an area of some controversy. In general, properly performed, FNAB does not pose a significant risk for seeding a tumor, but retinoblastoma is a notable exception. FNAB of a possible retinoblastoma lesion, if indicated, should be performed by an *ophthalmic oncologist* with ample experience in making the diagnosis and performing the procedure.

The cells obtained through FNAB can be processed through cytospin of fluid or preparation of a cell block (Fig 4-7). Cell block allows the pathologist to employ special stains, immunohistochemistry, in situ hybridization, microarray, and gene expression profiling, if needed.

Some orbital surgeons have used FNAB in the diagnosis of orbital lesions, especially presumed metastases to the orbit and optic nerve tumors. However, because it is difficult to make several passes at different angles through an intraorbital tumor, FNAB of orbital masses may not adequately sample representative areas of the tumor. Specific indications for when and when not to perform intraocular or intraorbital FNAB are beyond the scope of this discussion, but some of these indications are discussed in Part II of this book, Intraocular Tumors: Clinical Aspects. Ophthalmic FNAB should be performed only when an ophthalmic pathologist or cytologist experienced in the preparation and interpretation of these specimens is available.

Cohen VM, Dinakaran S, Parsons MA, Rennie IG. Transvitreal fine needle aspiration biopsy: the influence of intraocular lesion size on diagnostic biopsy result. *Eye.* 2001;15(Pt 2): 143–147.

Frozen Section

Permanent sections (tissue that is processed after fixation through alcohols and xylenes, embedded in paraffin, and sectioned) are always preferred in ophthalmic pathology because of the inherent small size of samples. If the lesion is too small, it could be lost during frozen sectioning. A frozen section (tissue that is snap-frozen and immediately sectioned in a cryostat) is indicated when the results of the study will affect management of the patient in the operating room. For example, the most frequent indication for a frozen

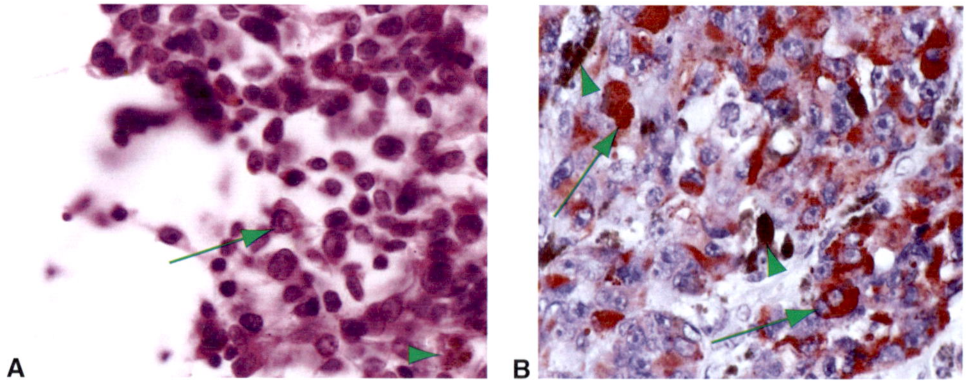

Figure 4-7 Fine-needle aspiration biopsy (FNAB) of choroidal tumor. **A,** Cytologic liquid-based preparation displays prominent nucleoli *(arrow)* and some brown pigment *(arrowhead)* suggestive of melanoma. **B,** Cell block of the aspirated cells, stained with HMB-45 using a red chromogen, is positive, confirming the diagnosis of melanoma. Notice the difference between the red chromogen *(arrows)* and the brown melanin *(arrowheads)*. *(Courtesy of Patricia Chévez-Barrios, MD.)*

section is to determine whether the resection margins are free of tumor, especially in eyelid carcinomas. Appropriate orientation of the specimen, correlated with documentation (through drawings of the excision site, labeled margins, or margins of the excised tissue that are tagged with sutures or other markers), is crucial when tissue is submitted for margin evaluation.

Two techniques are used for assessing the margins in eyelid carcinomas (basal cell carcinoma, squamous cell carcinoma, and sebaceous carcinoma): routine frozen sections and Mohs micrographic surgery. Mohs surgery preserves tissue while obtaining free margins. Eyelid lesions, especially those located in the canthal areas, require tissue conservation to maintain adequate cosmetic and functional results. Other frequent indications for frozen sections are to determine whether the surgeon has obtained, through biopsy, representative material for diagnosis (especially metastasis) and to submit fresh tissue for flow cytometry and molecular genetics (eg, cancers). Frozen sections are a time-intensive and costly process and should be used with discretion.

It is considered inappropriate to order frozen sections and then to proceed with a case before receiving the results from the pathologist. To ensure adequate understanding of the case and facilitate the best possible results for the patient, the surgeon should communicate with the pathologist ahead of time if a frozen section is anticipated.

Chévez-Barrios P. Frozen section diagnosis and indications in ophthalmic pathology. *Arch Pathol Lab Med.* 2005;129(12):1626–1634.

CHAPTER 5

Conjunctiva

Topography

The conjunctiva is a mucous membrane lining the posterior surface of the eyelids and the anterior surface of the globe as far as the limbus. It can be subdivided into *palpebral, forniceal, bulbar,* and *caruncular* sections. The conjunctiva consists of epithelium and underlying stroma. The epithelium is nonkeratinizing stratified squamous, with goblet cells. The conjunctival epithelium is continuous with the corneal epithelium, but the latter has no goblet cells. In the forniceal and bulbar areas, the conjunctival epithelium is flat and regular, while in the palpebral area, it exhibits ridges (Fig 5-1A, B). The goblet cells of the epithelium are most numerous in the fornices and plica semilunaris (Fig 5-1C, D). Beneath the epithelium is the conjunctival stroma, or *substantia propria,* which is thickest in the fornices and thinnest covering the tarsus. Constituents of this stromal layer include loosely arranged collagen fibers; vessels; lymphatics; nerves; occasional accessory lacrimal glands; and resident lymphocytes, plasma cells, macrophages, and mast cells. In places, the lymphocytes are organized into lymphoid follicles, and this *conjunctiva-associated lymphoid tissue (CALT)* is an example of *mucosa-associated lymphoid tissue (MALT)* (see the section Lymphocytic Lesions). The bulbar portion of the substantia propria fuses with the underlying *Tenon capsule.* In the medial canthal area, the conjunctiva forms a vertical fold, the *plica semilunaris,* and medial to this is the *caruncle.* The stroma of the caruncle is the only part of the conjunctiva that (like skin) also contains sebaceous glands and hair follicles (Fig 5-1E). See BCSC Section 2, *Fundamentals and Principles of Ophthalmology,* and Section 8, *External Disease and Cornea,* for further discussion.

Congenital Anomalies

Choristomas

A choristoma is a benign, congenital proliferation of histologically mature tissue elements not normally present at the site of occurrence. This heterotopic congenital lesion results from normal tissue migrating to or remaining in an abnormal location during embryogenesis (hence the derivation from the Greek word for "separated mass"). Examples include

- limbal dermoid
- lipodermoid (or dermolipoma)
- ectopic lacrimal gland

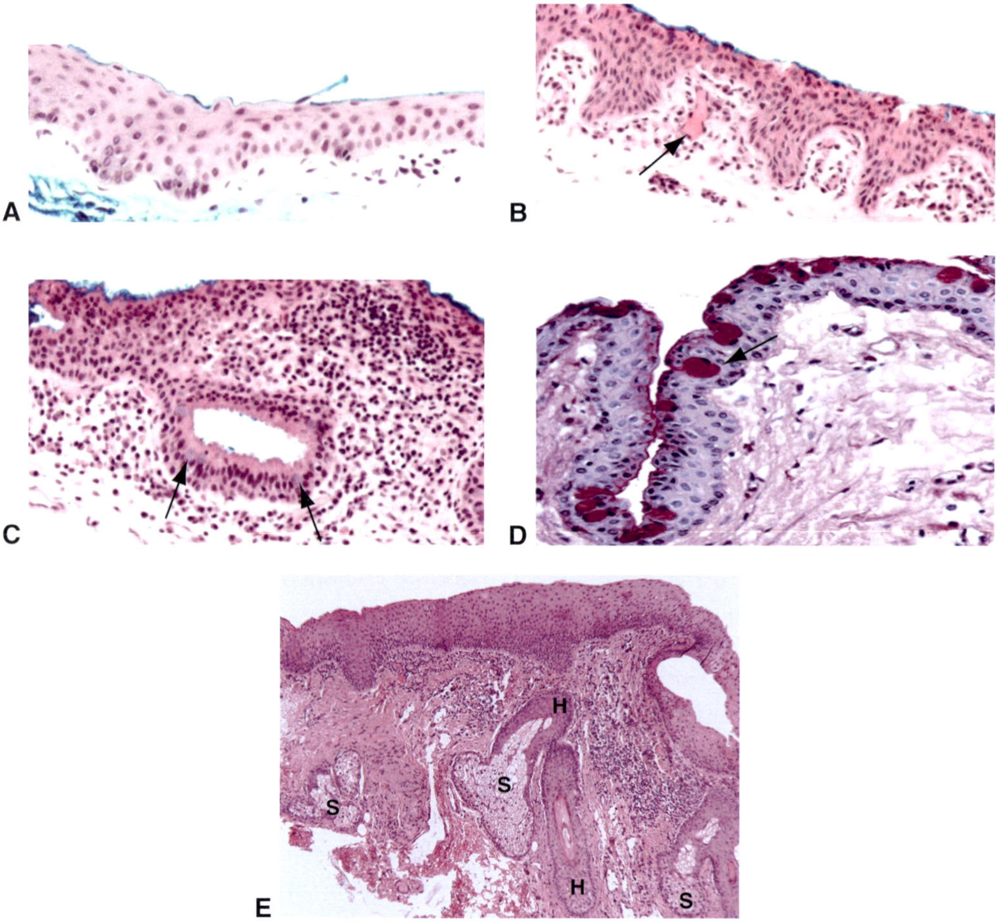

Figure 5-1 **A,** Epibulbar conjunctiva with regular, nonkeratinizing stratified squamous epithelium. **B,** Palpebral conjunctiva with epithelial ridges. Stroma contains vessels and inflammatory cells *(arrow)*. **C,** Conjunctiva at the fornix may contain pseudoglands of Henle, infoldings of conjunctiva with abundant goblet cells *(arrows)*. **D,** Periodic acid–Schiff (PAS) stain highlights the mucin in goblet cells *(arrow)*. **E,** Caruncular conjunctiva, containing sebaceous glands *(S)* and hair follicles *(H)*. *(Parts A–D courtesy of Patricia Chévez-Barrios, MD; part E courtesy of George J. Harocopos, MD.)*

- episcleral osseous choristoma and osseocartilaginous choristoma
- complex choristoma

Dermoids are firm, dome-shaped, white-yellow papules typically at or straddling the limbus, most commonly in the inferotemporal quadrant (Fig 5-2A, B). They may also involve the central cornea. Size varies from a few millimeters to more than 1 cm. Dermoids may occur in isolation or, particularly when bilateral, as a manifestation of a congenital complex such as Goldenhar syndrome (oculoauriculovertebral dysgenesis, characterized by epibulbar dermoid, upper eyelid coloboma, preauricular skin tags, and vertebral anomalies) or linear nevus sebaceous syndrome (an oculoneurocutaneous disorder). A dermoid often contains dermal adnexal structures. The surface epithelium may or may not be keratinized (Fig 5-2C).

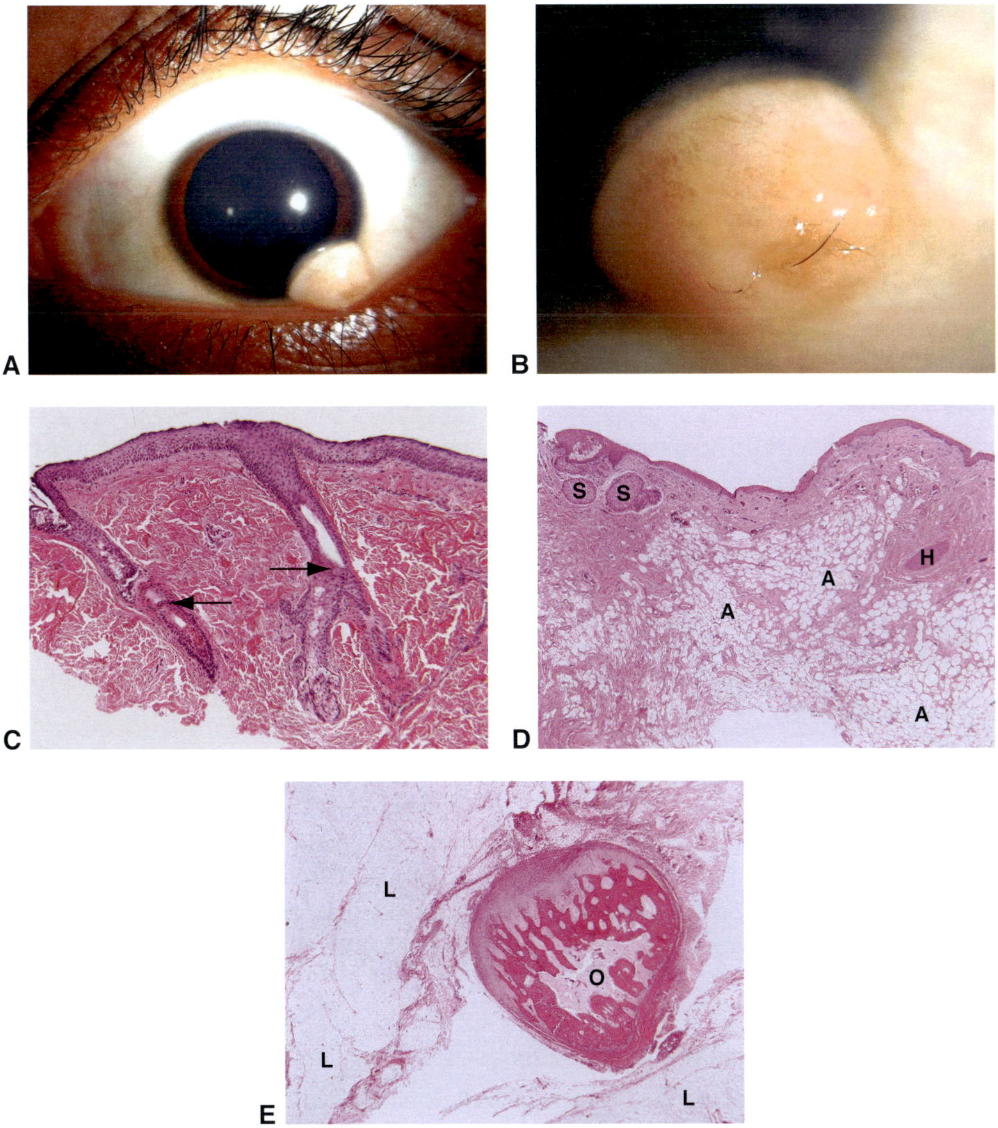

Figure 5-2 Ocular surface choristomas. **A,** Limbal dermoid, clinical appearance. **B,** Higher magnification shows hairs emanating from the dermoid. **C,** Histology shows keratinized epithelium, dense stroma, and sebaceous glands with hair follicles *(arrows)*. **D,** A lipodermoid differs from a dermoid in that significant amounts of mature adipose tissue *(A)* are present. This lipodermoid also contains dermal adnexal structures, including sebaceous glands *(S)* and hair follicles *(H)*. **E,** An osseous choristoma contains bone, and complex choristomas combine features of multiple types of choristomas, in this case osseous *(O)* plus lipodermoid *(L)*. *(Parts A and B courtesy of Morton E. Smith, MD; parts C–E courtesy of George J. Harocopos, MD.)*

Lipodermoids (or dermolipomas) occur more frequently in the superotemporal quadrant toward the fornix and may extend posteriorly into the orbit. As a result of its adipose tissue component, a lipodermoid is softer and yellower than a dermoid (Fig 5-2D). Dermal adnexal structures may or may not be present. Lipodermoids, like dermoids, may be associated with Goldenhar syndrome or linear nevus sebaceous syndrome.

Osseous choristomas contain bone. *Complex choristomas* combine features of multiple types of choristomas, for example, dermoid or lipodermoid plus osseous choristoma (Fig 5-2E). Clinically, they are often indistinguishable from dermoids or lipodermoids. See BCSC Section 6, *Pediatric Ophthalmology and Strabismus,* and Section 8, *External Disease and Cornea.*

Hamartomas

Hamartomas, like choristomas, are benign, congenital proliferations; but in contrast to choristomas, they are abnormal overgrowths of mature tissue normally present at that site (hence the derivation from the Greek word for "mistake mass"). In the conjunctiva, the most common variety of hamartoma is a *capillary hemangioma,* although this hamartoma most often involves the eyelid and may involve the orbit (see Chapter 13). Some consider hemangiomas to be true (acquired) neoplasms.

Inflammations

Because the conjunctiva is an exposed surface, a variety of organisms, allergens, and toxic agents can initiate an inflammatory response known as *conjunctivitis.* The response can be subdivided according to the time frame of symptoms and signs (acute or chronic); according to the appearance of the conjunctiva (papillary, follicular, or less commonly, granulomatous); or according to etiology (infectious, noninfectious). See BCSC Section 6, *Pediatric Ophthalmology and Strabismus,* and Section 8, *External Disease and Cornea,* for additional discussion.

Papillary Versus Follicular Conjunctivitis

Most cases of conjunctivitis may be categorized as either papillary or follicular, according to the macroscopic and microscopic appearance of the conjunctiva (Fig 5-3). Neither type is pathognomonic for a particular disease entity. *Papillary conjunctivitis* shows a cobblestone arrangement of flattened nodules with central vascular cores (Fig 5-4). It is most commonly associated with an allergic immune response, as in vernal and atopic keratoconjunctivitis, or it is a response to a foreign body such as a contact lens or ocular prosthesis. Papillae coat the tarsal surface of the upper eyelid and may reach large size *(giant papillary conjunctivitis).* Limbal papillae may occur in vernal keratoconjunctivitis *(Horner-Trantas dots).* The histologic appearance of papillary conjunctivitis is identical, regardless of the cause: closely packed, flat-topped projections, with numerous eosinophils, lymphocytes, plasma cells, and mast cells in the stroma surrounding a central vascular channel.

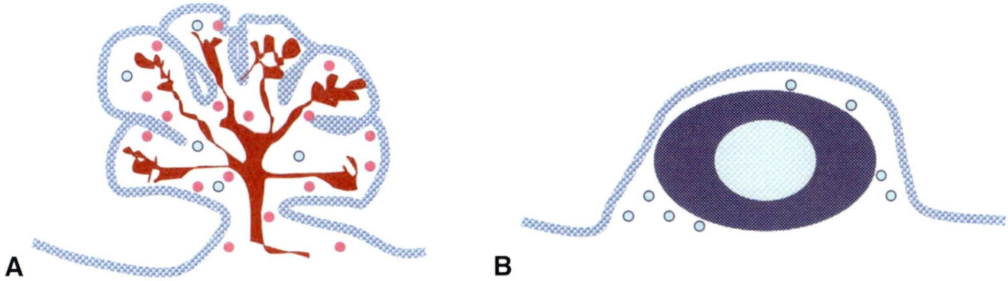

Figure 5-3 Schematic representation of papillary and follicular conjunctivitis. **A,** In papillary conjunctivitis, the conjunctival epithelium *(checkered blue)* covers fibrovascular cores with blood vessels *(red)*, and the stroma contains eosinophils *(pink circles)* and lymphocytes and plasma cells *(blue circles)*. **B,** In follicular conjunctivitis, the conjunctival epithelium covers lymphoid follicles, which have a paler germinal center surrounded by a darker corona *(central pale blue surrounded by dark blue)*, and the surrounding stroma contains lymphocytes and plasma cells *(small blue circles)*. *(Courtesy of Patricia Chévez-Barrios, MD.)*

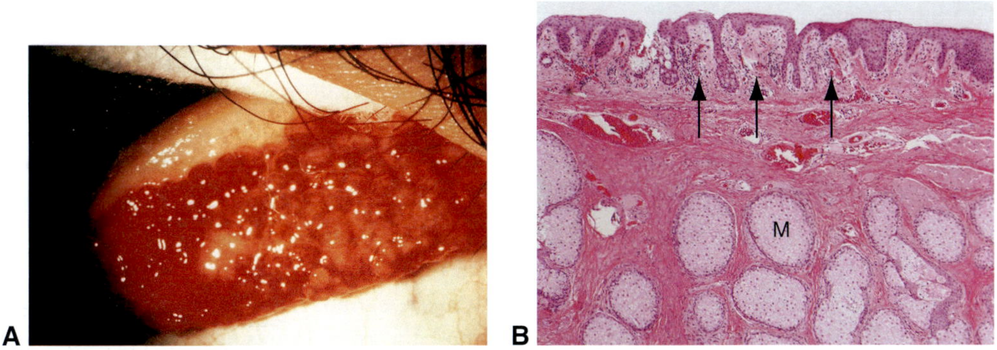

Figure 5-4 Papillary conjunctivitis. **A,** Clinical appearance. Papillae efface the normal palpebral conjunctival surface and form a confluent cobblestone pattern. **B,** Low-power photomicrograph exhibits the closely packed, flat-topped papillae with central fibrovascular cores *(arrows)*. The normal meibomian glands *(M)* of the tarsus are also shown. *(Part A courtesy of Harry H. Brown, MD; part B courtesy of George J. Harocopos, MD.)*

Follicular conjunctivitis (Fig 5-5) is seen in a variety of conditions, including inflammation caused by pathogens such as viruses; atypical bacteria; and toxins, including topical medications (glaucoma medications, especially brimonidine, or over-the-counter ophthalmic decongestants). In contrast to papillae, follicles are small, dome-shaped nodules without a prominent central vessel. Accordingly, whereas a papilla clinically appears more red on its surface and more pale at its base, a follicle appears more pale on its surface and more red at its base. Histologically, a lymphoid follicle is situated in the subepithelial region and consists of a *germinal center,* containing immature, proliferating lymphocytes; and surrounding *corona,* containing mature lymphocytes and plasma cells. The follicles in follicular conjunctivitis are typically most prominent in the inferior palpebral and forniceal conjunctiva.

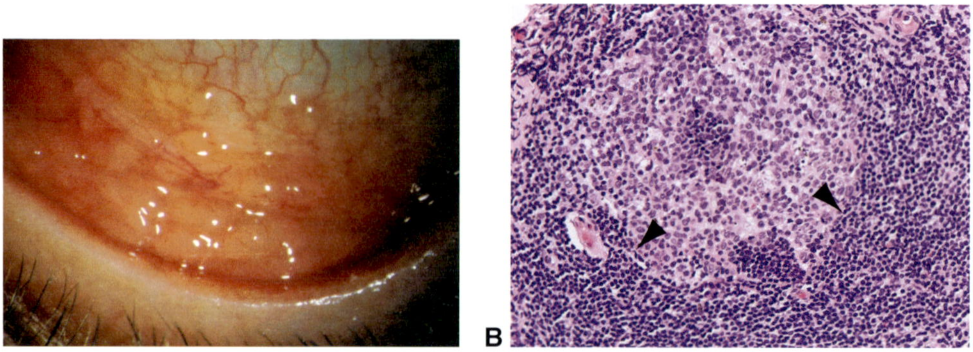

Figure 5-5 Follicular conjunctivitis. **A,** Clinical photograph showing follicles. **B,** High-power photomicrograph shows lymphoid follicle with boundary between germinal center and corona *(arrowheads).* Note the paler, relatively larger, immature lymphocytes in the germinal center, as compared to the darker, small, mature lymphocytes and plasma cells in the corona. *(Part A courtesy of Anthony J. Lubniewski, MD; part B courtesy of George J. Harocopos, MD.)*

Granulomatous Conjunctivitis

Though less common than papillary or follicular conjunctivitis, granulomatous conjunctivitis does occur. Clinically, the nodular elevations observed in granulomatous conjunctivitis may be difficult to distinguish from follicles, but clinical history and other systemic symptoms may point to the diagnosis. Granulomatous conjunctivitis in association with preauricular lymphadenopathy is known as *Parinaud oculoglandular syndrome.* Bacteria such as *Bartonella henselae* (cat-scratch disease) and *Francisella tularensis* (tularemia), mycobacteria (eg, tuberculosis), and treponemes (eg, syphilis) are possible causes. The diagnosis can be made by serology, culture, polymerase chain reaction (PCR), or a combination of these. If conjunctival biopsy is performed, the granulomas in infectious granulomatous conjunctivitis will typically demonstrate central necrosis (caseation). The bacteria may be demonstrated with Gram, acid-fast, or Warthin-Starry stains, depending on the organism.

There are also noninfectious causes of granulomatous conjunctivitis. *Sarcoidosis* may involve all ocular tissues, including the conjunctiva. It manifests as small, tan nodules, primarily within the forniceal conjunctiva (Fig 5-6). The nodules are often present even in the absence of an obvious conjunctivitis, that is, in noninjected, asymptomatic eyes. Conjunctival biopsy can be a simple, expedient way of providing diagnostic confirmation of this systemic disease. Histologically, noncaseating granulomatous "tubercles" (round to oval aggregates of epithelioid histiocytes) are present within the conjunctival stroma with a variable, but usually minimal, cuff of lymphocytes and plasma cells. Multinucleated giant cells may or may not be present within the granulomas. Central necrosis is not characteristic and, if present, should suggest infectious causes of granulomatous inflammation. The diagnosis of sarcoidosis is tenable only when supported by clinical findings and after other causes of granulomatous inflammation have been excluded by histochemical stains and/or by culture. See also Chapter 12 in this volume and BCSC Section 9, *Intraocular Inflammation and Uveitis.*

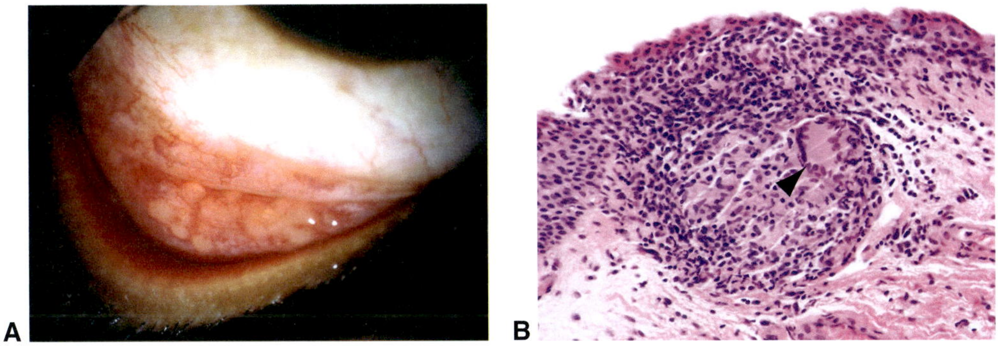

Figure 5-6 Sarcoidosis. **A,** Clinical appearance of sarcoid granulomas of the conjunctiva. **B,** Histology shows noncaseating granulomatous tubercle, with pale-staining histioctyes, including a multinucleated giant cell *(arrowhead)*. Note the minimal surrounding cuff of lymphocytes and plasma cells. *(Courtesy of George J. Harocopos, MD.)*

As an exposed surface, the conjunctiva is vulnerable to contact with foreign bodies. Some may be transient and/or inert, whereas others may become embedded and incite a foreign-body reaction, identifiable histologically as a granuloma surrounding the foreign object. Multinucleated giant cells are common. Viewing the tissue section under polarized light may be helpful in identifying the offending foreign material (Fig 5-7).

Infectious Conjunctivitis

A wide variety of pathogens may infect the conjunctiva, including viruses, bacteria, atypical bacteria (eg, chlamydiae), fungi, and parasites. The most common offending agents in children are bacterial *(Haemophilus influenzae, Streptococcus pneumoniae)* and, in adults, viral; the usual culprits are adenovirus and the herpesviruses (simplex and zoster). Viral infections, in addition to inciting a follicular conjunctivitis, often affect the cornea,

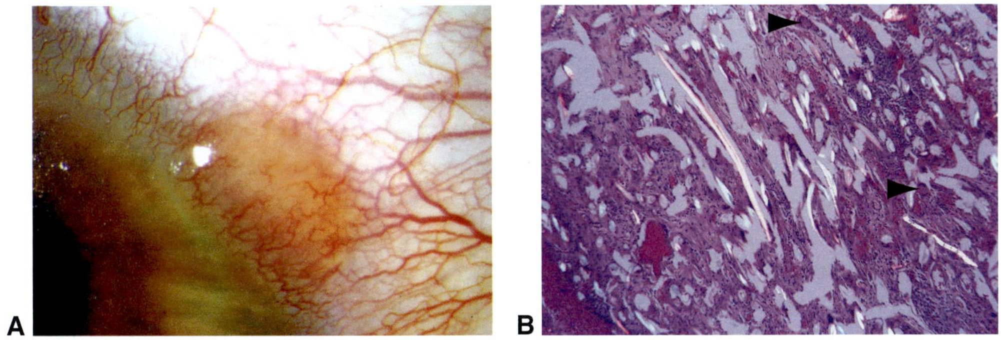

Figure 5-7 Conjunctival foreign-body granuloma. **A,** Clinical appearance on the bulbar conjunctiva. **B,** Histologic analysis of the specimen from a different patient under polarized light shows multiple foreign fibers of various colors, with surrounding foreign-body granulomatous reaction, including multiple giant cells *(arrowheads)*. *(Part A courtesy of Anthony J. Lubniewski, MD; part B courtesy of George J. Harocopos, MD.)*

resulting in ulcers in herpetic disease (see Chapter 6) and subepithelial infiltrates in adenoviral disease. Specific diagnosis of infectious conjunctivitis may be made based on clinical history and examination (typically sufficient for viral disease), or it may require Gram stain/culture, PCR, or serology, depending on the organism. In cases of diagnostic uncertainty or cases unresponsive to initial treatment, exfoliative (ie, impression) cytology of ocular surface epithelium or tissue biopsy may be helpful in establishing a definitive diagnosis.

Chlamydiae are obligate intracellular pathogens that may cause follicular conjunctivitis. *Chlamydia trachomatis* is a major cause of ocular infection (trachoma), particularly in the Middle East. Serotypes A, B, and C are associated with trachoma; serotypes D through K cause neonatal and adult inclusion conjunctivitis. Exfoliative cytology of ocular surface epithelium (Giemsa stain) or tissue biopsy may demonstrate these intracellular organisms (Fig 5-8).

When the conjunctiva alone is infected, fungi are rarely the inciting pathogen. Fungal ocular surface infections typically involve the cornea (see Chapter 6).

Microsporida, a group of obligate intracellular parasites, may cause conjunctivitis, keratitis, or keratoconjunctivitis, particularly in patients with acquired immunodeficiency syndrome (AIDS). *Rhinosporidium seeberi,* which may cause an isolated conjunctivitis (typically affects the palpebral/forniceal conjunctiva), is seen most often in areas such as India and Southeast Asia but has also been reported in the southeastern United States. Infection is typically associated with exposure to stagnant water. This organism was initially classified as a fungus but has been reclassified as a protozoon. The protozoon *Acanthamoeba* occasionally causes an isolated conjunctivitis but typically also infects the cornea (see Chapter 6). This diagnosis should be considered in chronic unilateral conjunctivitis unresponsive to standard therapy; exfoliative cytology may be helpful in establishing the diagnosis.

Noninfectious Conjunctivitis

As discussed previously, most papillary conjunctivitis, some forms of granulomatous conjunctivitis, and toxic follicular conjunctivitis are associated with noninfectious etiologies. See the sections Papillary Versus Follicular Conjunctivitis and Granulomatous Conjunctivitis for specific examples.

Ocular cicatricial pemphigoid (OCP) is a form of cicatrizing conjunctivitis that is of autoimmune etiology. It typically also involves other mucous membranes and sometimes involves the skin. When this diagnosis is suspected clinically, conjunctival biopsy is performed to establish the diagnosis. Half of the specimen should be submitted in formalin for routine histology, and half submitted in Michel medium or saline for immunofluorescence analysis. Histology shows bullae of the epithelium and a subepithelial band of chronic inflammatory cells, predominantly plasma cells (Fig 5-9). Immunofluorescence demonstrates IgG, IgM, and/or IgA immunoglobulins, and/or complement (C3) positivity in the epithelial basement membrane zone. The clinician must bear in mind that the sensitivity of immunofluorescence may be as low as 50% (particularly in long-standing cases with severe cicatrization). Thus, a negative result does not rule out the possibility of OCP. See also BCSC Section 8, *External Disease and Cornea.*

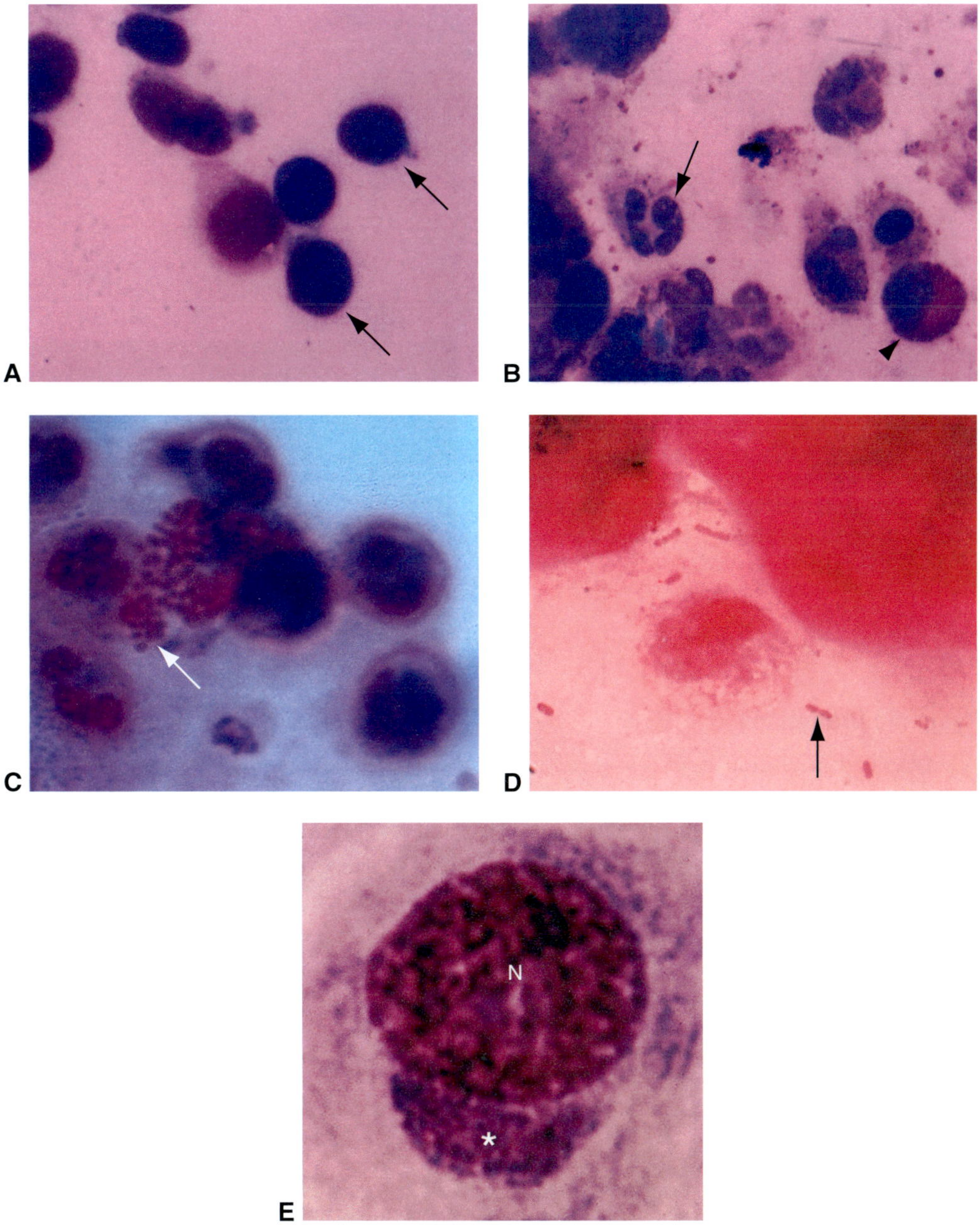

Figure 5-8 Exfoliative conjunctival cytology. **A,** Lymphocytes *(arrows)* predominate in viral conjunctivitis. **B,** A mixture of neutrophils *(arrow)* and eosinophils *(arrowhead)* is typical of vernal conjunctivitis. **C,** Gram stain reveals the polymorphonuclear leukocyte response to gonococcal conjunctivitis. Note the intracellular gram-negative diplococci *(arrow)*. **D,** A case of *Moraxella lacunata* angular conjunctivitis demonstrating the bacilli, which often are found in pairs *(arrow)*. **E,** *Chlamydia,* conjunctival scraping, Giemsa stain. The cytoplasmic inclusion body *(asterisk)*, composed of multiple chlamydial organisms, can be seen capping the nucleus *(N)*. A distinct space separates the inclusion body from the nuclear chromatin.

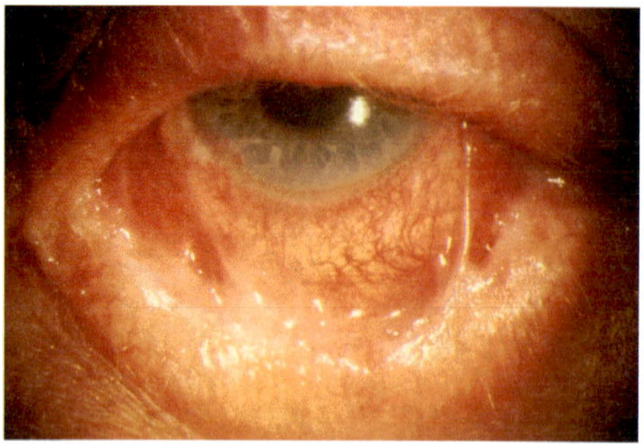

A

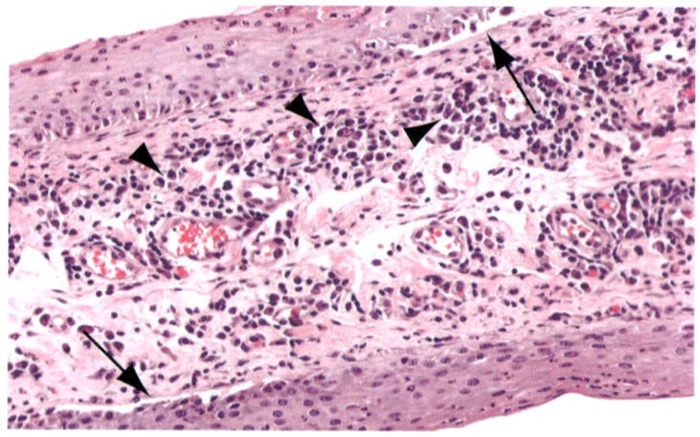

B

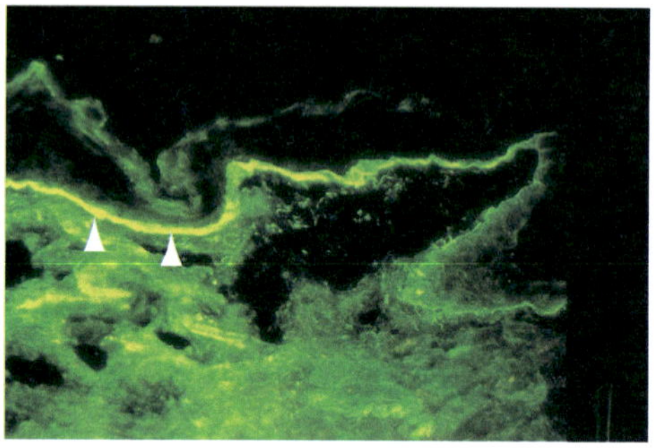

C

Figure 5-9 Ocular cicatricial pemphigoid (OCP). **A,** Clinical appearance. **B,** Histology shows epithelial bullae *(arrows)* and dense plasma cell infiltrate in the substantia propria *(arrowheads)*. **C,** Immunofluorescent staining of the epithelial basement membrane *(arrowheads)* in OCP. *(Part A courtesy of Andrew J.W. Huang, MD; part B courtesy of George J. Harocopos, MD.)*

Pyogenic Granuloma

A pyogenic granuloma appears as a reddish nodular elevation on the ocular surface, typically occurring in association with a chalazion (on the palpebral conjunctiva), or at a site of prior accidental or surgical trauma. Classic examples of the latter include a site of strabismus surgery (at the muscle insertion), retinal surgery, or enucleation. The name of this condition is somewhat of a misnomer because the lesion is not necrotic, nor is it a true granuloma. Rather, it consists of granulation tissue, that is, a pedunculated mass composed of a mixture of acute and chronic inflammatory cells, with proliferating capillaries that classically form a "spoke-wheel" pattern (Fig 5-10).

Degenerations

Pinguecula and Pterygium

A *pinguecula* is a small, yellowish nodule, often bilateral, situated at the nasal and/or temporal limbus (Fig 5-11A). It is a manifestation of actinic damage (exposure to sunlight) and is therefore more common with advancing years. Pingueculae are typically asymptomatic and may generally be observed. On histology, the stromal collagen shows fragmentation and basophilic degeneration called *elastotic degeneration* because the degenerated collagen stains positively with histochemical stains for elastic fibers such as the Verhoeff–van Gieson (VVG) stain (Fig 5-11B, C). See Chapter 6 for a discussion of actinic keratopathy, which may be regarded as the corneal analogue of pinguecula.

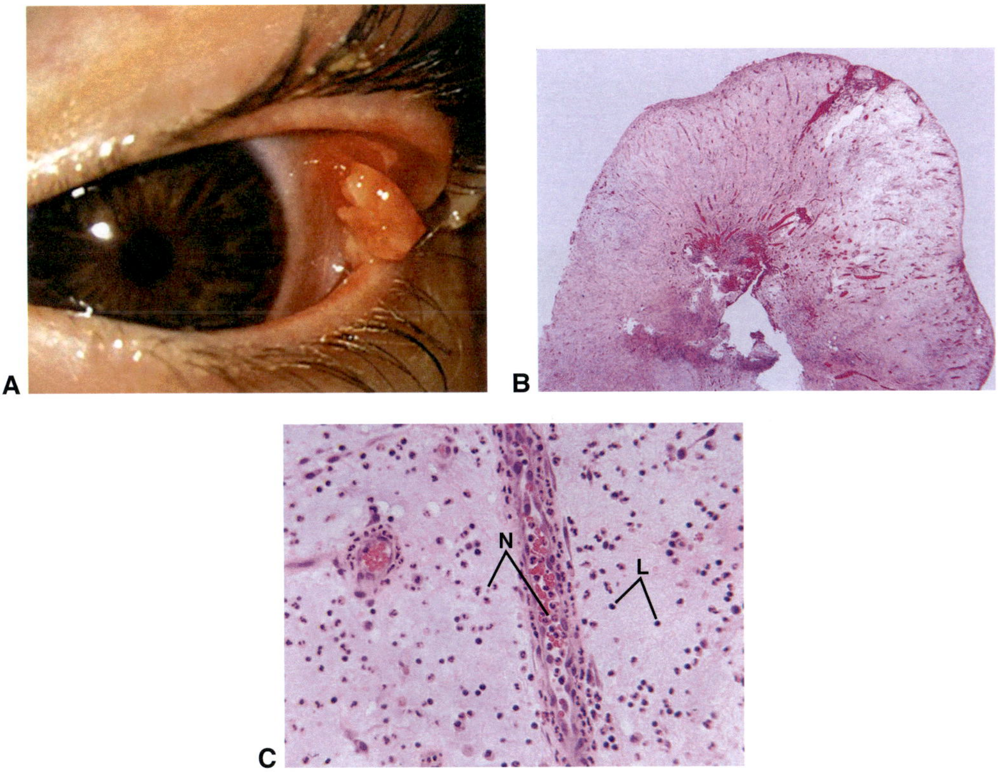

Figure 5-10 Pyogenic granuloma. **A,** Clinical appearance, at a site of prior strabismus surgery. **B,** Histology at low magnification shows a pedunculated mass of granulation tissue, with a "spoke-wheel" vascular pattern. **C,** High magnification shows a mixture of acute and chronic inflammatory cells: note neutrophils *(N)*, both within the lumen of blood vessels and also infiltrating the tissue; chronic inflammatory cells are also present, predominantly lymphocytes *(L)* in this field. *(Part A courtesy of Gregg T. Lueder, MD; parts B and C courtesy of George J. Harocopos, MD.)*

A *pterygium* has similar etiology and location, but it differs from a pinguecula in that it exhibits prominent vascularity and also encroaches onto the cornea in a winglike fashion (Fig 5-12A). Pterygia are excised when they threaten the visual axis, thereby becoming visually significant, or when they cause chronic irritation. Histology typically shows elastotic degeneration, as in a pinguecula, but also shows prominent blood vessels, correlating with the vascularity seen clinically (Fig 5-12B, C), and variable degrees of chronic inflammation. So-called *recurrent pterygia* may completely lack the histologic feature of elastotic degeneration and are more accurately classified as an exuberant fibroconnective tissue response.

In pingueculae and pterygia, the overlying epithelium may exhibit mild squamous metaplasia, for example, loss of goblet cells and surface keratinization. Some studies have demonstrated that there is abnormal expression of Ki-67 (a proliferation marker) and of tumor suppressor genes such as *p53* and *p63,* as well as loss of heterozygosity and microsatellite instability. Thus, as with actinic damage to the skin, there is always the potential

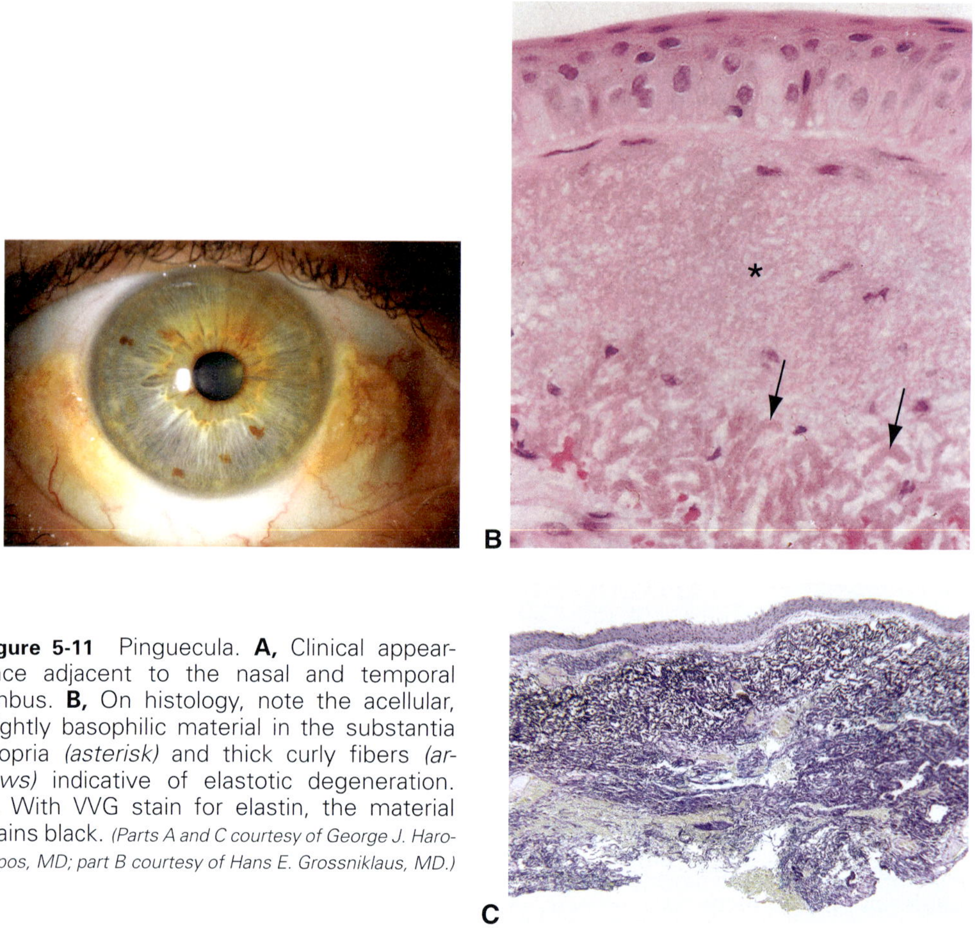

Figure 5-11 Pinguecula. **A,** Clinical appearance adjacent to the nasal and temporal limbus. **B,** On histology, note the acellular, slightly basophilic material in the substantia propria *(asterisk)* and thick curly fibers *(arrows)* indicative of elastotic degeneration. **C,** With VVG stain for elastin, the material stains black. *(Parts A and C courtesy of George J. Harocopos, MD; part B courtesy of Hans E. Grossniklaus, MD.)*

for future malignant transformation, although this occurs only rarely in association with pingueculae and pterygia. When conjunctival squamous neoplasia does arise, however, it often occurs overlying an area of preexisting elastotic degeneration. If features such as epithelial hyperplasia, nuclear hyperchromasia and pleomorphism, and excessive mitotic figures are identified in an excised pinguecula or pterygium, then a diagnosis of ocular surface squamous neoplasia should be assigned (see the section "Ocular surface squamous neoplasia" under Squamous Lesions). See also BCSC Section 8, *External Disease and Cornea.*

Dong N, Li W, Lin H, et al. Abnormal epithelial differentiation and tear film alteration in pinguecula. *Invest Ophthalmol Vis Sci.* 2009;50(6):2710–2715.

Amyloid Deposits

Amyloid deposition in the conjunctiva is most commonly an idiopathic, primary localized process seen in healthy young and middle-aged adults. Less often, it occurs secondary to preexisting, long-standing inflammation, such as with trachoma (ie, secondary localized amyloidosis). Occasionally, conjunctival amyloidosis may occur secondary to a systemic

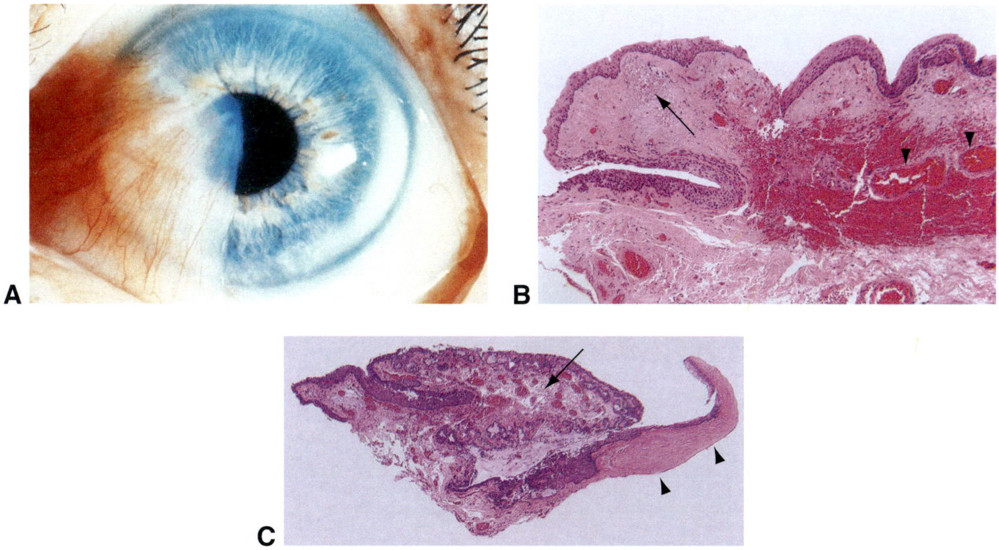

Figure 5-12 Pterygium. **A,** Clinical appearance. **B,** Histologically, a focus of elastotic degeneration is present *(arrow)*, as well as prominent blood vessels *(arrowheads)*, with surgically induced hemorrhage. **C,** In this case, the conjunctival and corneal portions of the pterygium are evident. Note the prominent blood vessels in the conjunctival portion *(arrow)*, and the destruction of the Bowman layer by ingrowth of fibroconnective tissue in the corneal portion *(arrowheads)*. *(Part A courtesy of Hans E. Grossniklaus, MD; parts B and C courtesy of George J. Harocopos, MD.)*

disease such as multiple myeloma. Localized or systemic amyloidosis may also involve the orbit. Clinically, conjunctival amyloidosis typically presents as a salmon-colored nodular elevation (Fig 5-13). The color may resemble the "salmon patch" appearance of a lymphoid lesion (discussed later). Histologically, amyloid appears as eosinophilic, extracellular deposits within the stroma, sometimes demonstrating a perivascular distribution. On Congo red stain, under standard light, amyloid deposits appear orange; but when viewed with polarized light and a rotating polarization filter, they exhibit birefringence with dichroism. That is, they change from orange to apple green as the filter is rotated. Other useful staining methods include crystal violet and the fluorescent stain thioflavin T. Electron microscopy shows characteristic fibrils (see Chapter 10, Fig 10-11). In localized amyloidosis, local clonal proliferations of plasma cells have been demonstrated, and it is thought that locally secreted monoclonal immunoglobulins are the precursors of biochemically identified immunoglobulin-derived amyloid proteins. See Chapter 6 of this volume for examples of primary and secondary localized amyloidosis of the cornea and BCSC Section 8, *External Disease and Cornea.*

Kaplan B, Martin BM, Cohen HI, et al. Primary local orbital amyloidosis: biochemical identification of the immunoglobulin light chain κIII subtype in a small formalin fixed, paraffin wax embedded tissue sample. *J Clin Pathol.* 2005;58(5):539–542.

Epithelial Inclusion Cyst

A conjunctival epithelial inclusion cyst may form at a site of prior accidental or surgical trauma (eg, after strabismus surgery, retinal surgery, or enucleation). Clinically, the lesion

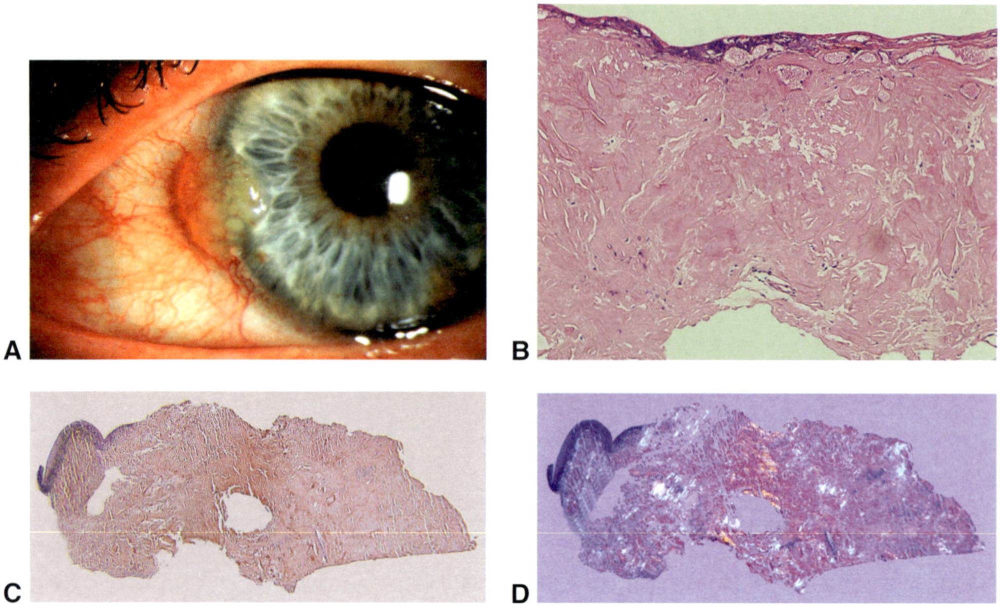

Figure 5-13 Conjunctival amyloidosis. **A,** Clinical appearance at the limbus and adjacent bulbar conjunctiva. **B,** On histology, note the diffuse extracellular amorphous eosinophilic material throughout the substantia propria. **C,** Congo red stain, under standard light, highlights the amyloid orange. **D,** On Congo red stain under polarization, amyloid exhibits birefringence with dichroism (orange and apple-green colors). *(Parts A, C, and D courtesy of George J. Harocopos, MD; part B courtesy of Shu-Hong Chang, MD.)*

appears as a transparent, cystic elevation on the ocular surface. There may be associated injection (Fig 5-14). Histology shows a cystic space lined by conjunctival epithelium, located in the substantia propria. The lumen may be empty or may contain inspissated proteinaceous material and cellular debris.

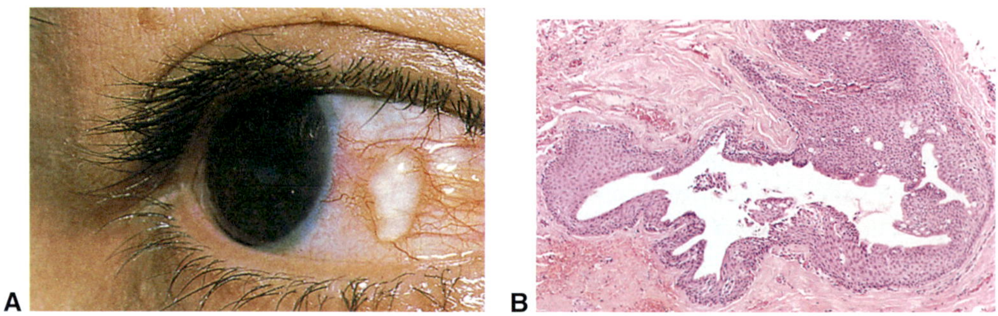

Figure 5-14 Epithelial inclusion cyst. **A,** Clinical appearance. **B,** The cyst is lined by nonkeratinizing, stratified squamous epithelium, characteristic of conjunctiva.

Neoplasia

Squamous Lesions

Squamous papillomas

The most common ocular surface neoplasms are those of the squamous family. *Squamous papillomas* may be divided clinically into pedunculated and sessile subtypes.

Pedunculated papillomas are exophytic, pink-red, strawberry-like papillary growths (Fig 5-15A) that occur more commonly in children, in whom multiple lesions often exist. They are associated with human papillomavirus (HPV) subtypes 6 and 11. The histologic examination of a pedunculated papilloma demonstrates papillary fibrovascular fronds covered by hyperplastic squamous epithelium (Fig 5-15B). Goblet cells may be present as in normal conjunctival epithelium. If there is overlying tear-film disruption resulting in exposure, the number of goblet cells may be reduced and the surface keratinized. Neutrophils may be seen within the epithelium, and a chronic inflammatory infiltrate may occupy the stroma, to varying degrees, which may be indicative of eye rubbing. Pedunculated papillomas exhibit benign behavior. They may spontaneously involute over months or years, and a small, nonirritating papilloma may be observed. Excisional biopsy may be performed for an irritating or cosmetically objectionable papilloma or if the diagnosis is in doubt.

Sessile papillomas occur more commonly in adults, arising on the bulbar conjunctiva, especially adjacent to the limbus. They may be difficult to distinguish clinically from ocular surface squamous neoplasia (see the following discussion). In sessile papillomas, the distinction between truly "benign" and "premalignant" is often not clear-cut. Sessile papillomas are associated with HPV subtypes 16 and 18, the same subtypes associated

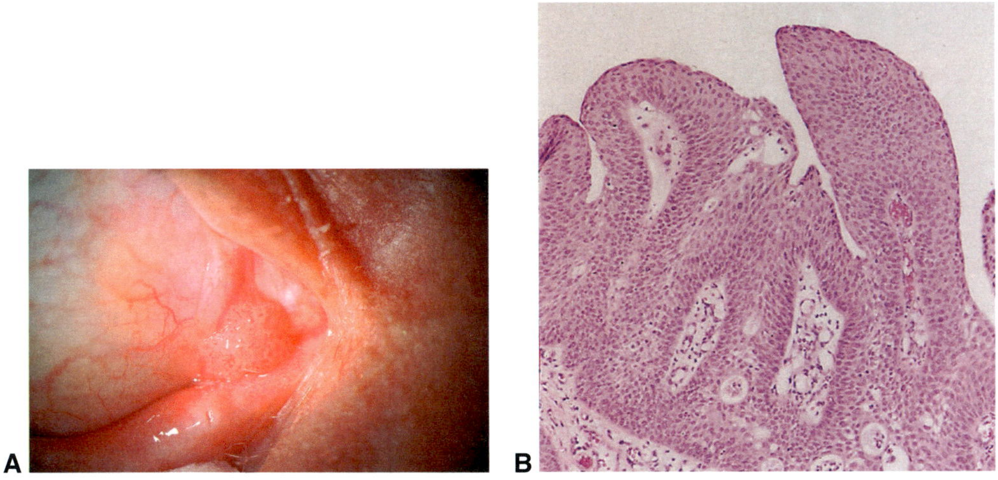

Figure 5-15 Squamous papilloma. **A,** Clinical appearance at the caruncle. **B,** The epithelium is hyperplastic, draped over fibrovascular cores. *(Part A courtesy of Robert H. Rosa, Jr, MD.)*

with squamous neoplasia. Worrisome clinical features suggestive of transformation into neoplasia would include leukoplakia (white surface) and inflammation. Sessile papillomas may be observed closely if there are no suspicious features, but biopsy is often required for histologic diagnosis. Histologically, a sessile papilloma exhibits a broad base (as opposed to the more narrow base seen in a pedunculated papilloma) and lacks the fingerlike projections seen in a pedunculated papilloma. The epithelium exhibits hyperplasia, but the individual cells should appear normal. If there are features such as nuclear hyperchromasia and pleomorphism, altered cell polarity, and abundant mitotic figures, then a diagnosis of ocular surface squamous neoplasia should be made.

Ocular surface squamous neoplasia

Ocular surface squamous neoplasia (OSSN) typically arises adjacent to the limbus, over a preexisting pinguecula, that is, over an area of solar elastosis, similar to actinic keratoses of the skin. Ultraviolet light (UV) exposure, especially in individuals with light skin pigmentation, is a known risk factor for OSSN, and the prevalence of OSSN is higher in equatorial regions of the world. UV-associated mutations in tumor suppressor genes such as *p53* have been demonstrated in OSSN, and hereditary deficiency of DNA repair such as in xeroderma pigmentosum increases the risk of OSSN formation. OSSN is also associated with HPV infection, subtypes 16 and 18, as well as with human immunodeficiency virus (HIV) infection. HIV-associated OSSN is especially common in sub-Saharan Africa, and HIV should be suspected in any patient with OSSN younger than 50 years. Non–HIV-related immunosuppression is also a risk factor for OSSN. Other risk factors include older age and smoking.

The clinical appearance of OSSN is characterized by epithelial thickening, and the lesion may extend onto the peripheral cornea. There may be a prominent "corkscrew" vascular pattern, or the surface may appear gelatinous or leukoplakic, indicative of surface keratinization (Fig 5-16). Surface keratinization is not pathognomonic for OSSN and may be seen over any elevated lesion not covered adequately by the tear film; however, it is very commonly seen in OSSN and must therefore arouse suspicion. The adjacent conjunctiva may appear injected, with prominent "feeder" vessels leading to the lesion.

Histologically, the epithelium exhibits hyperplasia, loss of goblet cells, loss of normal cell polarity, nuclear hyperchromasia and pleomorphism, and mitotic figures. There is often surface keratinization, correlating with the leukoplakia observed clinically. Dyskeratosis (non-surface cells producing keratin) may also be seen. A chronic inflammatory response is often present in the substantia propria.

The most important assessment to be made histologically in OSSN is whether the neoplasia is contained by the basement membrane (ie, intraepithelial or in situ) or whether neoplastic cells have traversed the epithelial basement membrane and invaded the stroma. For lesions contained by the basement membrane, the term *conjunctival intraepithelial neoplasia (CIN)* may be used. The neoplasia may be graded as mild, moderate, or severe, according to the degree of cellular atypia (although this grading does not necessarily have clinical utility in terms of prognosis). In cases with the most severe atypia, full-thickness involvement of the epithelium is seen, often with squamous eddies or keratin whorls/pearls. For these more advanced lesions, the term *squamous carcinoma in situ*

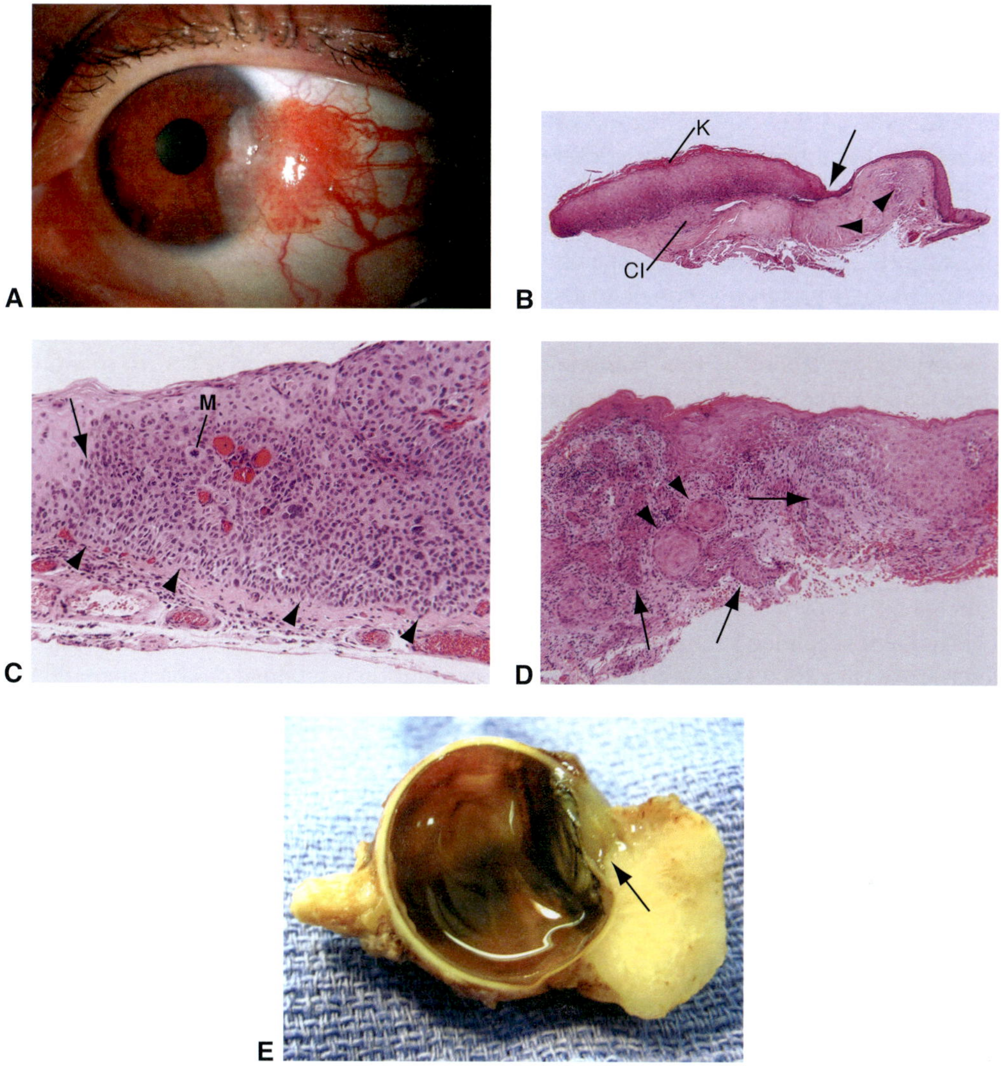

Figure 5-16 Ocular surface squamous neoplasia (OSSN). **A,** Clinical appearance: note the "corkscrew" vascular pattern of the conjunctival portion and leukoplakia of the corneal portion. Also note feeder vessels. **B,** Note the sharp demarcation *(arrow)* between normal and abnormal epithelium in OSSN. The epithelium is hyperplastic, with surface keratinization *(K)*. With the basement membrane intact, a diagnosis of conjunctival intraepithelial neoplasia (CIN) is made. There is a chronic inflammatory response in the substantia propria *(CI)*. Also note areas of elastotic degeneration in the substantia propria *(arrowheads)*, indicating that the lesion arose over a pinguecula. **C,** High magnification (different patient) shows transition zone where neoplasia begins *(arrow)*. To the right of the arrow, the epithelium exhibits mild keratinization, hyperplasia, nuclear hyperchromasia, loss of goblet cells, altered cellular polarity, significant pleomorphism, full-thickness involvement, and mitotic figures *(M)*. The basement membrane is intact *(arrowheads)*, with an underlying chronic inflammatory response. **D,** In invasive squamous carcinoma, tongues of epithelium violate the basement membrane and invade the stroma *(arrows)*, with squamous eddies *(arrowheads)*. **E,** Gross photograph of squamous carcinoma invading the limbus and anterior chamber angle through a previous surgical incision *(arrow)*. *(Part A courtesy of Vahid Feiz, MD; parts B–E courtesy of George J. Harocopos, MD.)*

may be used. If, however, the neoplastic cells have invaded the stroma, then the diagnosis is *invasive squamous cell carcinoma* (Fig 5-17; see Fig 5-16). Clinically, the term *CIN* has fallen out of favor in preference to the more general term *OSSN*, because it is not possible to determine on clinical examination whether stromal invasion has occurred. *CIN* should be regarded as a histologic term, reserved for noninvasive lesions. Invasion through the sclera or cornea and intraocular spread are uncommon complications of invasive squamous carcinoma. When there is intraocular spread, it often occurs at the site of a previous surgical procedure, such as cataract surgery. However, intraocular invasion may also occur through previously nonviolated sclera, especially in immunosuppression-related cases and cases occurring in ozone-depleted areas, as these cases tend to be more aggressive. Although regional lymph node metastasis is not as common as it is with squamous carcinomas of the skin or other sites, dissemination and death can occur.

Mucoepidermoid carcinoma and *spindle cell carcinoma* are rare variants of squamous cell carcinoma. Both entities are more aggressive neoplasms with higher rates of recurrence and intraocular spread.

Treatment options for suspected squamous neoplasms of the ocular surface include excisional biopsy with 3–4 mm margins and cryotherapy to the edges of excision; or topical chemotherapy with interferon (IFN) alfa-2b, 5-fluorouracil (5-FU), or mitomycin C (MMC). For specimen submission, the lesion should be placed flat on filter paper and allowed to dry for 30–60 seconds (so that its flat orientation is retained on the paper and the lesion is not folded over onto itself), and then the paper with specimen is gently placed in a formalin jar. It is ideal for the surgeon to mark 2 adjacent margins with different-colored sutures and to include a diagram depicting this orientation on the pathology requisition form. The status of the lateral and deep margins is important for prognosis.

See the appendix for the American Joint Committee on Cancer (AJCC) definitions and staging of squamous carcinoma of the conjunctiva. See also BCSC Section 8, *External Disease and Cornea.*

Sudesh S, Rapuano CJ, Cohen EJ, Eagle RC Jr, Laibson PR. Surgical management of ocular surface squamous neoplasms: the experience from a cornea center. *Cornea.* 2000;19(3):278–283.

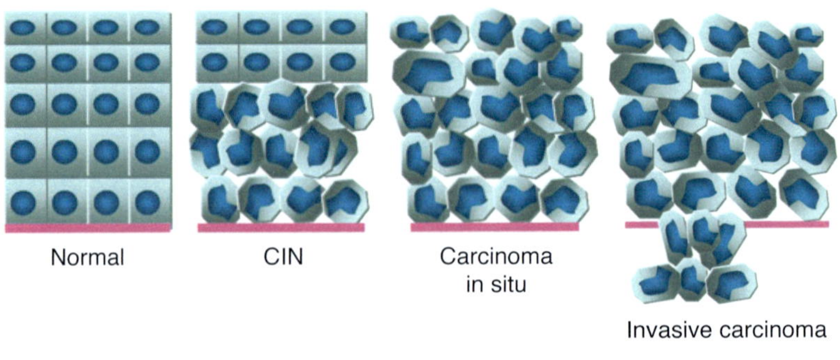

Figure 5-17 Schematic representation of the progression of OSSN. The first panel represents normal epithelium with basement membrane *(pink line).* In conjunctival intraepithelial neoplasia (CIN), a portion of the epithelium is replaced with dysplastic cells. Carcinoma in situ is the complete replacement of epithelium by dysplastic cells, with the basement membrane still intact. In invasive squamous cell carcinoma, note the invasion through the basement membrane into the stroma. *(Courtesy of Patricia Chévez-Barrios, MD.)*

Table 5-1 Clinical Comparison of Ocular Surface Melanocytic Lesions

Lesion	Onset	Size/Pattern	Location	Malignant Potential
Conjunctival nevus	Youth	Small, usually unilateral	Conjunctiva	Yes, but low (conjunctival melanoma)
Ocular and oculodermal melanocytosis	Congenital	Patchy or diffuse; usually unilateral	Under conjunctiva (episclera/sclera)	Yes (uveal melanoma)
Benign acquired melanosis (BAM)	Young adulthood	Patchy or diffuse; bilateral	Conjunctiva	None to minimal
Primary acquired melanosis (PAM)	Middle age	Diffuse; usually unilateral	Conjunctiva; mainly bulbar	Yes (conjunctival melanoma)

Melanocytic Lesions

Table 5-1 summarizes key clinical features of ocular surface melanocytic lesions.

Melanocytic nevi

As with hemangiomas, *melanocytic nevi* are classified by some authors as hamartomas and by others as neoplasms, with this distinction resting upon whether the lesion is congenital or acquired. Conjunctival melanocytic nevi usually appear on the bulbar conjunctiva in childhood. Analogous to cutaneous melanocytic nevi, conjunctival nevi undergo evolutionary changes. In the initial junctional phase, nevus cells are arranged in nests *(theques)* at the interface (junction) between the epithelium and the substantia propria. As the nevus evolves, the nests descend into the substantia propria and may lose connection with the epithelium. Nevi residing exclusively at the epithelial–stromal junction are called *junctional nevi,* whereas nevi exclusively in the substantia propria are termed *subepithelial* or *stromal nevi;* nevi with both junctional and subepithelial components are designated *compound nevi.* Epithelial inclusion cysts are often encountered within compound nevi. The presence of these cysts, in conjunction with melanocytes exhibiting a nested pattern, is a histologic feature of a benign lesion (Fig 5-18). Nevi also occur fairly commonly in the caruncle. Nevi in the caruncle and on the bulbar conjunctiva may be nonpigmented *(amelanotic),* in which case they have a pinkish appearance and the diagnosis may be more challenging clinically. The pigmentation of a nevus may increase during puberty, at which point the lesion may be first noticed by the patient or parents. Nevi occur only rarely in the palpebral conjunctiva; pigmented lesions in this area are more likely to represent intraepithelial melanosis or melanoma.

Nevi can be further categorized, for example, into Spitz nevus, halo nevus, and blue nevus. A blue nevus is a dark blue-gray to blue-black nevus in which the melanocytes are located in the deep stroma and have spindly morphology, similar to that of nevus cells seen in the uveal tract. Ocular, dermal, and oculodermal melanocytosis are forms of blue nevi typically seen unilaterally in darkly pigmented (eg, African, Hispanic, Asian) individuals. In *ocular melanocytosis,* the nevus is located in the deep episclera and sclera, resulting in a slate-gray appearance to the ocular surface (Fig 5-19), and also in the uveal tract, often resulting in iris heterochromia; the conjunctiva (epithelium and substantia propria)

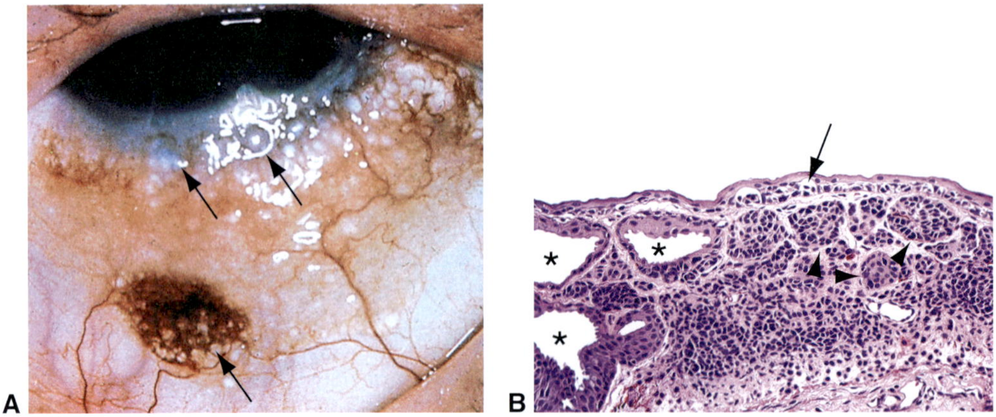

Figure 5-18 Conjunctival melanocytic nevus. **A,** Clinical appearance, with characteristic cystic areas *(arrows)*. **B,** On histology, the melanocytes are round, oval, or pear-shaped cells, mostly arranged in nests *(arrowheads)*. Melanocytes are present at the epithelial–stromal junction *(arrow)*; hence, this is a compound nevus. Note the epithelial inclusion cysts *(asterisks)* within the lesion, correlating with the clinical appearance. *(Part B courtesy of George J. Harocopos, MD.)*

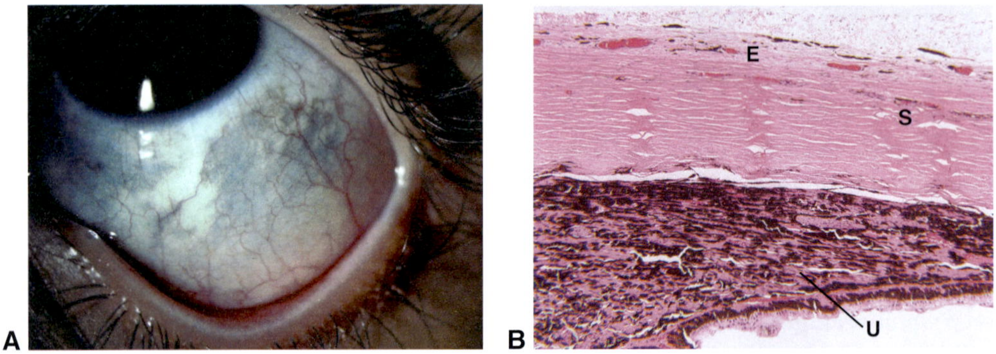

Figure 5-19 Ocular melanocytosis. **A,** Clinical appearance. **B,** Histology shows an abnormally increased population of melanocytes in the deep episclera *(E)*, sclera *(S)*, and uveal tract *(U)*. *(Part A courtesy of Gabriela M. Espinoza, MD; part B courtesy of George J. Harocopos, MD.)*

is uninvolved. In *dermal melanocytosis,* the nevus is located in the periocular skin. Dermal melanocytosis may also occur in conjunction with orbital melanocytosis, that is, *dermal orbital melanocytosis. Oculodermal melanocytosis,* also known as *nevus of Ota,* combines the features of ocular and dermal melanocytosis. Although these conditions are rare in lightly pigmented individuals, it is these individuals who are at risk for malignant transformation. When transformation into melanoma occurs, it is generally seen in the uveal tract; cutaneous, conjunctival, orbital, and meningeal melanomas are rare. Recent studies have shown that nevi of Ota manifest the same mutation in the G protein α-subunit gene *(GNAQ)* as primary ciliochoroidal and central nervous system melanomas. Patients with ocular and oculodermal melanocytosis (regardless of race) are also at increased risk for secondary glaucoma.

Intraepithelial melanosis

Intraepithelial melanosis of the conjunctiva may be divided into 2 categories: *benign acquired melanosis (BAM)* and *primary acquired melanosis (PAM)*. BAM appears as bilateral, flat patches of brown pigmentation with irregular margins, in individuals with dark skin pigmentation (Fig 5-20). BAM typically involves the bulbar conjunctiva and limbus. Streaks and whorls of melanotic pigmentation may extend onto the peripheral cornea, called *striate melanokeratosis.* The caruncle and palpebral conjunctiva may also be involved. The term *BAM* is appropriate for these lesions because they are almost always benign, with an exceedingly low rate of malignant transformation. Histologically, BAM consists of a lentiginous proliferation of benign-appearing melanocytes along the basal epithelial layer.

In contrast, PAM is most often unilateral, generally occurring in individuals with lighter skin. The clinical appearance is otherwise similar to that of BAM (Fig 5-21). PAM most commonly presents in middle-aged adults. It may occasionally be amelanotic. The lesion may remain stable or grow slowly over a period of 10 or more years. It may be difficult to predict clinically in any given patient whether PAM is likely to progress to melanoma, and thus the recommendations regarding when to observe versus perform biopsy are controversial. Retrospective data suggest that the number of clock-hours of conjunctiva involved may help predict the risk of malignant transformation: lesions less than 1 clock-hour in extent have a low chance of progressing to malignancy, whereas lesions involving 3 clock-hours or more have a greater than 20% chance of malignant transformation. Lesions less than 1 clock-hour may therefore be observed, and biopsy should be considered for lesions at least 3 clock-hours in size. In addition, involvement of the caruncle, fornix, or palpebral conjunctiva may prompt biopsy, because malignant transformation in these regions of the conjunctiva would be associated with a worse prognosis (discussed later).

The technique for excisional biopsy and specimen submission of PAM is similar to that described earlier for squamous lesions. MMC may also be considered as primary therapy in extensive cases; however, the efficacy of this treatment remains to be proven in a large clinical series.

A 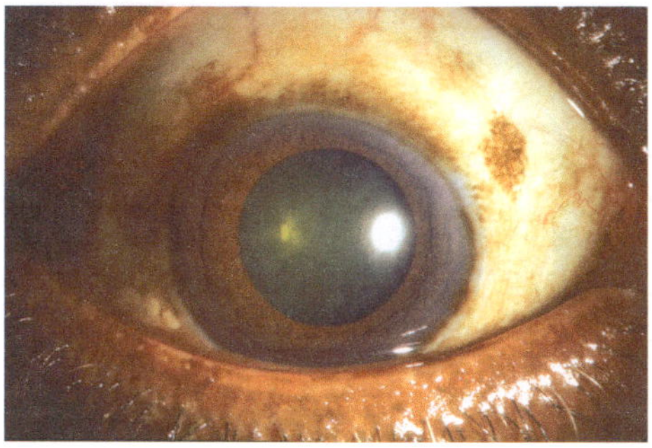

B 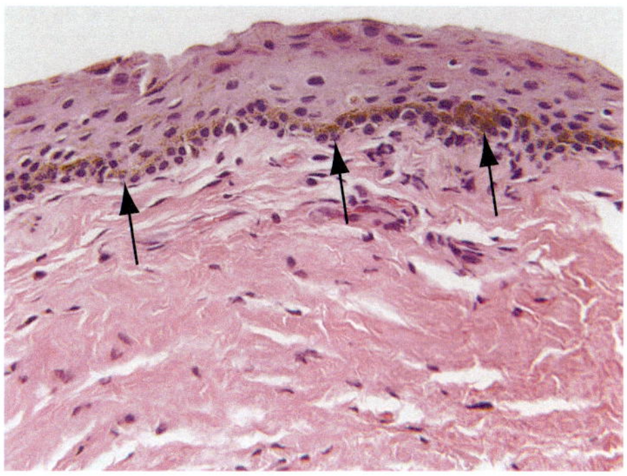

Figure 5-20 Benign acquired melanosis. **A,** Clinical appearance. **B,** Histology shows a proliferation of melanocytes confined to the basal layer of the epithelium *(arrows).* The melanocytes are small, with no cellular atypia. *(Courtesy of George J. Harocopos, MD.)*

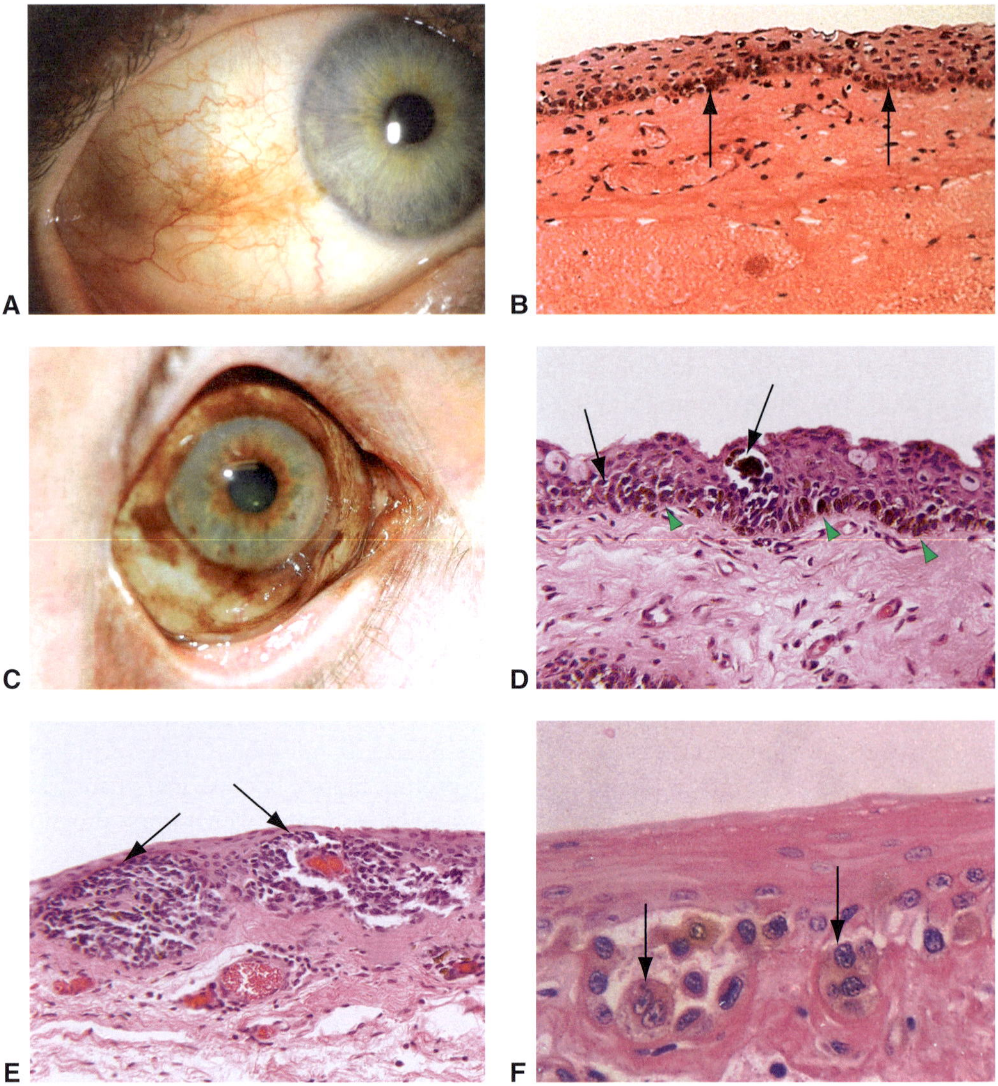

Figure 5-21 Primary acquired melanosis (PAM). **A,** Clinical appearance of mild PAM, involving only about 1 clock-hour of conjunctiva adjacent to the limbus. This lesion is unlikely to harbor atypia and may be observed. **B,** Histology of PAM without atypia. The melanocytic proliferation is confined to the basal layer of the epithelium *(arrows),* and there is no cellular atypia. **C,** Clinical appearance of extensive PAM, involving much of the ocular surface, including the caruncle, as well as palpebral conjunctiva and eyelid margin nasally. This lesion likely harbors atypia and warrants biopsy. **D,** Histology of PAM with mild to moderate atypia. Most of the melanocytic proliferation is located in the basal epithelial layer *(arrowheads)*, and the melanocytes are small, without prominent nucleoli. However, some melanocytes are seen in the more superficial epithelium *(arrows)*; also note the white spaces around many of the melanocytes, indicating discohesiveness. The patient is at low to moderate risk for transformation to melanoma. **E,** Histology of PAM with severe atypia. The melanocytic proliferation *(arrows)* involves most of the epithelial thickness. (In this case, the lesion is minimally pigmented.) **F,** Higher magnification of PAM with severe atypia (different patient), showing epithelioid melanocytes *(arrows)* within the epithelium. These latter two patients are at significant risk for progression to melanoma. *(Parts A, D, and E courtesy of George J. Harocopos, MD; part C courtesy of Vahid Feiz, MD.)*

Histologic criteria have been developed to identify patients at high risk for malignancy. *PAM without atypia,* essentially histologically identical to BAM, denotes a lentiginous proliferation of melanocytes without atypical features, confined to the basal epithelial layer. PAM without atypia does not progress to melanoma. In *PAM with atypia,* melanocytes migrate into the more superficial epithelium *(pagetoid spread)* and exhibit discohesiveness; a portion of the cells often exhibit epithelioid morphology, with large hyperchromatic nuclei and prominent nucleoli. Mitotic figures may be present. A chronic inflammatory response may be present in the substantia propria. As with squamous lesions, the atypia may be graded as mild, moderate, or severe, and full-thickness replacement of the epithelium may be termed *melanoma in situ.* In PAM with mild atypia, only a few melanocytes will be seen extending into the more superficial epithelium; there is minimal, if any, risk of malignant transformation. With moderate or greater atypia, the risk of malignant transformation correlates with the degree of atypia. PAM with atypia is similar histologically to lentigo maligna of the skin. The current dermatologic literature, however, has largely discarded the term *lentigo maligna* in favor of the term *melanoma in situ,* whereas for conjunctiva, many ophthalmic pathologists prefer to reserve the term *melanoma in situ* for only the most severe lesions with full-thickness epithelial involvement. Note that lentigo maligna of the eyelid skin is sometimes seen in continuity with PAM of the palpebral conjunctiva.

Melanoma

Approximately 50%–70% of cases of *conjunctival melanoma* arise from PAM with atypia (Fig 5-22); the remainder develop either from a nevus (a few percent) or de novo. Melanomas are usually nodular growths with vascularity that may involve any portion of the conjunctiva. The nodule may be pigmented but may be amelanotic, even if arising from pigmented PAM. Histologically, the cellular morphology in melanomas may range from spindle to epithelioid, similar to that in melanomas of the uveal tract. In more aggressive lesions, mitotic figures may be identified. Immunohistochemical stains for melanocytes such as Melan-A red, MART-1, and HMB-45 may help to identify problematic cases as melanocytic. Conjunctival melanomas are more akin to cutaneous melanomas than to uveal melanomas in behavior; that is, metastasis generally occurs by lymphatic spread rather than hematogenously. Typically, metastases first develop in preauricular, submandibular, or cervical lymph nodes, and the tumor may metastasize to the lungs, liver, brain, bone, and skin. Unfavorable clinical and histologic prognostic factors in conjunctival melanoma include

- nonepibulbar location, that is, caruncular, forniceal, or palpebral or involvement of the eyelid skin or orbit
- greater tumor thickness
- scleral invasion
- positive lateral margin of excision

The treatment of conjunctival melanoma is surgical (see BCSC Section 8, *External Disease and Cornea,* Chapter 8). The overall mortality rate from conjunctival melanoma ranges from approximately 15% to 30% in published studies (somewhat lower than the overall mortality rate from cutaneous melanoma).

A B C
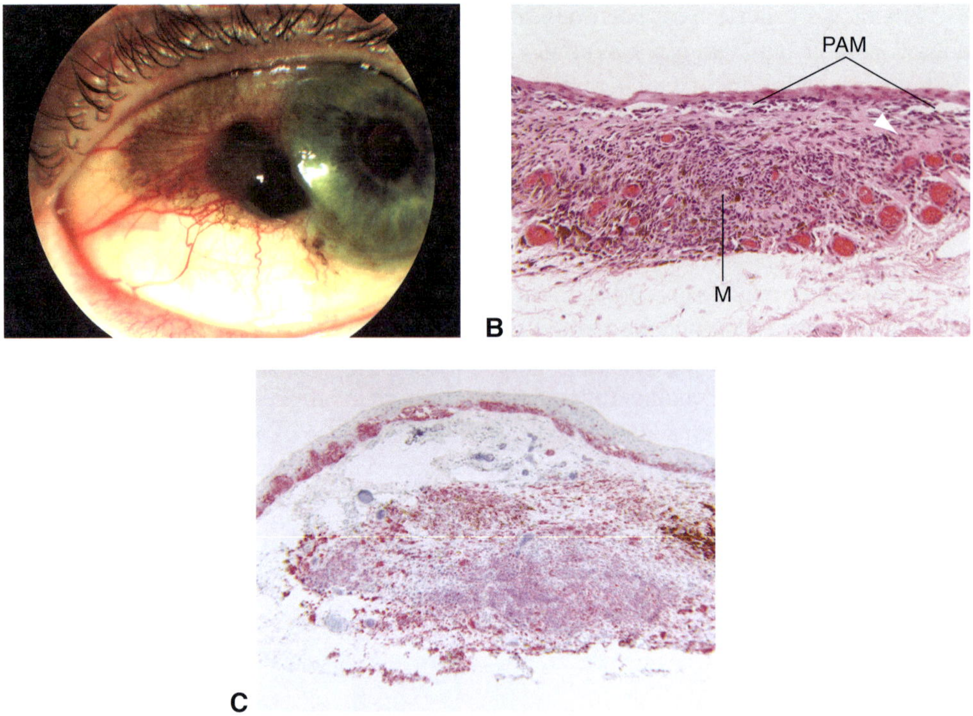

Figure 5-22 Melanoma arising from PAM. **A,** Clinical appearance. Note the elevated melanoma nodule adjacent to the limbus arising from a background of PAM (diffuse, flat, brown pigmentation). Also note prominent vascularity. **B,** On histology, melanoma *(M)* is seen arising from PAM, with *arrowhead* indicating the track of invasion. **C,** Melan-A red immunostain highlights melanocytes, confirming the diagnosis of melanoma arising from PAM. *(Part A courtesy of Morton E. Smith, MD; parts B and C courtesy of George J. Harocopos, MD.)*

Occasionally, melanoma of the uveal tract that has eroded through the anterior sclera will present initially as an episcleral/conjunctival mass. This possibility should be considered especially for a pigmented or amelanotic episcleral nodule overlying the ciliary body (ie, intercalary location), with no surrounding PAM (Fig 5-23). A complete dilated funduscopic examination should always be performed in any patient with a conjunctival mass.

In rare instances, conjunctival melanoma may represent a metastasis from cutaneous melanoma or from another site. In these cases, there is generally a known history of prior primary melanoma elsewhere, and it can be seen histologically that the melanoma is not arising from PAM.

See the appendix for the AJCC definitions and staging of conjunctival melanoma. See also BCSC Section 8, *External Disease and Cornea.*

Shields JA, Shields CL, Mashayekhi A, et al. Primary acquired melanosis of the conjunctiva: risks for progression to melanoma in 311 eyes. The 2006 Lorenz E. Zimmerman lecture. *Ophthalmology.* 2008;115(3):511–519.

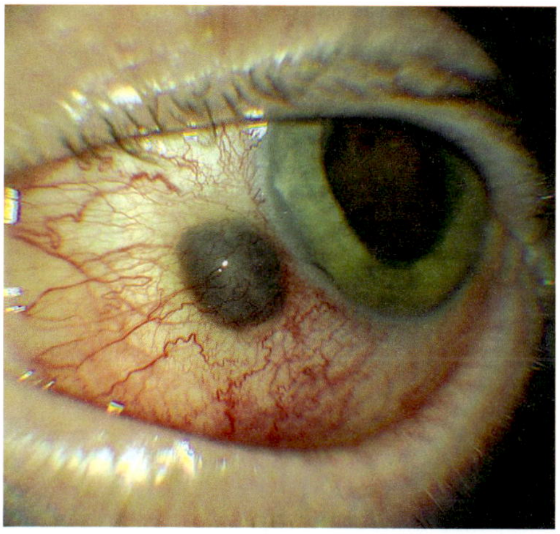

Figure 5-23 Melanoma of the ciliary body with extrascleral extension, presenting as an ocular surface mass. Note that there is no PAM surrounding the nodule, a clue that the lesion might have an intraocular origin. Also note that the lesion does not obscure the overlying conjunctival vessels. This indicates that the lesion is deep to the conjunctiva. *(Courtesy of J. William Harbour, MD.)*

Lymphocytic Lesions

The normal conjunctiva is an example of mucosa-associated lymphoid tissue (MALT), and a few small follicles are often visible clinically in the normal inferior fornix. As described previously, the normal lymphoid follicle consists of a germinal center and surrounding corona (see Fig 5-5). The corona is further subdivided into marginal and mantle zones, although these are not well delineated histologically without the use of special stains.

Occasionally in asymptomatic patients (generally children or adolescents), numerous, prominent follicles may be incidentally found in the inferior fornix bilaterally, a condition called *benign lymphoid folliculosis.* Lymphoid follicles of the palpebral/forniceal conjunctiva may also become more prominent and increase in number when associated with conjunctival inflammation, that is, follicular conjunctivitis (discussed earlier).

Lymphoid tissue may proliferate in the conjunctiva abnormally, often in the absence of inflammation, and this lymphoid hyperplasia may be benign or malignant. Clinically, both benign and malignant lymphoproliferative lesions of the conjunctiva have a salmon-pink appearance with a smooth surface and are usually soft (Fig 5-24A, B). Both benign and malignant lesions may be unilateral or bilateral. Lymphocytic lesions are often seen in the inferior fornix but may also be seen on the bulbar, tarsal, or caruncular conjunctiva. A lymphocytic lesion involving the forniceal conjunctiva or caruncle may also have an orbital component. As benign and malignant lymphocytic lesions of the conjunctiva may appear similar clinically, incisional biopsy is generally required to make a precise diagnosis.

For biopsy of suspected lymphoid lesions of the conjunctiva, 4–5 mm of tissue is generally sufficient, and the biopsy may usually be performed in the office with topical or subconjunctival anesthetic. The specimen should be submitted in formalin for routine H&E sections and immunohistochemistry. If possible, an additional 4–5 mm of tissue may be harvested and submitted in saline or special flow cytometry medium, on ice.

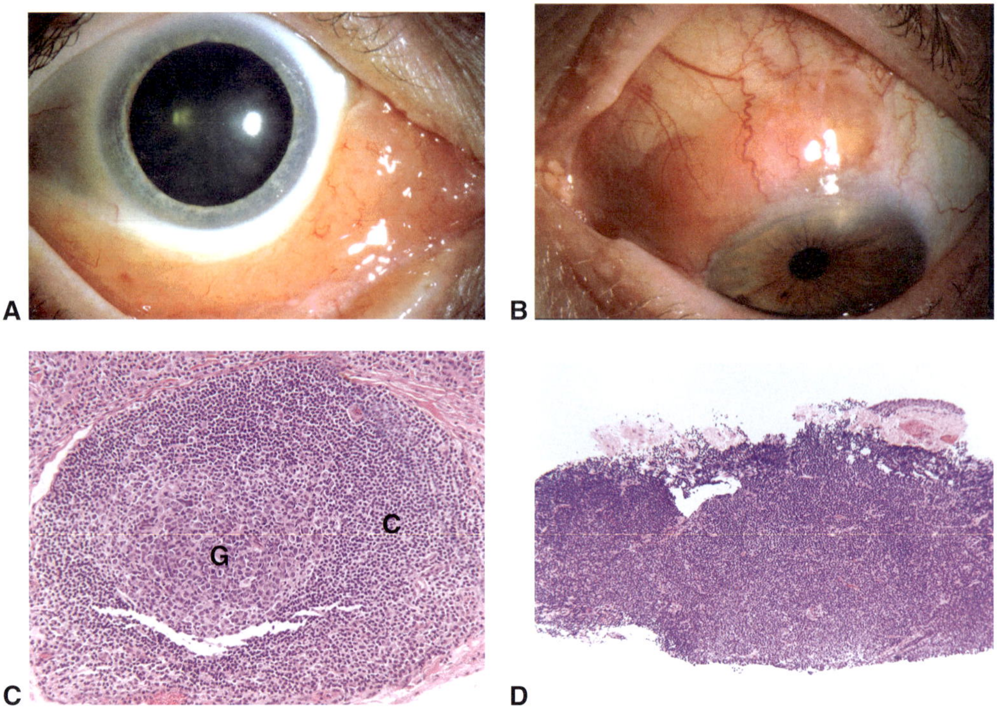

Figure 5-24 Lymphocytic lesions of the conjunctiva. **A,** Clinical appearance ("salmon patch") in the inferior fornix. **B,** Clinical appearance on the bulbar conjunctiva. **C,** Histology of benign lymphoid hyperplasia, showing normal follicular architecture, with well-defined germinal center *(G)* and corona *(C)*. **D,** Histology of lymphoma, showing a sheet of lymphocytes infiltrating the substantia propria, without well-defined follicles. *(Part A courtesy of Anthony J. Lubniewski, MD; part B courtesy of Anjali K. Pathak, MD; parts C and D courtesy of George J. Harocopos, MD.)*

Histologic features favoring a diagnosis of *benign lymphoid hyperplasia* on routine H&E sections include the presence of normal-appearing lymphoid follicles with distinct germinal centers and with small, mature coronal lymphocytes (Fig 5-24C). In contrast, *lymphoma* often demonstrates a solid sheet of lymphocytes in the substantia propria, without well-defined follicles (Fig 5-24D). However, most conjunctival lymphomas are low grade, and these low-grade malignant lesions are sometimes difficult to differentiate from benign lesions on H&E sections. Immunohistochemistry, flow cytometry, and other techniques are useful diagnostically, as discussed later. Also, it should be noted that some patients with "benign" lymphoid hyperplasia eventually develop lymphoma.

Lymphoma

The most common form of lymphoma of the conjunctiva (and also of the orbit), seen in over half of cases, is *extranodal marginal zone lymphoma* (formerly known as *MALToma*), so named because the pathogenesis involves expansion of the follicle's marginal zone. *Extranodal* refers to the site of the tumor being somewhere other than a lymph node. Conjunctival marginal zone lymphoma may be unilateral or bilateral and often presents in the forniceal conjunctiva but may present on the bulbar conjunctiva. This is a form of low-grade B-cell lymphoma, and histology shows small lymphocytes (Fig 5-25).

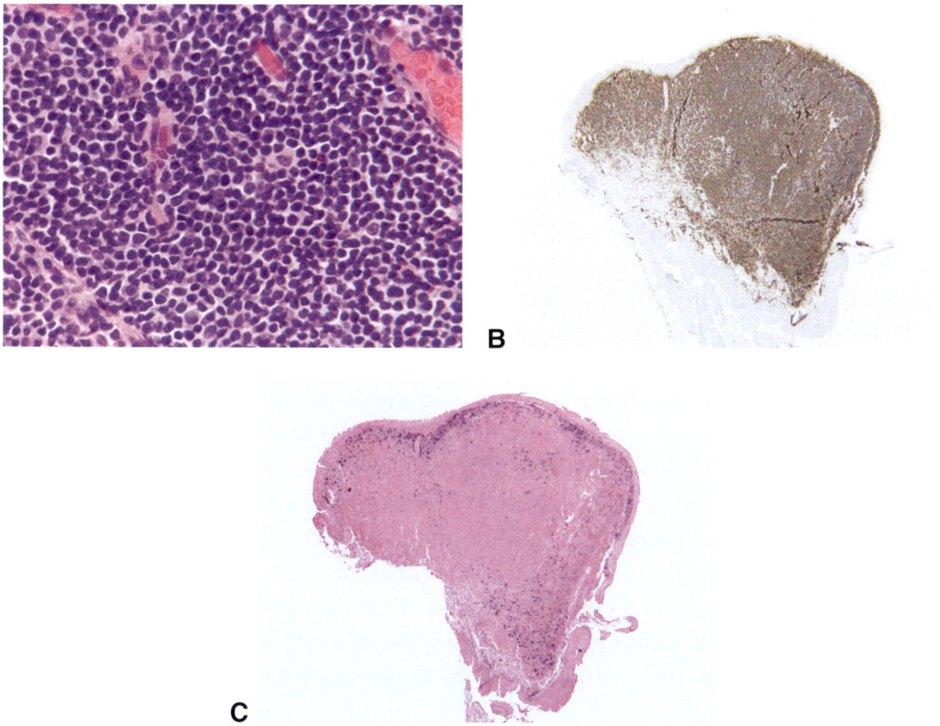

Figure 5-25 Histology of marginal zone lymphoma. **A,** Higher magnification of the same case shown in Fig 5-24D, showing small lymphocytes. **B,** CD20 immunostain *(brown)* for B cells, staining positive in the vast majority of the lymphocytes. **C,** In situ hybridization (ISH) for λ light chain, exhibiting prominent positivity *(blue cells),* confirming λ clonality and establishing the diagnosis of marginal zone lymphoma. *(Courtesy of George J. Harocopos, MD.)*

Immunohistochemistry for B-cell and T-cell markers demonstrates a preponderance of B cells, although a variable proportion of normal T cells will be present. Tissue in situ hybridization (ISH) for immunoglobulin light chains often demonstrates B-cell monoclonality by revealing either κ or λ light-chain predominance. However, ISH is not as sensitive as flow cytometry for detecting κ or λ clonality, and thus flow cytometry is especially useful in cases that fail to show clonality by ISH. Another technique to detect clonality, which can be performed on fresh or formalin-fixed tissue, is IgH (immunoglobulin heavy chain) gene rearrangement testing by PCR. In addition, fluorescence in situ hybridization (FISH) may be performed on fresh or formalin-fixed tissue to test for specific genetic translocations. The t(3;14) translocation, involving the *FOXP1* gene, and other translocations have been described in marginal zone lymphoma; and various translocations have been found in other forms of conjunctival lymphoma. Interestingly, the same translocation may be associated with more than one type of lymphoma.

Other forms of conjunctival lymphoma include follicular lymphoma (arising from the germinal center) and, less commonly, mantle cell lymphoma (which arises from the mantle zone). Also less common in the conjunctiva are diffuse large B-cell lymphoma, Burkitt lymphoma, Hodgkin lymphoma, and plasmacytoma. T-cell lymphomas are rare. High-grade lymphomas such as diffuse large B-cell lymphoma are readily recognized as malignant by virtue of their nuclear features ("coarse clumping" chromatin pattern, that is, multiple nucleoli) and high mitotic rate. Large B-cell lymphoma is relatively rare in the conjunctiva and is more commonly seen in the central nervous system and vitreous (see Chapters 10 and 20 of this volume).

Approximately two-thirds of conjunctival lymphomas are localized to the conjunctiva and *not* associated with systemic disease. In contrast, nearly two-thirds of lymphomas arising in the preseptal skin eventually show evidence of systemic involvement. However, the likelihood of systemic involvement varies according to the type of lymphoma; that is, marginal zone lymphoma presenting on the conjunctiva has been estimated in some studies to be localized in up to 90% of cases, whereas mantle cell lymphoma often has systemic involvement. The vast majority of cases of conjunctival marginal zone lymphoma present initially to the ophthalmologist, with no known systemic disease; the frequency of known preexisting systemic disease is greater with higher-grade lymphomas. Any patient presenting with conjunctival lymphoma must be referred to an oncologist for a systemic workup.

The treatment of conjunctival lymphoma depends on the presence or absence of systemic involvement. When disease is localized to the conjunctiva, the mainstay of treatment is orbital radiation; in cases with systemic involvement, the treatment is chemotherapy. See Chapter 8 in BCSC Section 8, *External Disease and Cornea,* and Section 7, *Orbit, Eyelids, and Lacrimal System,* for additional discussion. Interestingly, some case series have provided evidence of an infectious trigger *(Chlamydia psittaci)* for conjunctival lymphoma, for example, by demonstrating chlamydial DNA in a high proportion of cases of marginal zone lymphoma. Less common microbial associations with conjunctival/orbital lymphoma include *Chlamydia pneumoniae, Chlamydia trachomatis,* and *Helicobacter pylori,* the latter being more commonly associated with gastric lymphoma. Accordingly, cases of regression have been reported with oral doxycycline treatment. Viruses such as hepatitis C and Epstein-Barr have also been implicated in lymphoproliferative disorders.

The overall prognosis in conjunctival lymphoma is good, given that most cases are low-grade neoplasms. However, the prognosis in any given case depends on the subtype of lymphoma, because this has bearing on the likelihood of systemic disease. In the absence of systemic involvement, the remission rate at 10 years is 75%–100% for patients treated with radiation therapy; with systemic involvement, disease-free survival at 5 years is only 20%. Lymphoma-related death is significantly associated with advanced clinical stage and age older than 60 years. The extent of *p53* positivity (tumor suppressor gene) and MIB-1 positivity (cell proliferation marker) has also been shown to affect prognosis, although these stains are not routinely obtained in all cases. The average time frame for relapse of marginal zone lymphoma is more than 5 years after initial remission. Thus, these patients require long-term (over 5 years) follow-up.

See the appendix for the AJCC staging.

Shields CL, Shields JA, Carvalho C, Rundle P, Smith AF. Conjunctival lymphoid tumors: clinical analysis of 117 cases and relationship to systemic lymphoma. *Ophthalmology.* 2001;108(5):979–984.

Swerdlow SH, Campo E, Harris NL, et al. *WHO Classification of Tumours of Haematopoietic and Lymphoid Tissues.* 4th ed. Lyon, France: IARC; 2008.

Glandular Lesions

Oncocytoma is a benign proliferation of apocrine or accessory lacrimal gland epithelium, that is, an adenoma. It typically arises in the caruncle, although it may occasionally be seen elsewhere on the conjunctiva. Oncocytoma most commonly occurs in elderly women. Clinically, it appears as a tan to reddish, vascularized nodule (Fig 5-26). When this lesion is seen clinically, the differential diagnosis typically includes squamous, melanocytic, and lymphocytic lesions, as well as amyloid. Histologically, the lesion is composed of proliferating epithelial cells, similar in appearance to apocrine (gland of Moll) epithelium, around glandlike spaces. Because of the cystic appearance of these spaces, the term *apocrine cystadenoma* is also used to describe this lesion. The epithelial cells exhibit distinctive eosinophilic cytoplasm; hence, this lesion is also referred to as *oxyphilic (eosinophilic) cystadenoma.* Malignant apocrine neoplasms may also occur but are very rare.

Other Neoplasms

Virtually any neoplasm that can occur in the orbit may occasionally arise in the conjunctiva, including neural, muscular, vascular, and fibrous tumors. Metastatic lesions to the conjunctiva are rare but may occur. See Chapter 14 of this volume. See also BCSC Section 8, *External Disease and Cornea,* and Section 7, *Orbit, Eyelids, and Lacrimal System.*

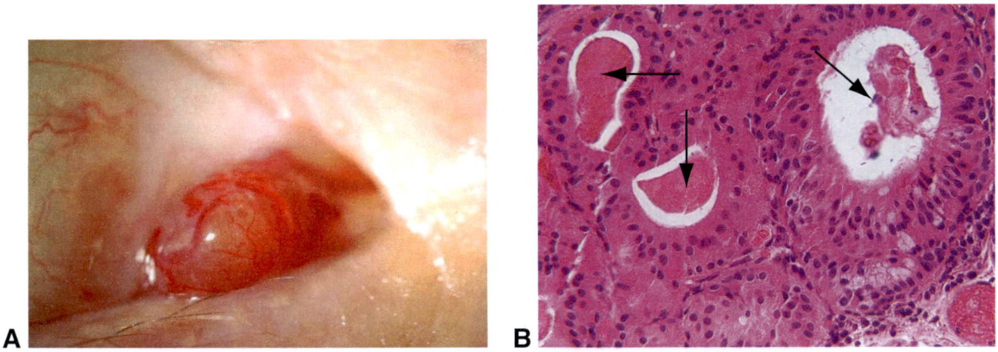

Figure 5-26 Oncocytoma. **A,** Clinical appearance at the caruncle. **B,** Histology shows proliferation of glandular epithelial cells, with deeply eosinophilic cytoplasm. Some of the cells surround protein-filled lumina *(arrows). (Part A courtesy of Mark J. Mannis, MD; part B courtesy of George J. Harocopos, MD.)*

CHAPTER 6

Cornea

Topography

The normal cornea is composed of 5 layers: epithelium, Bowman layer, stroma, Descemet membrane, and endothelium (Fig 6-1). See BCSC Section 2, *Fundamentals and Principles of Ophthalmology,* and Section 8, *External Disease and Cornea,* for a discussion of the embryology, structure, and physiology of the cornea.

The corneal *epithelium* is nonkeratinized, stratified squamous, ranging between 5 and 7 cell layers in thickness. The epithelial basement membrane is thin and is best seen with periodic acid–Schiff (PAS) stain. The basement membrane is more easily visualized when it becomes pathologically thickened, such as in anterior basement dystrophy (ie, map-dot-fingerprint dystrophy) or secondary to endothelial decompensation.

The *Bowman layer* is located immediately beneath the epithelial basement membrane. It is also known as the Bowman "membrane," but this term may be misleading because this layer is not a true basement membrane; that is, it is not elaborated by the epithelial cells. Rather, it is more properly regarded as the most anterior layer of the stroma. The Bowman layer is acellular and is composed of irregularly arranged collagen fibrils. It is not restored after injury but is replaced by fibroconnective scar tissue.

The corneal *stroma* makes up 90% of the total corneal thickness. It consists of collagen-producing keratocytes, collagenous lamellae, and proteoglycan ground substance. The elongated collagenous lamellae are regularly arranged in a precise orientation to yield transparency, allowing for the orderly passage of light through the cornea.

The next layer, the *Descemet membrane,* is the basement membrane elaborated by the corneal endothelium. The production of Descemet membrane begins during fetal development and continues throughout adulthood. The thickness of this membrane may increase further in endothelial disease states. The Descemet membrane (like the epithelial basement membrane) is a true basement membrane, composed primarily of type IV collagen, and is strongly PAS-positive.

The corneal *endothelium* is composed of a single layer of cells. The cells appear mostly hexagonal *en face,* such as on confocal microscopy. In a histologic cross-section of the cornea, the endothelial cells have a cuboidal appearance. The primary function of the endothelium is to maintain corneal clarity by pumping water from the corneal stroma. The number of endothelial cells gradually decreases with age, and endothelial cell loss is accelerated in endothelial disease states. Human endothelial cells cannot regenerate; so as

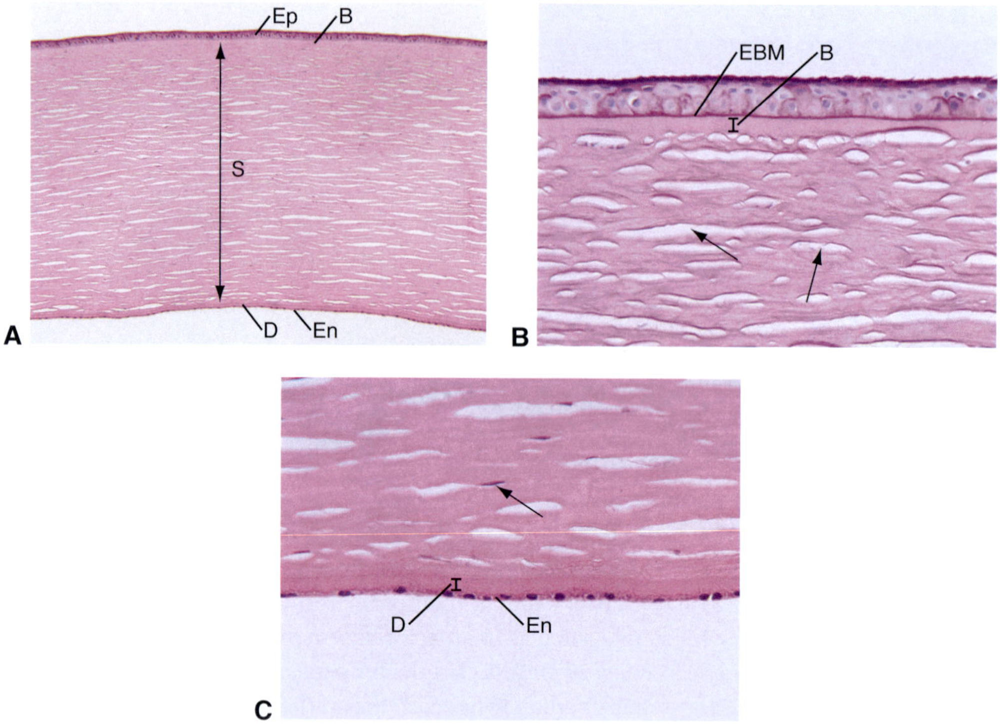

Figure 6-1 Normal cornea. **A,** The cornea is composed of epithelium *(Ep),* the Bowman layer *(B),* stroma *(S),* the Descemet membrane *(D),* and endothelium *(En).* **B,** On higher magnification, PAS stain highlights the epithelial basement membrane *(EBM),* distinguishing it from the Bowman layer *(B).* Because of dehydration of the tissue during processing for paraffin embedding, multiple areas of separation (clefts) of the stromal lamellae are evident *(arrows).* If the stromal clefts are absent, corneal edema or fibrosis is suspected (the former if the cornea is thick, and the latter if thin). This is an example of a meaningful artifact. **C,** Higher magnification (H&E stain) also delineates Descemet membrane *(D)* and endothelium *(En).* The keratocyte nuclei *(arrow)* are apparent. (Note that PAS stain also highlights Descemet membrane.) *(Courtesy of George J. Harocopos, MD.)*

the endothelial cell number declines, the remaining cells flatten and elongate to provide coverage of the posterior corneal surface.

Introduction to Corneal Pathology

Corneal specimens are among the most common specimens seen by the ophthalmic pathologist. In the pathology laboratory, specimens submitted from penetrating keratoplasty are referred to as corneal "buttons." The most common indications for keratoplasty are listed in Table 6-1 and are discussed later in this chapter. In recent years, alternatives to penetrating surgery have become more widely utilized for certain corneal conditions in which only some of the corneal layers are diseased. For example, if the anterior cornea is diseased but the endothelium is healthy, then deep anterior lamellar keratoplasty (DALK) may be an option. On the other hand, if only the endothelium is diseased, then

Table 6-1 Most Common Indications for Keratoplasty

Fuchs endothelial dystrophy
Pseudophakic/aphakic bullous keratopathy
Keratoconus
Visually significant corneal opacity (eg, following infectious keratitis, especially herpetic)
Failure of an existing corneal graft

endokeratoplasty may be an option (eg, Descemet stripping endothelial keratoplasty [DSEK], in which only Descemet membrane and endothelium are removed). Examples of specimens from these procedures are shown in their corresponding sections.

Congenital Anomalies

Congenital Hereditary Endothelial Dystrophy

There are 2 forms of *congenital hereditary endothelial dystrophy (CHED),* with both forms causing bilateral corneal edema. The autosomal recessive form, the more common of these, is apparent at birth, accompanied by nystagmus, but nonprogressive. The autosomal dominant form is apparent within the first few years of life, not accompanied by nystagmus, but progressive (Fig 6-2A). The genetic loci for the autosomal dominant and recessive forms of CHED have been mapped to 20p11.2-q11.2 and 20p13, respectively. Despite their clinical differences, the 2 forms of CHED appear similar histologically. The corneal stroma is diffusely edematous, accounting for the marked increase in thickness observed clinically. The Descemet membrane appears thickened, without guttae (Fig 6-2B). Endothelial cell loss may be diffuse or focal. The histologic findings overall are very similar

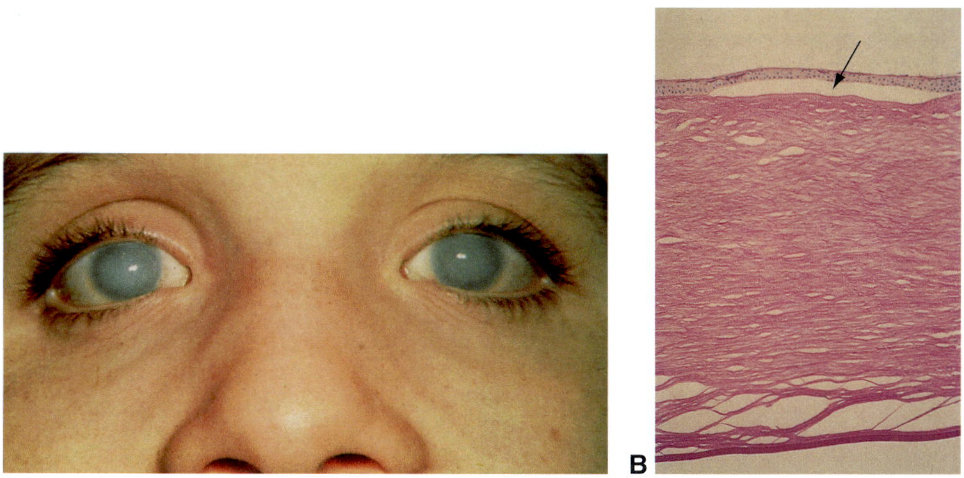

A B

Figure 6-2 Congenital hereditary endothelial dystrophy. **A,** Clinical appearance with bilateral corneal clouding. **B,** Note diffuse edema, with bullous keratopathy *(arrow).* The Descemet membrane is diffusely thickened, without guttae, and endothelial cells are absent. *(Courtesy of Hans E. Grossniklaus, MD.)*

to those seen in pseudophakic/aphakic bullous keratopathy. The primary abnormality in CHED is thought to be a degeneration of endothelial cells during or after the fifth month of gestation. No systemic abnormalities are consistently associated with CHED. See also BCSC Section 8, *External Disease and Cornea.*

Klintworth GK. The molecular genetics of the corneal dystrophies—current status. *Front Biosci.* 2003;8:d687–713.

Posterior Polymorphous Dystrophy

Posterior polymorphous dystrophy (Fig 6-3) is another endothelial dystrophy that may be inherited in autosomal dominant or recessive fashion, with the mutation mapped to 20q11. In this condition, the endothelium has epithelial-like characteristics. These include multilayering, which may be seen histologically on routine light microscopy, and microvilli, which are best demonstrated on electron microscopy. The total number of endothelial cells may be decreased. Variable thickening of the Descemet membrane and guttae may be observed. There may also be secondary glaucoma, either open-angle or associated with iridocorneal adhesions. The resultant corneal clouding is typically central, but the degree of opacification varies greatly, with some patients never requiring corneal transplantation and others requiring keratoplasty in childhood or even infancy. See also BCSC Section 8, *External Disease and Cornea.*

Dermoid

Dermoid, a type of choristoma that may involve the cornea, is discussed in Chapter 5 (see Fig 5-2). Dermoids are typically located at the limbus but may involve the central cornea. See also BCSC Section 6, *Pediatric Ophthalmology and Strabismus.*

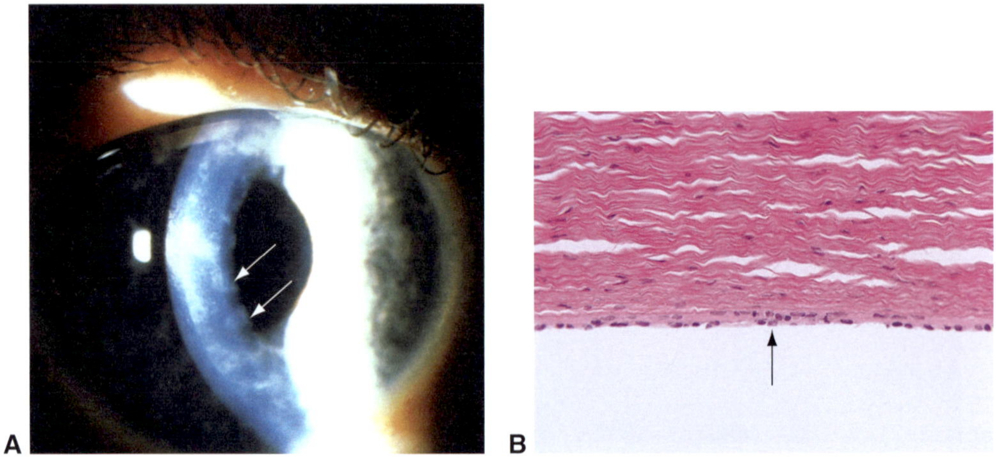

Figure 6-3 Posterior polymorphous dystrophy. **A,** Clinical appearance, showing nummular opacities *(arrows)* on the endothelial surface. **B,** Note multilayering of endothelial cells *(arrow)*. *(Part A courtesy of Andrew J.W. Huang, MD; part B courtesy of George J. Harocopos, MD.)*

Peters Anomaly

Peters anomaly represents the more severe end of the spectrum of anterior segment dysgenesis syndromes, in which neural crest migration, with respect to angle development and cleavage of the lens from the corneal endothelium, does not occur properly. This anomaly is typically bilateral and sporadic, although autosomal dominant and recessive modes of inheritance have also been reported. In this anomaly, there is a localized defect in the central or paracentral portion of the Descemet membrane, known as *internal ulcer of von Hippel,* at the edges of which, typically, are iris strands adherent to the posterior corneal surface. In the most severe form of Peters anomaly, the lens is also adherent to the posterior corneal surface. These defects result in variable degrees of corneal clouding, often requiring corneal transplantation (Fig 6-4).

A related entity in the spectrum of anterior segment dysgenesis syndromes is *sclerocornea.* Whereas the corneal clouding in Peters anomaly is central, the clouding in

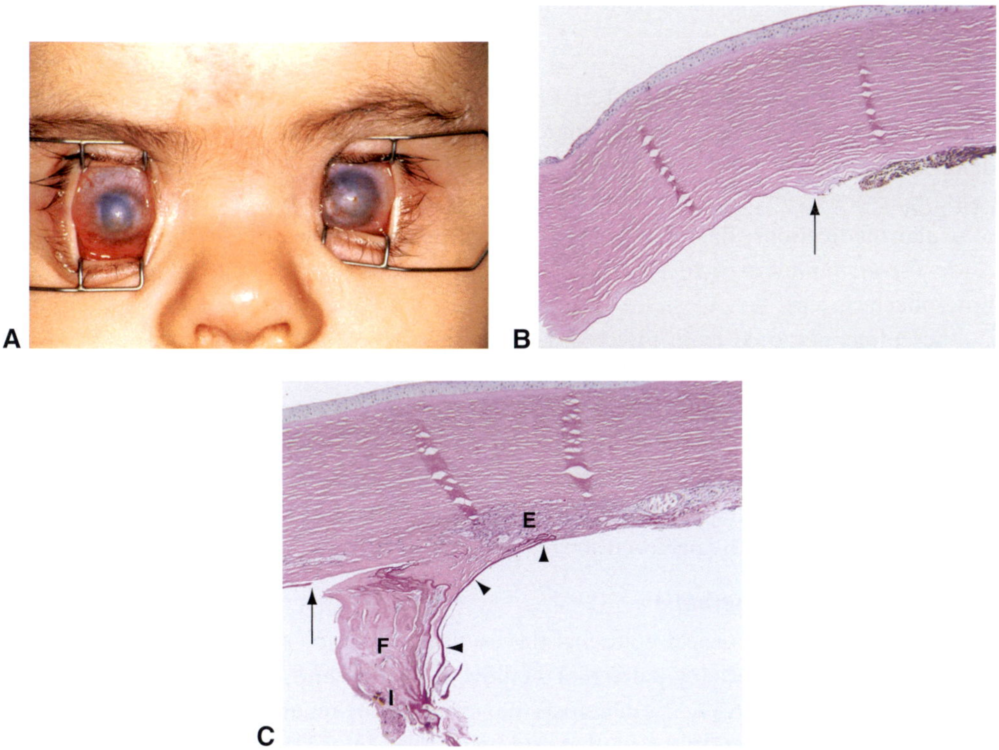

Figure 6-4 Peters anomaly. **A,** Clinical appearance. Note the central corneal opacities, diffuse corneal clouding, and vascularization. **B,** PAS stain demonstrates internal ulcer of von Hippel. The Descemet membrane trails off at the edge of the internal ulcer *(arrow).* Iris tissue *(to the right of the arrow)* adheres to the posterior corneal surface at the edge of the internal ulcer. Also note endothelial cell loss. **C,** Severe case showing lens tissue adherent to posterior corneal surface. The *arrow* marks the edge of the internal ulcer. Note lens capsule *(arrowheads),* swollen lens epithelial cells *(E),* lens fibers *(F),* and iris tissue with melanin pigment *(I).* *(Part A courtesy of Andrew J.W. Huang, MD; parts B and C courtesy of George J. Harocopos, MD.)*

sclerocornea is typically peripheral, although it may involve the entire cornea. The limbus is usually poorly defined, and vessels that are extensions of scleral, episcleral, and conjunctival vessels extend across the cornea. The most common ocular association is cornea plana, found in 80% of cases. Histologically, stromal vascularization and disorderly stromal lamellae of variable thickness may be present, correlating with the peripheral clouding seen clinically. Histologic findings similar to those of Peters anomaly are typically present. See also BCSC Section 8, *External Disease and Cornea,* and Section 6, *Pediatric Ophthalmology and Strabismus.*

Inflammations

Infectious Keratitis

The cornea may be affected by infectious processes caused by a number of different microbial agents. Severe inflammation can lead to corneal necrosis, ulceration, and perforation. See also BCSC Section 8, *External Disease and Cornea.*

Bacterial infections

Corneal infections caused by bacterial agents often follow a disruption in the corneal epithelial integrity resulting from contact lens wear, trauma, alteration in immunologic defenses (eg, use of topical or systemic immunosuppressives), antecedent corneal disease (eg, dry eye, exposure keratopathy), ocular medication toxicity, or contamination of ocular medications. Bacterial organisms commonly involved in corneal infections include *Pseudomonas aeruginosa, Staphylococcus aureus, Streptococcus pneumoniae,* and Enterobacteriaceae.

Scrapings obtained from infected corneas show collections of neutrophils admixed with necrotic debris. The presence of organisms may be demonstrated on Gram stain. Culture is helpful for accurate identification of specific organisms and for assessment of antibiotic sensitivities. Following sterilization of the ulcer with antibiotic therapy, penetrating keratoplasty may be required in cases of visually significant corneal scarring. Keratoplasty is sometimes required urgently in the acute phase of infection, for example, for perforation or impending perforation (Fig 6-5).

Herpes simplex virus keratitis

Usually a self-limited corneal epithelial disease, herpes simplex virus keratitis is characterized by a linear arborizing pattern of shallow ulceration and swelling of epithelial cells called a *dendrite* (Fig 6-6A). The diagnosis may generally be made clinically. Corneal scrapings obtained from a dendrite and prepared using the Giemsa stain reveal the presence of intranuclear viral inclusions. Viral culture, antigen detection, or polymerase chain reaction (PCR) techniques may be helpful in atypical cases. A dendrite is associated with subepithelial infiltration by chronic inflammatory cells and loss of the Bowman layer. Stromal and/or disciform keratitis (Fig 6-6B) may accompany or follow epithelial infection, leading to stromal scarring and possibly vascularization. Histologically, chronic inflammatory cells and blood vessels may be seen tracking between stromal lamellae, that is, *interstitial keratitis*

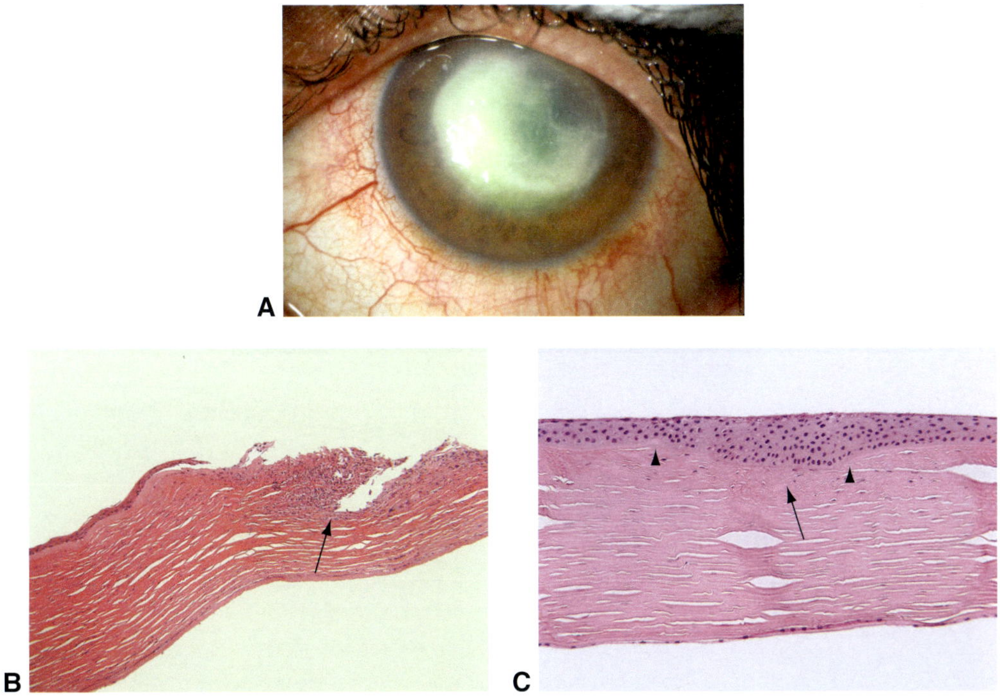

Figure 6-5 Bacterial ulcer. **A,** Clinical appearance of pseudomonal ulcer. **B,** In this patient, penetrating keratoplasty was performed during the acute phase of infection. On H&E stain, the corneal button shows ulcerative keratitis, with stromal necrosis and neutrophilic infiltration *(arrow)*. **C,** Keratoplasty specimen (different patient) showing scar from healed keratitis. Note loss of the Bowman layer *(between arrowheads)* and stromal thinning/fibrosis *(arrow)*, with compensatory epithelial thickening. *(Part A courtesy of Andrew J.W. Huang, MD; parts B and C courtesy of George J. Harocopos, MD.)*

(Fig 6-6C) (discussed later). Endotheliitis may also occur, with a granulomatous reaction at the level of the Descemet membrane (Fig 6-6D), which corresponds to *disciform keratitis* clinically. Visually significant corneal scarring from herpetic keratitis is the single most common infection-related indication for penetrating keratoplasty. Postherpetic neurotrophic keratopathy may result from corneal hypoesthesia or anesthesia and is characterized histologically by a featureless corneal stroma with a paucity of keratocytes (Fig 6-6E).

Fungal keratitis

Mycotic keratitis is often a complication of trauma, especially involving plant or vegetable matter, or microtrauma related to contact lens wear. Corticosteroid use, especially topical, is another major risk factor. Unlike most bacteria, fungi are able to penetrate the cornea and extend through the Descemet membrane into the anterior chamber. The most common organisms are the septated, filamentous fungi *Aspergillus* and *Fusarium* and the yeast *Candida; Mucor* (nonseptated, filamentous) is less common. Culture, particularly on Sabouraud agar, is helpful for accurate identification of specific organisms and for assessment of antifungal sensitivities. When culture is negative and organism identity remains

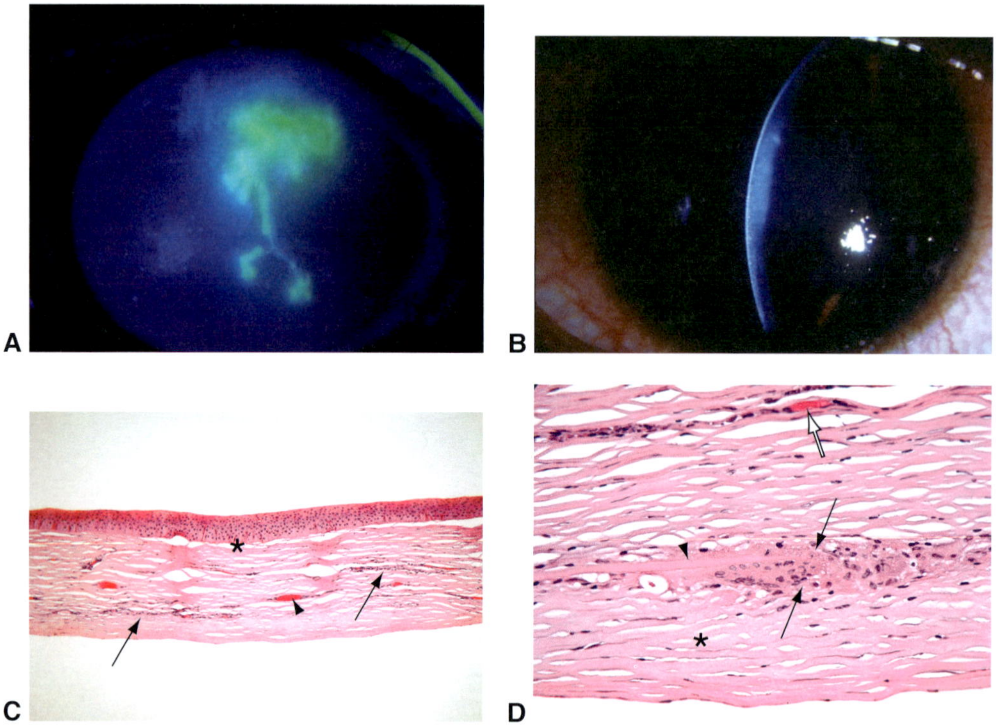

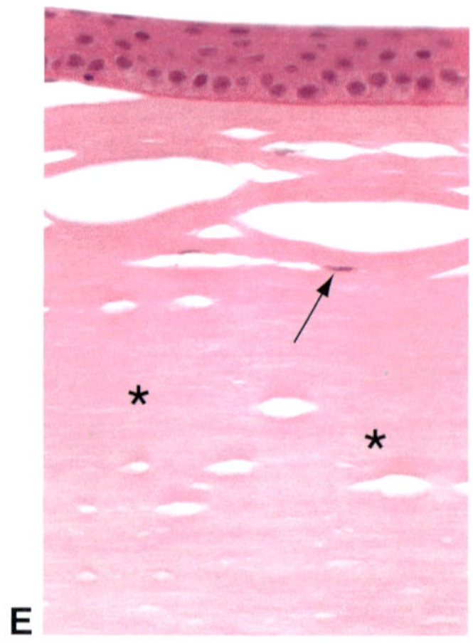

Figure 6-6 Herpes simplex virus keratitis. Clinical photographs depicting dendritic **(A)** and stromal/disciform **(B)** keratitis. **C,** Histology of corneal button shows stromal keratitis with loss of the Bowman layer *(asterisk)*, stromal scarring and vascularization *(arrowhead)*, and scattered chronic inflammatory cells *(arrows)*. **D,** Higher-power photomicrograph shows granulomatous reaction *(between arrows)* in the region of Descemet membrane *(arrowhead)*. Note the fibrous retrocorneal membrane *(asterisk)*, scattered chronic inflammatory cells, and blood vessel *(open arrow)*. **E,** Postherpetic neurotrophic keratopathy. Photomicrograph shows featureless corneal stroma *(asterisks)* with only rare keratocytes *(arrow)*. *(Parts A and B courtesy of Anthony J. Lubniewski, MD; parts C and D courtesy of Tatyana Milman, MD; part E courtesy of Robert H. Rosa, Jr, MD.)*

elusive, corneal biopsy may be considered, for both histologic evaluation and PCR. Many fungi can be seen in tissue sections with the use of special stains such as Grocott-Gomori methenamine–silver nitrate (GMS) or PAS (Fig 6-7). Fungi (eg, *Mucor*) are sometimes apparent on routine H&E sections.

Acanthamoeba keratitis

Acanthamoeba protozoa most commonly cause infection in soft contact lens wearers who do not take appropriate precautions in cleaning and sterilizing their lenses or whose

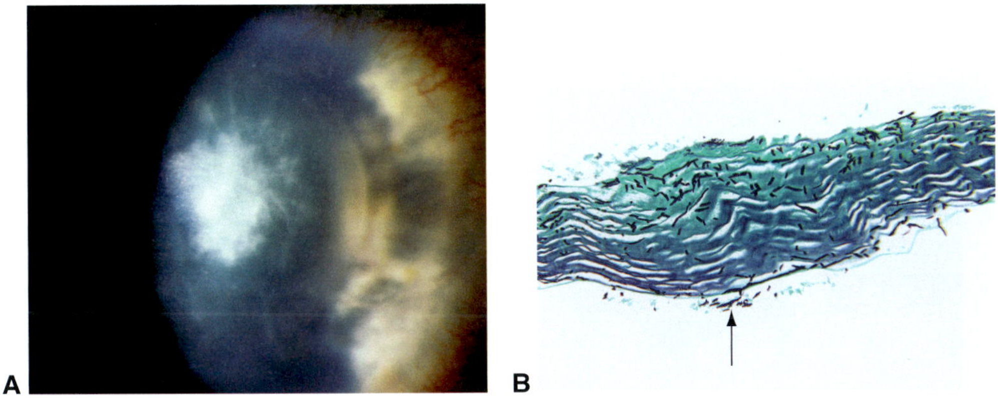

Figure 6-7 *Fusarium* keratitis. **A,** Clinical photograph shows gray-white, dry-appearing stromal infiltrate with feathery margins. **B,** Grocott-Gomori methenamine–silver nitrate (GMS) stain of corneal button demonstrates fungal hyphae *(black).* Note that fungi have penetrated through the Descemet membrane *(arrow). (Part A courtesy of Andrew J.W. Huang, MD; part B courtesy of George J. Harocopos, MD.)*

lenses come into contact with contaminated stagnant water (eg, as found in hot tubs and ponds). The most frequently involved species are *Acanthamoeba castellani* and *Acanthamoeba polyphagia.* Patients presenting with *Acanthamoeba* keratitis usually have severe eye pain. Clinically, radial keratoneuritis and, in late stages, a ring infiltrate may be present (Fig 6-8A). Special culture techniques and media, including nonnutrient blood agar layered with *Escherichia coli,* are required to grow *Acanthamoeba.* In later stages of disease, the organisms penetrate into deeper layers of the stroma and may be difficult to isolate from superficial scraping. Confocal microscopy may be useful for demonstrating the organisms. Scrapings, biopsy specimens, or corneal buttons may show cysts and trophozoites (Fig 6-8B). The organisms may generally be visualized with routine H&E sections but may be more easily seen with PAS stain. Calcofluor white or acridine orange stain may also be used.

Infectious crystalline keratopathy

Infectious crystalline keratopathy (ICK) typically occurs in patients on long-term topical corticosteroid therapy, as, for example, following penetrating keratoplasty. The infection typically arises along a suture track. The most common etiologic microorganism is viridans group (α-hemolytic) Streptococci, although a host of other organisms have been reported, including bacteria and fungi. It is thought that chronic immunosuppression, combined with properties of the organism's glycocalyx that sequester the organism from the immune system, promote growth of the organism in this condition. No true crystals are involved; rather, this condition derives its name from the crystalloid appearance of the opacity seen clinically (Fig 6-9A). The overlying epithelium is often intact, making diagnosis challenging in the early stages of the disease and also making the organism difficult to culture. In many cases, the diagnosis is missed clinically and is made histologically after failure of a corneal graft. On histology, colonies of bacteria are present within the interlamellar spaces of the stroma. The inflammatory cell infiltrate is typically insignificant,

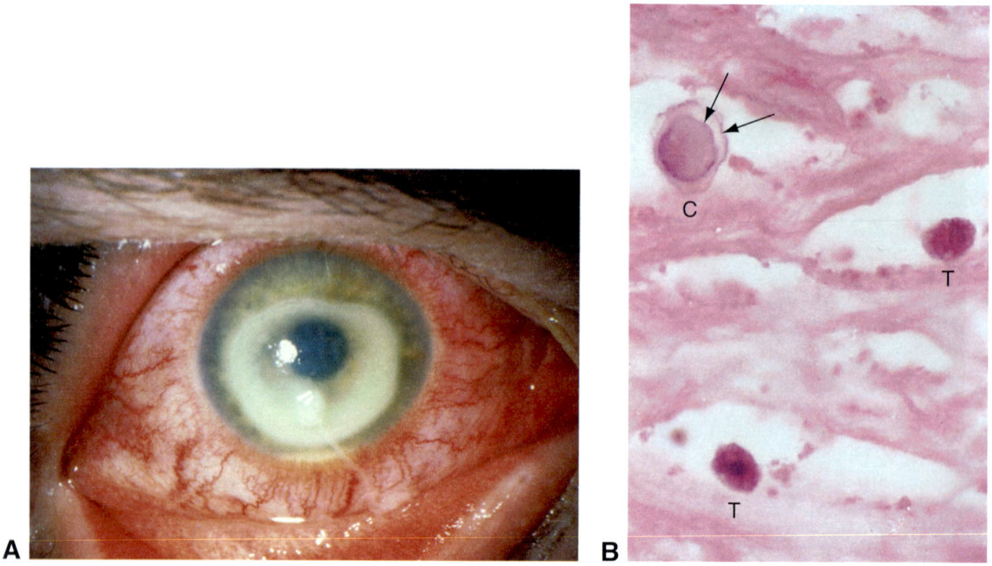

Figure 6-8 *Acanthamoeba* keratitis. **A,** Clinical photograph depicting ring infiltrate and small hypopyon. **B,** Note the cyst *(C)* and trophozoite *(T)* forms. The cyst has a double wall, that is, endocyst and exocyst *(arrows)*. *(Part A courtesy of Sander Dubovy, MD.)*

although in some cases ICK is associated with an adjacent corneal ulcer. The organisms may sometimes be apparent on H&E stain but may be more easily seen on Gram stain or, for some species, on GMS or PAS stain (Fig 6-9B).

Interstitial keratitis

Interstitial keratitis (IK) refers to nonsuppurative inflammatory cell infiltration in the interlamellar spaces of the corneal stroma, often with vascularization, and typically with an

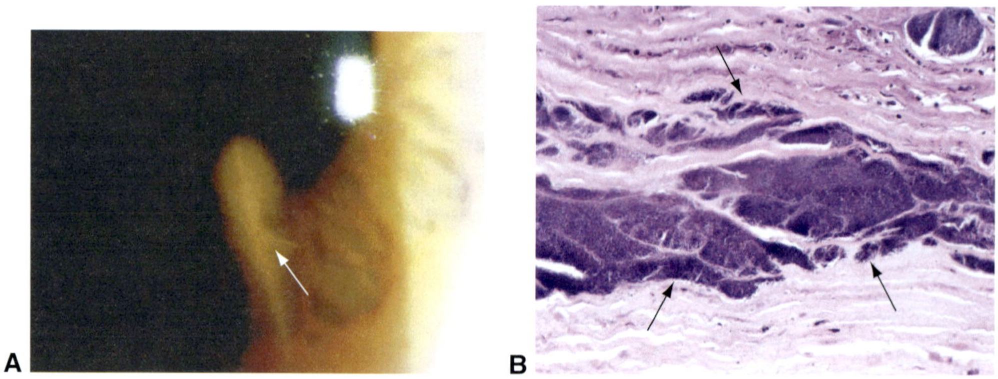

Figure 6-9 Infectious crystalline keratopathy. **A,** Clinical photograph depicting crystalloid-appearing (or "fernlike") stromal infiltrate *(arrow)*, with intact overlying epithelium. The infection arose along a suture track following repair of a corneal laceration. **B,** Gram stain demonstrates colonies of gram-positive cocci interposed between stromal collagen lamellae *(arrows)*. *(Part A courtesy of Anthony J. Lubniewski, MD; part B courtesy of Morton E. Smith, MD.)*

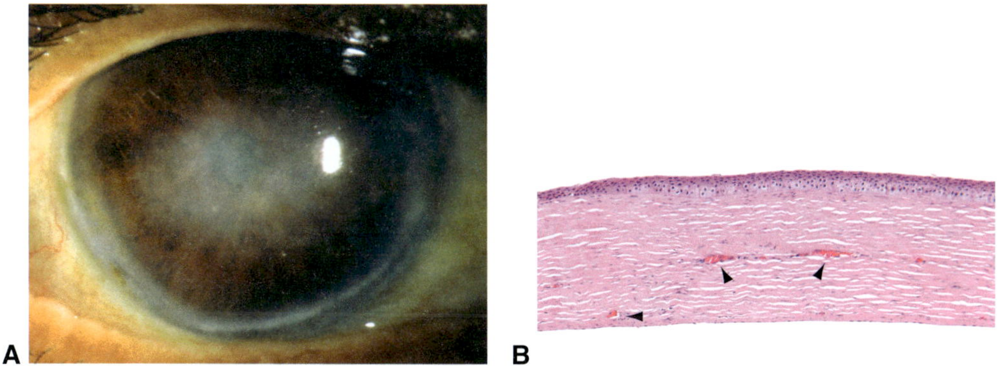

Figure 6-10 Interstitial keratitis of congenital syphilis. **A,** Clinical photograph depicting stromal opacity, with intact overlying epithelium. **B,** Histology shows vascularization *(arrowheads)* in the midstroma and deep stroma, with surrounding chronic inflammatory cells tracking along the interlamellar spaces. Note the intact epithelium. Corneal thickness measured less than 400 μm, indicative of visually significant stromal fibrosis. *(Part A courtesy of Anthony J. Lubniewski, MD; part B courtesy of George J. Harocopos, MD.)*

intact overlying epithelium. Transplacental infection of the fetus by *Treponema pallidum* (congenital syphilis) may cause IK (Fig 6-10). These changes are thought to result from an immunologic response to infectious microorganisms or their antigens. Chronic/recurrent IK may lead to stromal scarring.

Although congenital syphilis represents the "classic" cause of IK, the single most common etiologic agent of IK is herpes (see Fig 6-6). Other causative organisms of IK include *Mycobacterium tuberculosis, Mycobacterium leprae, Borrelia burgdorferi,* and Epstein-Barr virus.

Noninfectious Keratitis

Corneal inflammation can also be caused by noninfectious agents. For example, autoimmune diseases, especially rheumatoid arthritis and graft-vs-host disease, may be associated with sterile corneal ulceration. Topical medication toxicity (eg, overuse of topical anesthetics, nonsteroidal anti-inflammatory drugs [NSAIDs], or antivirals) may also result in corneal melting. On histology, such cases often appear similar to infectious ulcerations on H&E sections, but no organisms are demonstrated on special stains. See also BCSC Section 8, *External Disease and Cornea.*

Degenerations and Dystrophies

Degenerations

Corneal degenerations are secondary changes that occur in previously normal tissue. They are often associated with aging, are not inherited, and are not necessarily bilateral. See also BCSC Section 8, *External Disease and Cornea.*

Salzmann nodular degeneration

Salzmann nodular degeneration is a noninflammatory corneal degeneration that may occur secondary to long-standing keratitis or may be idiopathic. It may be bilateral and is more commonly seen in middle-aged and older women, often in association with blepharitis. Gray-white or bluish flat or raised lesions are present where the eyelid margin contacts the cornea in primary gaze and/or in the central and paracentral cornea (Fig 6-11A). Histologic examination discloses irregular epithelial thickness and replacement of the Bowman layer with disorganized collagenous tissue (Fig 6-11B). Thickening of the epithelial basement membrane may also be seen.

Calcific band keratopathy

Seen clinically as a band-shaped calcific plaque in the interpalpebral zone and typically sparing the most peripheral clear cornea, band keratopathy is characterized by the deposition of calcium at the level of the Bowman layer and the anterior stroma. The calcium deposits appear as basophilic granules in H&E sections; the presence of calcium can be further confirmed by the use of special stains such as alizarin red or von Kossa stain (Fig 6-12). Band keratopathy may develop after any chronic local corneal disease, following prolonged chronic inflammation (especially in eyes with a history of chronic juvenile idiopathic arthritis–associated uveitis and in blind, painful eyes), and, less commonly, in association with systemic hypercalcemic states.

Actinic keratopathy

Also known as *spheroidal degeneration* or *Labrador keratopathy,* actinic keratopathy involves elastotic degeneration of corneal collagen similar to that seen in pingueculae, pterygia, and solar elastosis of the skin. This condition may be caused by prolonged exposure to solar (actinic) irradiation. It may also be caused by corneal inflammation, sometimes in association with calcific band keratopathy. The actinic damage usually occurs within the interpalpebral fissure. Clinical examination discloses translucent, golden-brown spheroidal deposits in the superficial cornea (Fig 6-13A). H&E-stained sections show basophilic globules beneath the epithelium in the region of the Bowman layer and the anterior

A B
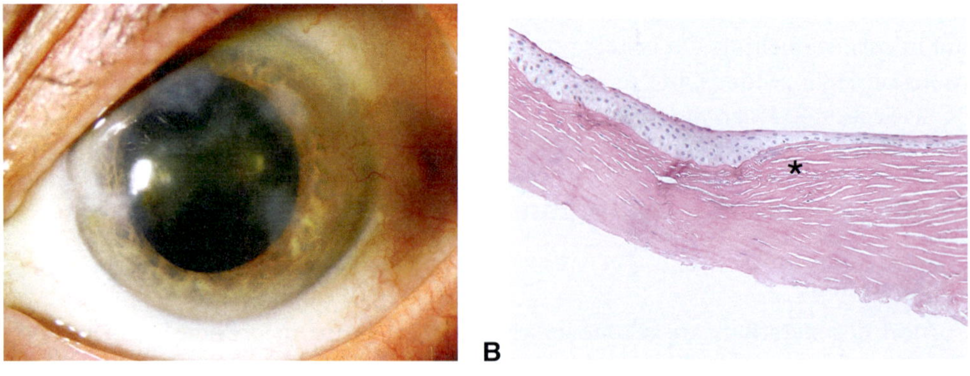

Figure 6-11 Salzmann nodular degeneration. **A,** Clinical appearance. Note the gray-white corneal opacities. **B,** Histology of superficial keratectomy specimen (PAS stain) shows irregular epithelial thickness and diffuse loss of the Bowman layer, with this layer replaced by disorganized collagenous tissue *(asterisk)*. *(Courtesy of George J. Harocopos, MD.)*

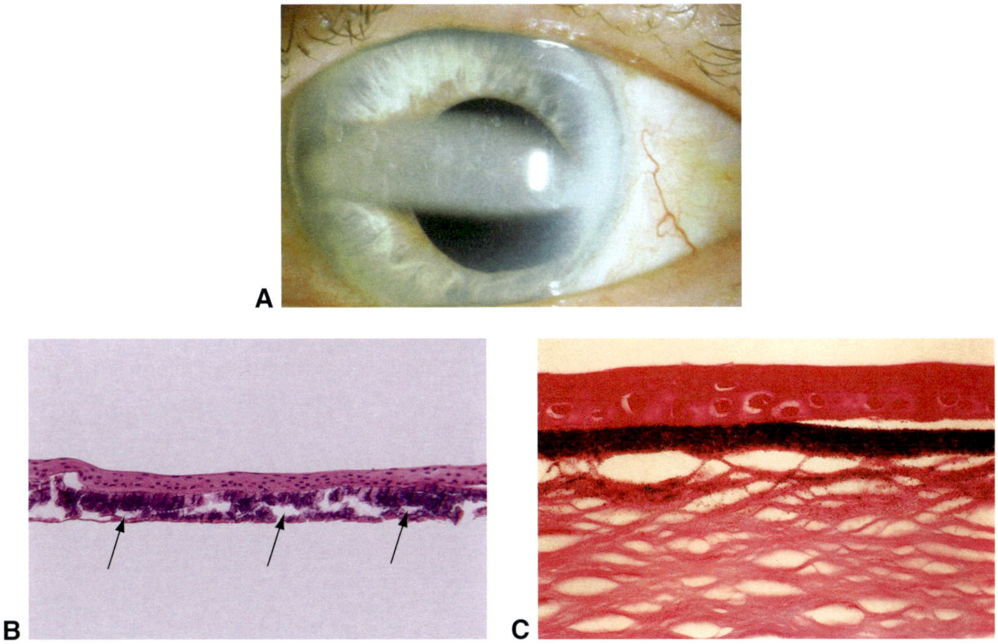

Figure 6-12 Calcific band keratopathy. **A,** Clinical appearance. **B,** Calcific keratopathy may be treated with epithelial scraping and chelation with ethylenediaminetetraacetic acid (EDTA "scrub"). The calcium is deposited at the level of the Bowman layer *(arrows),* appearing deeply basophilic (purple) on H&E stain. **C,** Calcium deposits appear black on von Kossa stain. *(Part A courtesy of Anthony J. Lubniewski, MD; part B courtesy of George J. Harocopos, MD; part C courtesy of Hans E. Grossniklaus, MD.)*

stroma (Fig 6-13B). The deposits stain black with special stains for elastin, such as the Verhoeff–van Gieson (VVG) stain.

Pannus

Pannus refers to the growth of fibrovascular or fibrous tissue between the epithelium and the Bowman layer (Fig 6-14). The Bowman layer may be disrupted. Pannus is frequently seen in cases of chronic corneal edema or following prolonged corneal inflammation.

Bullous keratopathy

Intraocular surgery, most commonly cataract surgery, invariably results in some loss of corneal endothelial cells. In cases of extensive endothelial cell loss, the cornea may decompensate postoperatively, either early in the postoperative period or years later, after more endothelial cells are lost with age. When the endothelium begins to decompensate, Descemet folds and stromal edema occur, followed by intracellular epithelial edema and, ultimately, separation of the epithelium from the Bowman layer. Small separations are referred to as "microcysts"; these may coalesce to form large separations, known as *bullae.* In more advanced cases of bullous keratopathy, as in Fuchs endothelial dystrophy (discussed later), secondary epithelial basement membrane changes and fibrous pannus may be seen. The Descemet membrane may be thickened, but it typically does not show guttae (Fig 6-15). Although bullous keratopathy is more commonly seen after cataract surgery,

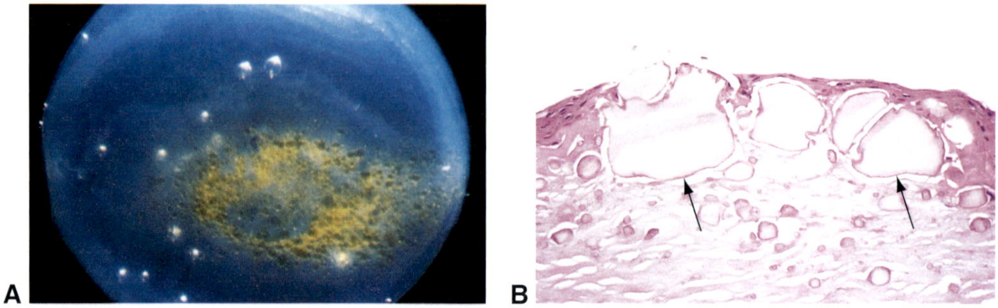

Figure 6-13 Actinic keratopathy (spheroidal degeneration). **A,** Gross appearance of corneal button. The air bubbles are artifacts. **B,** Histology shows lightly staining basophilic globules *(arrows)* in the epithelium and superficial stroma. *(Courtesy of Hans E. Grossniklaus, MD.)*

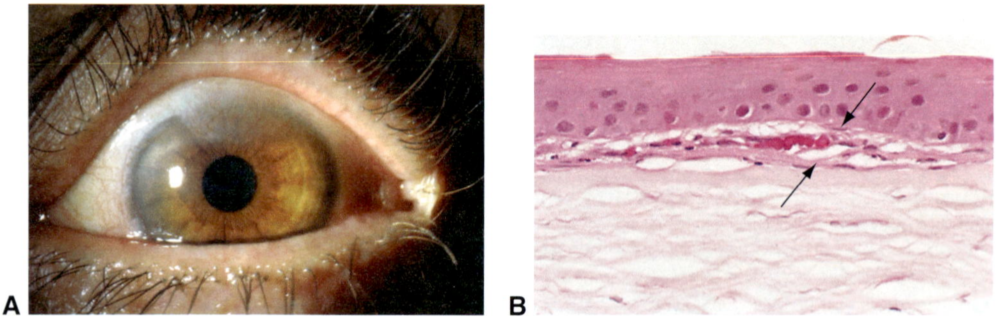

Figure 6-14 Fibrovascular pannus. **A,** Clinical appearance on the superior cornea. **B,** Fibrovascular pannus *(between arrows)* is interposed between the epithelium and the Bowman layer. *(Part A courtesy of George J. Harocopos, MD.)*

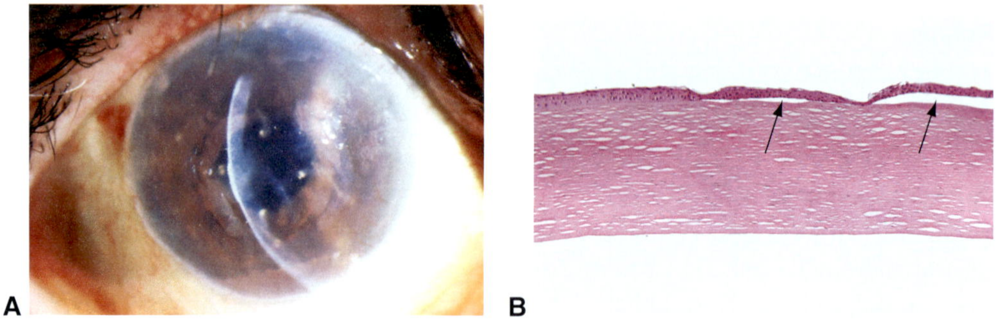

Figure 6-15 Pseudophakic bullous keratopathy. **A,** Clinical appearance of severe bullous keratopathy associated with an anterior chamber lens implant. **B,** Corneal button from penetrating keratoplasty. Note the subepithelial bullae *(arrows)*. Also note diffuse endothelial cell loss, without guttae of Descemet membrane. *(Part A courtesy of Andrew J.W. Huang, MD; part B courtesy of George J. Harocopos, MD.)*

in which case it is termed *pseudophakic* or *aphakic bullous keratopathy,* it may also be seen after other forms of intraocular surgery, for example, multiple glaucoma procedures or retinal detachment repair with silicone oil ("silicone oil keratopathy").

Corneal graft failure

Failure of an existing corneal graft is one of the most common indications for penetrating keratoplasty. The final common pathway of graft failure is endothelial cell loss. The endothelial cells of a graft may gradually decrease over time until failure occurs, or there may be an acute event resulting in endothelial cell loss, such as a rejection episode or ulcerative keratitis. When endothelial failure occurs, there is often associated bullous keratopathy. In about half of cases, a fibrous retrocorneal membrane is visualized (Fig 6-16). If the membrane is thick and contiguous with the corneal stroma in the region of an incision, then the membrane may be termed *fibrous downgrowth* or *ingrowth.* Less commonly, a graft may fail because of growth of surface epithelium through a poorly apposed wound and onto the retrocorneal surface, that is, *epithelial downgrowth* or *ingrowth.* The main risk factor for fibrous or epithelial downgrowth is multiple prior penetrating keratoplasties. Both types of downgrowth are very poor prognostic signs for graft survival and for general ocular health, as they are typically associated with secondary angle-closure glaucoma.

Keratoconus

Keratoconus is a bilateral noninflammatory condition characterized by central or inferocentral ectasia of the cornea, typically diagnosed during adolescence or young adulthood (Fig 6-17A). It is often sporadic, but family history is positive in some cases, thereby blurring the distinction between degeneration and dystrophy in this condition. Keratoconus can occur as an isolated finding, or it may be associated with other ocular disorders or with systemic conditions, including atopy, Down syndrome, and Marfan syndrome. The alteration in the normal corneal contour produces myopia and irregular astigmatism. In advanced disease, visually significant apical scarring develops, often requiring therapeutic keratoplasty. A small percentage of keratoconus patients develop a spontaneous break in Descemet membrane, resulting in acute corneal edema known as *corneal hydrops.*

Histologic findings in keratoconus include central stromal thinning and focal discontinuities in the Bowman layer. Apical anterior stromal fibrosis is often present (Fig 6-17B, C). Iron deposition in the basal epithelial layers at the base of the cone *(Fleischer ring)* can sometimes be demonstrated with Prussian blue stain (Fig 6-17D). In patients with a history of hydrops, a break in Descemet membrane may be observed (Fig 6-17E). Occasionally, amyloid material may accumulate in the anterior cornea in advanced keratoconus (an example of secondary localized amyloidosis).

Pellucid marginal degeneration is another ectatic disorder and is likely part of the same disease spectrum as keratoconus. The stromal thinning of pellucid marginal degeneration is typically more inferior than that of keratoconus.

Pigment deposits

Krukenberg spindle is seen in pigment dispersion syndrome, a form of secondary open-angle glaucoma typically occurring in young to middle-aged adults with myopia, associated

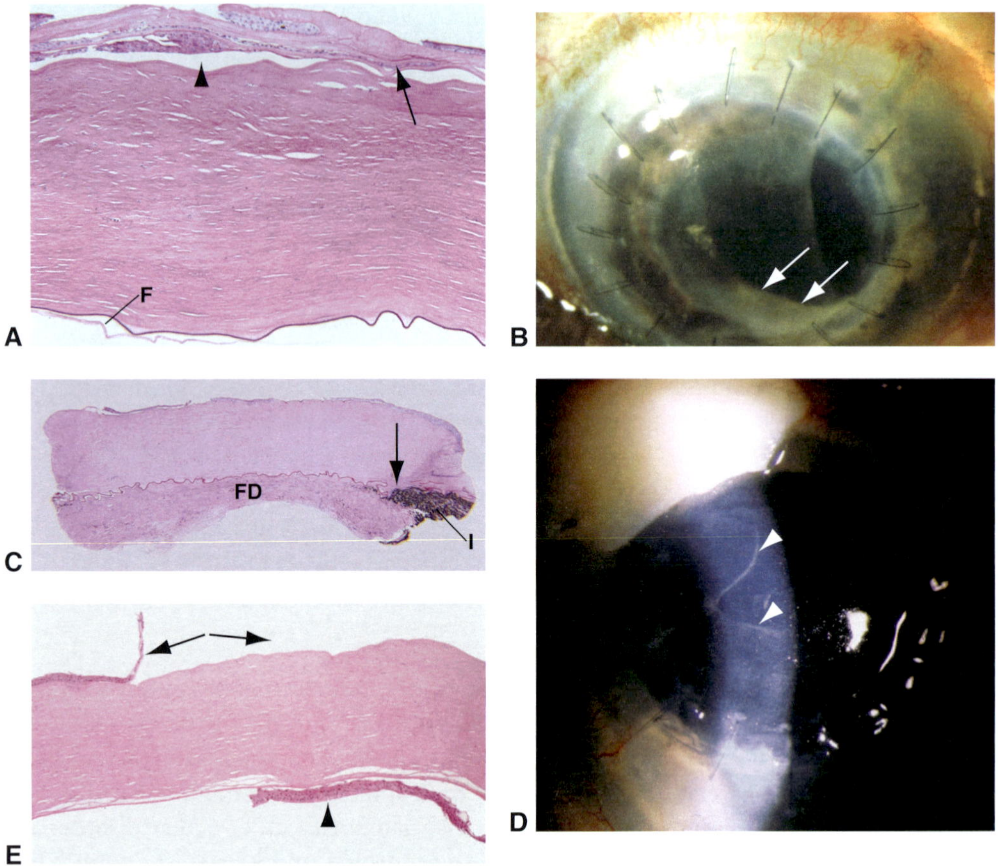

Figure 6-16 Corneal graft failure. **A,** PAS stain of corneal button, showing diffuse endothelial cell loss and fibrous retrocorneal membrane *(F)*. There is secondary bullous keratopathy *(arrowhead)* and epithelial basement membrane thickening/redundancy *(arrow)*. **B,** Clinical appearance of fibrous downgrowth *(arrows)*. **C,** PAS stain of corneal button (different patient) showing fibrous downgrowth *(FD)*. The continuity between the fibrous downgrowth and the corneal stroma may be seen through the break in Descemet membrane *(arrow)* at the graft–host interface. Also note peripheral anterior synechiae, with iris tissue *(I)* adherent to the fibrous membrane. **D,** Clinical appearance of epithelial downgrowth *(arrowheads)*. **E,** Histology of failed graft (different patient) with epithelial downgrowth *(arrowhead)* and diffuse endothelial cell loss. Also note secondary bullous keratopathy, with ruptured bulla *(arrows)*. *(Parts A, C, and E courtesy of George J. Harocopos, MD; parts B and D courtesy of Anthony J. Lubniewski, MD.)*

with posterior bowing of the midperipheral iris. The melanin pigment is located within the corneal endothelial cells and may also be found extracellularly on the posterior corneal surface (Fig 6-18). In pigment dispersion syndrome, melanin pigment is also seen in and around the endothelial cells lining the trabecular meshwork, correlating with the abnormally dark color of the meshwork observed gonioscopically (see Chapter 7, Fig 7-13). See also BCSC Section 10, *Glaucoma*.

Blood staining of the cornea may complicate hyphema when the intraocular pressure (IOP) is very high for a long duration; however, if the endothelium is compromised, blood

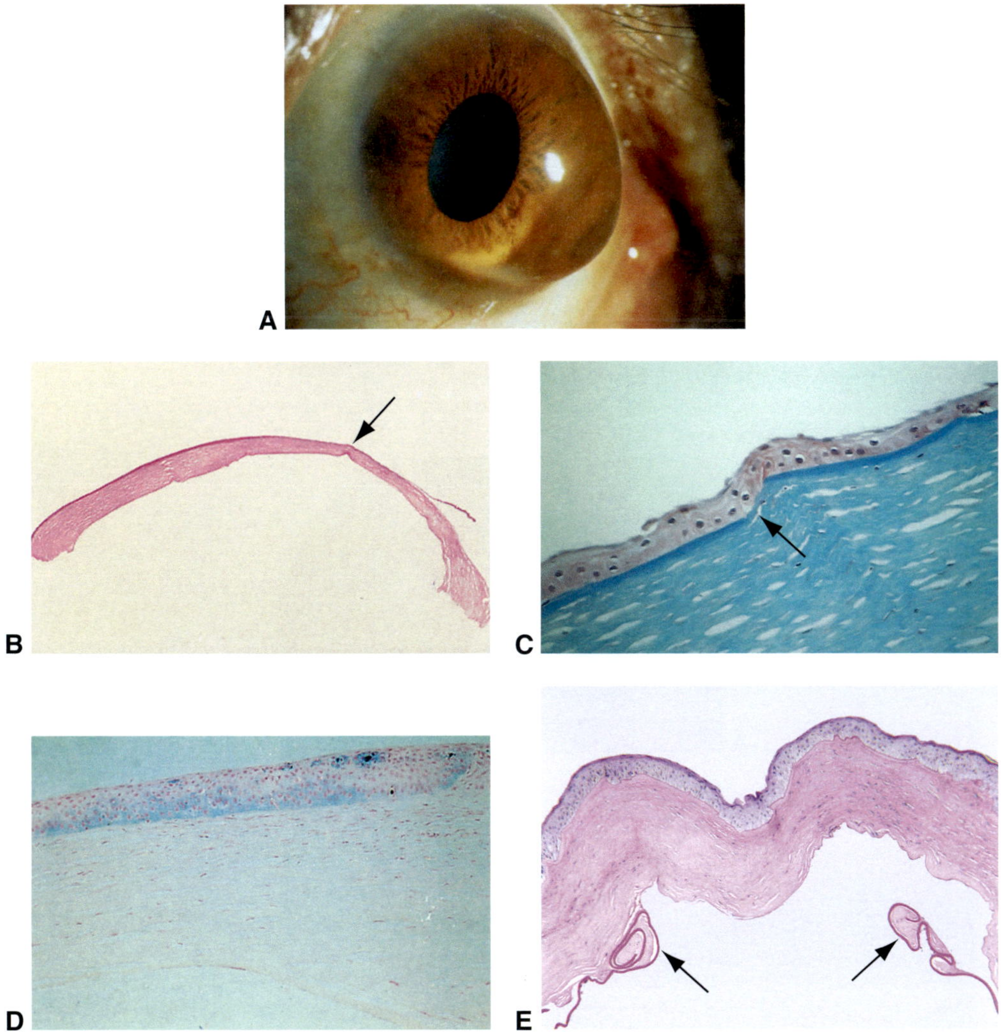

Figure 6-17 Keratoconus. **A,** Clinical appearance. **B,** Low-magnification view shows apical stromal thinning *(arrow).* **C,** Masson trichrome stain demonstrates focal disruption of the Bowman layer *(arrow).* **D,** Prussian blue stain demonstrates intraepithelial iron deposition (Fleischer ring). **E,** In a patient with prior hydrops, PAS stain highlights rupture of Descemet membrane, with rolled-up edges on either side *(arrows). (Part A courtesy of Sander Dubovy, MD; part C courtesy of Hans E. Grossniklaus, MD; part E courtesy of George J. Harocopos, MD.)*

staining can occur even at normal or low IOP (Fig 6-19). Histologically, red blood cells and their breakdown products (mostly hemoglobin and also small amounts of hemosiderin) are seen in the corneal stroma. The hemosiderin is located in the cytoplasm of keratocytes and may be demonstrated with iron stains such as Prussian blue.

Iron deposition in the corneal epithelium in keratoconus *(Fleischer ring)* was previously discussed (see Fig 6-17D).

See BCSC Section 8, *External Disease and Cornea,* for additional discussion of blood staining of the cornea as well as other forms of ocular surface iron lines.

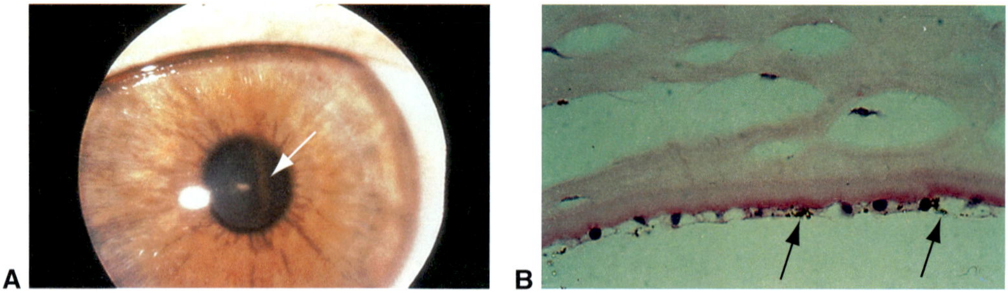

Figure 6-18 Krukenberg spindle. **A,** Clinical appearance of Krukenberg spindle *(arrow)*. **B,** Melanin pigment is found within the cytoplasm of endothelial cells *(arrows)*. *(Part A courtesy of L.J. Katz, MD; part B courtesy of Debra J. Shetlar, MD.)*

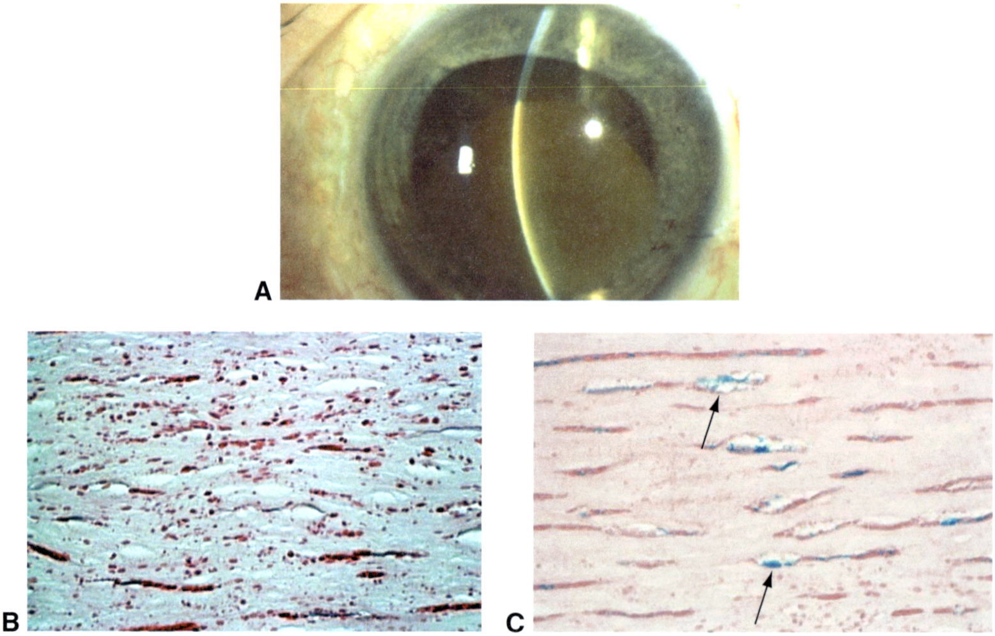

Figure 6-19 Corneal blood staining. **A,** Clinical appearance. **B,** Masson trichrome stain. The red particles represent erythrocytic debris and hemoglobin in the corneal stroma. **C,** An iron stain demonstrates hemosiderin *(arrows)*, confined to the stromal keratocytes. *(Part A courtesy of Anthony J. Lubniewski, MD; parts B and C courtesy of Hans E. Grossniklaus, MD.)*

Dystrophies

Dystrophies of the cornea are primary, generally inherited, bilateral disorders, categorized by the layer of the cornea most involved (ie, epithelial, stromal, endothelial). Keratoconus (previously discussed) may be considered a dystrophy, except that it is often sporadic and likely multifactorial in etiology. Only the most common corneal dystrophies are discussed in the following sections. See also BCSC Section 8, *External Disease and Cornea.*

Epithelial dystrophy

Also called *map-dot-fingerprint dystrophy, Cogan microcystic dystrophy, anterior basement membrane dystrophy (ABMD),* and *epithelial basement membrane dystrophy (EBMD),* epithelial dystrophy may be the most common of the corneal dystrophies seen by the comprehensive ophthalmologist (Fig 6-20). It is often sporadic but may be inherited in an autosomal dominant fashion. In this condition, the basement membrane is thickened and may extend into the epithelium (forming "map" and "fingerprint" lines). The intraepithelial basement membrane redundancies may encircle foci of epithelial cells, which may then degenerate, resulting in epithelial debris within cystoid spaces ("dots") (see Fig 6-20C). Patients with epithelial dystrophy often present with symptoms of recurrent erosion syndrome.

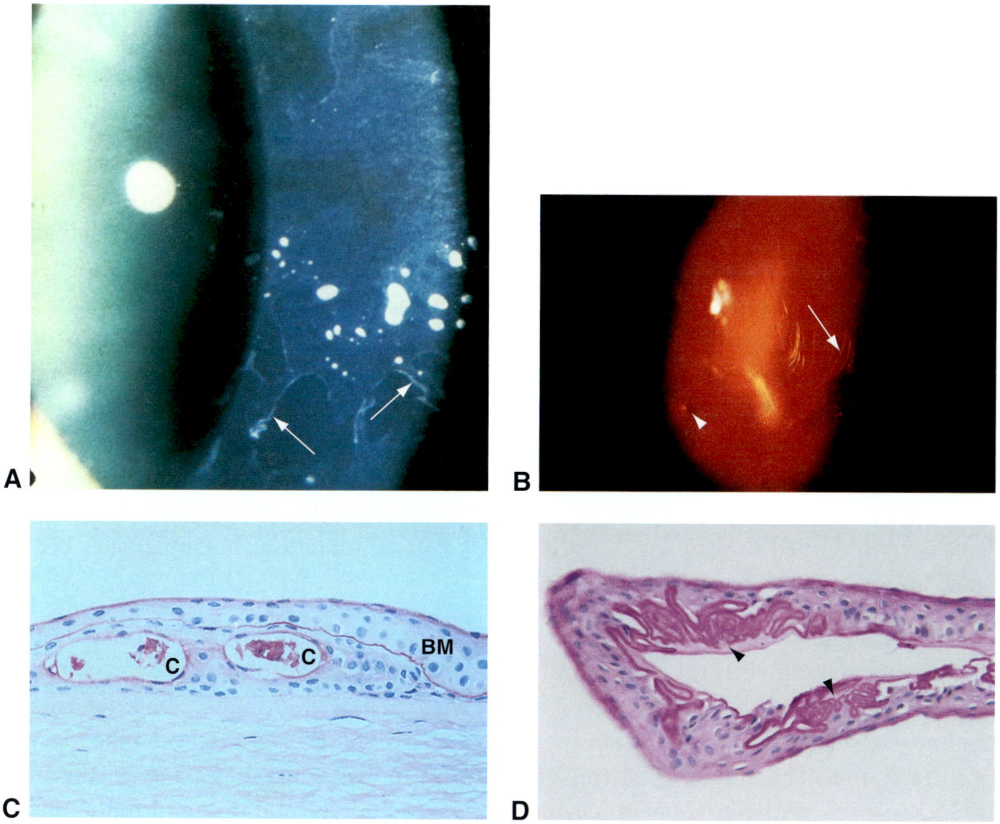

Figure 6-20 Epithelial basement membrane dystrophy (EBMD, map-dot-fingerprint dystrophy). **A,** Clinical appearance depicting fine, lacy opacities *(arrows).* **B,** Retroillumination demonstrating wavy lines *(arrow)* and dotlike lesions *(arrowhead).* **C,** The changes in primary map-dot-fingerprint dystrophy are essentially identical to those seen in cases of chronic corneal edema secondary to endothelial decompensation. Note the intraepithelial basement membrane *(BM)* and the degenerating epithelial cells trapped within cystoid spaces *(C).* **D,** When surgical treatment is required for EBMD, removal of abnormal epithelium (superficial keratectomy) may be performed, as in this case. PAS stain highlights numerous folds *(arrowheads)* in the epithelial basement membrane. *(Part A courtesy of Andrew J.W. Huang, MD; part D courtesy of George J. Harocopos, MD.)*

Stromal dystrophies

The corneal stromal dystrophies presented in the following subsections (macular, granular, lattice, Avellino) are all inherited disorders and may present with symptoms of decreased vision and recurrent erosion syndrome. All of the stromal dystrophies may recur in corneal grafts.

The genetics of the stromal dystrophies have become elucidated in recent years, enhancing our understanding of these disorders. At the same time, the genetic discoveries raise questions regarding the proper classification of the corneal dystrophies: the same dystrophy may be associated with multiple different mutations, while the same mutation may result in multiple different clinical phenotypes. The International Committee for Classification of Corneal Dystrophies (IC3D) was created for the purpose of devising a current, accurate, and uniform nomenclature. The information given in the following subsections reflects the current IC3D nomenclature. The IC3D classification is available on the website of The Cornea Society (www.corneasociety.org/ic3d).

Weiss JS, Møller HU, Lisch W, et al. The IC3D classification of the corneal dystrophies. *Cornea.* 2008;27(Suppl 2):S1–S80.

Macular dystrophy Macular dystrophy, an autosomal recessive stromal dystrophy, involves the entire cornea (ie, limbus to limbus) and may involve the full thickness of the cornea, including the endothelium. Clinically, it is characterized by poorly defined stromal lesions (focal opacities) with hazy intervening stroma. Mucopolysaccharide material is deposited both intracellularly and extracellularly in the corneal stroma (Fig 6-21). The material stains blue with alcian blue and colloidal iron stains, with the majority of mucopolysaccharide deposits seen in the interlamellar spaces and in keratocytes. Corneal thinning may occur as well. The number of endothelial cells may be decreased, and guttae may be seen in the Descemet membrane. Macular dystrophy is caused by mutations in the carbohydrate sulfotransferase 6 gene *(CHST6)* on chromosome 16 (16q22), which is responsible for the sulfation of keratan sulfate. Numerous different mutations in this gene have been described in macular dystrophy, with certain mutations having greater prevalence in specific regions of the world.

Granular dystrophy Granular dystrophy (type 1) is an autosomal dominant stromal dystrophy that involves the central cornea and has sharply defined lesions with clear intervening stroma (Fig 6-22). Histologically, irregularly shaped, well-circumscribed deposits of hyaline material are visible in the stroma. This material stains bright red with the Masson trichrome stain. The mutation causing granular dystrophy occurs in the *TGFβI* (βig-h3 = BIGH3 = keratoepithelin) gene on chromosome 5 (5q31). Several different mutations in this gene have been described in association with granular dystrophy.

Lattice dystrophy Lattice dystrophy (type 1) is an autosomal dominant stromal dystrophy that involves the central cornea and is characterized by refractile lines with hazy intervening stroma (Fig 6-23). This disorder is a form of primary localized amyloidosis, in which amyloid deposits may arise from epithelial cells and keratocytes. Histologically, the amyloid deposits are concentrated most heavily in the anterior stroma, but they may also occur in the subepithelial area and deeper stroma. The amyloid material stains positive (orange) with the Congo red stain on standard light microscopy, and under polarized

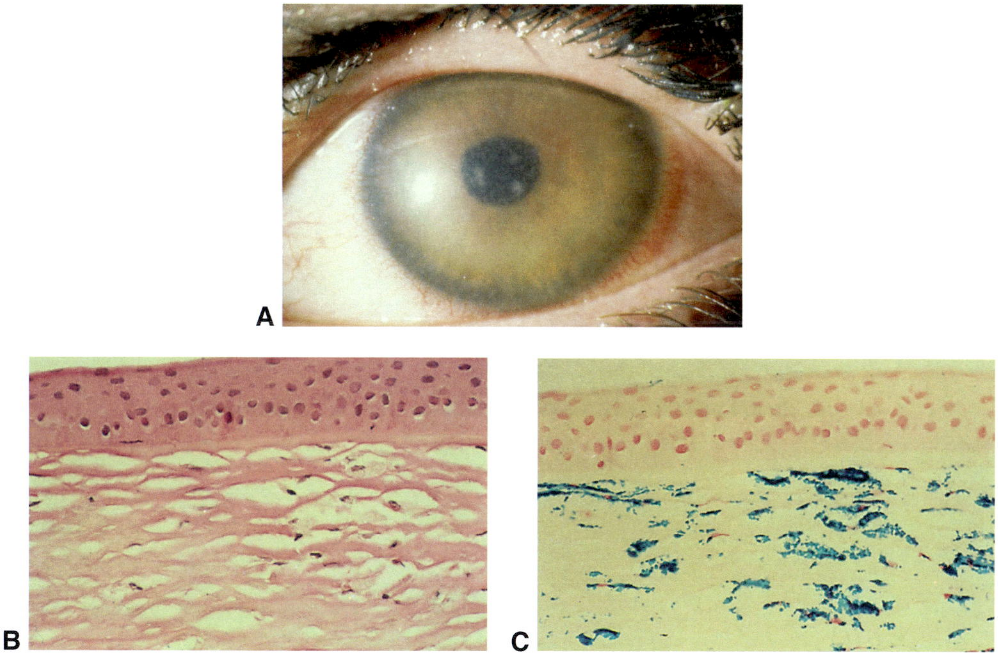

Figure 6-21 Macular dystrophy. **A,** Clinical appearance depicting diffusely hazy cornea with focal opacities. **B,** H&E stain. Note the clear spaces surrounding the keratocytes and in the stroma. **C,** Colloidal iron stains mucopolysaccharides in the keratocytes and stroma. *(Part A courtesy of Sander Dubovy, MD.)*

light, it exhibits birefringence with dichroism (orange and apple green). Amyloid demonstrates metachromasia with crystal violet stain. The fluorescent stain thioflavin T may also be used to demonstrate amyloid. As in granular dystrophy, several different mutations in the *BIGH3* gene on 5q31 have been reported to cause lattice dystrophy.

Avellino dystrophy Features of both granular and lattice dystrophy appear in Avellino dystrophy, first described in patients tracing their ancestry to Avellino, Italy. Histologically, both hyaline deposits (typical of granular dystrophy) and amyloid deposits (characteristic of lattice dystrophy) are present within the corneal stroma (Fig 6-24). This autosomal dominant dystrophy, like granular and lattice dystrophy, has been attributed to mutations in the *BIGH3* gene on 5q31. See Table 6-2 for a histologic comparison of macular, granular, lattice, and Avellino dystrophies.

Table 6-2 Histologic Differentiation of Macular, Granular, Lattice, and Avellino Dystrophies

Dystrophy	Trichrome	Alcian Blue	Congo Red	Birefringence
Macular	–	+	–	–
Granular	+	–	–	–
Lattice	–	–	+	+
Avellino	+	–	+	+

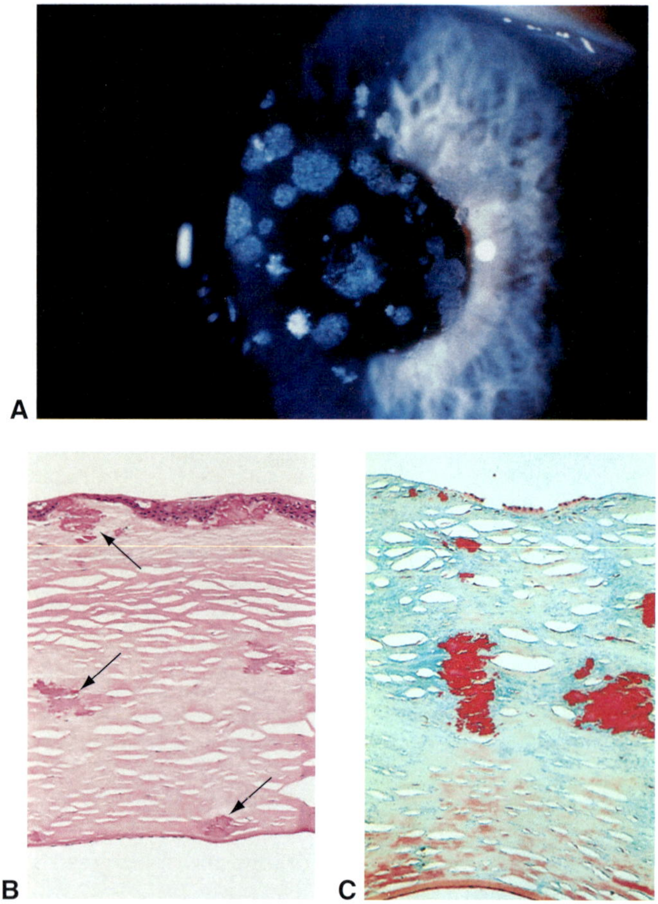

Figure 6-22 Granular dystrophy. **A,** Clinical appearance; note the clear intervening stroma. **B,** H&E stain. Note the eosinophilic deposits *(arrows)* at all levels of the corneal stroma. **C,** Masson trichrome stain. The stromal background stains blue, and the granular deposits stain brilliant red.

Endothelial dystrophy

Fuchs dystrophy is inherited in an autosomal dominant fashion or may be sporadic. It is one of the leading causes of bullous keratopathy (discussed earlier). Its defining characteristic is the presence of anvil-shaped excrescences of Descemet membrane, called *guttae,* which protrude into the anterior chamber or may be buried within a thickened Descemet membrane (Fig 6-25). Guttae may be recognized clinically in young adulthood, long before the cornea decompensates. Over time, progressive endothelial cell loss occurs, ultimately resulting in visually significant corneal edema and bullous keratopathy, typically in middle-aged to older individuals. As in bullous keratopathy from other causes, there are varying degrees of secondary epithelial basement membrane changes and subepithelial fibrosis, similar to changes seen in map-dot-fingerprint dystrophy. In cases of endothelial decompensation without extensive subepithelial fibrosis, endokeratoplasty rather than penetrating keratoplasty may be an alternative surgical option. Other endothelial

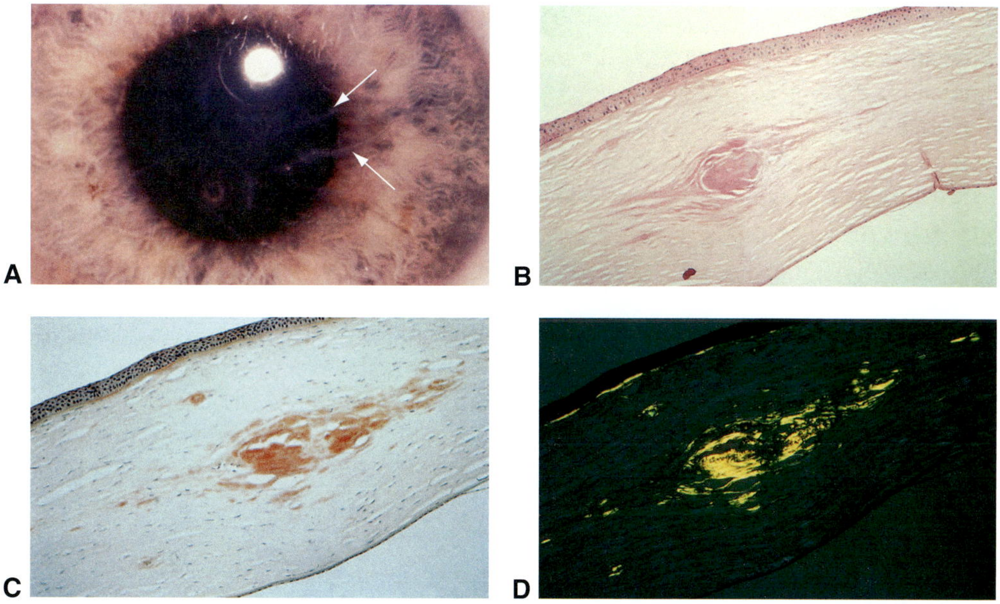

Figure 6-23 Lattice dystrophy. **A,** Clinical appearance with lattice lines *(arrows)*. **B,** H&E stain shows scattered fusiform, eosinophilic material deposited at all levels of the stroma. **C,** Congo red stain (orange) demonstrates that the fusiform deposits are amyloid. **D,** With Congo red stain, under polarized light, amyloid deposits exhibit birefringence and dichroism. *(Parts B–D courtesy of Hans E. Grossniklaus, MD.)*

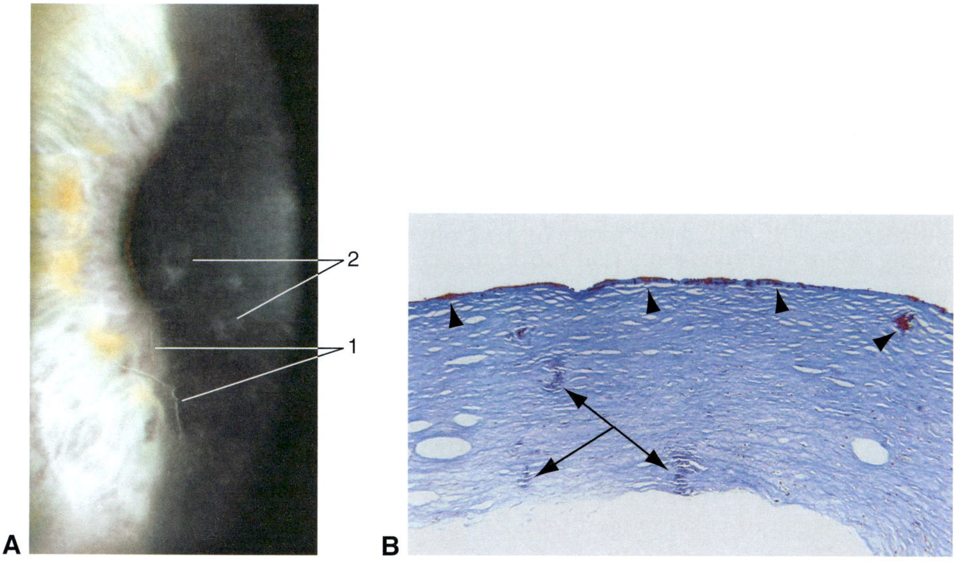

Figure 6-24 Avellino dystrophy. **A,** Clinical appearance, showing both lattice lines *(1)* and granular deposits *(2)*. **B,** Trichrome stain of deep anterior lamellar keratoplasty (DALK) button highlights hyaline deposits at the level of the Bowman layer and anterior stroma *(arrowheads)*. Other deposits at various levels of the stroma stain a darker blue than the stromal background *(triple arrow)*; these deposits were found on Congo red stain to be amyloid. *(Part A modified with permission from Krachmer JH, Palay DA.* Cornea Atlas. *2nd ed. Philadelphia: Mosby-Elsevier; 2006:163. Part B courtesy of George J. Harocopos, MD.)*

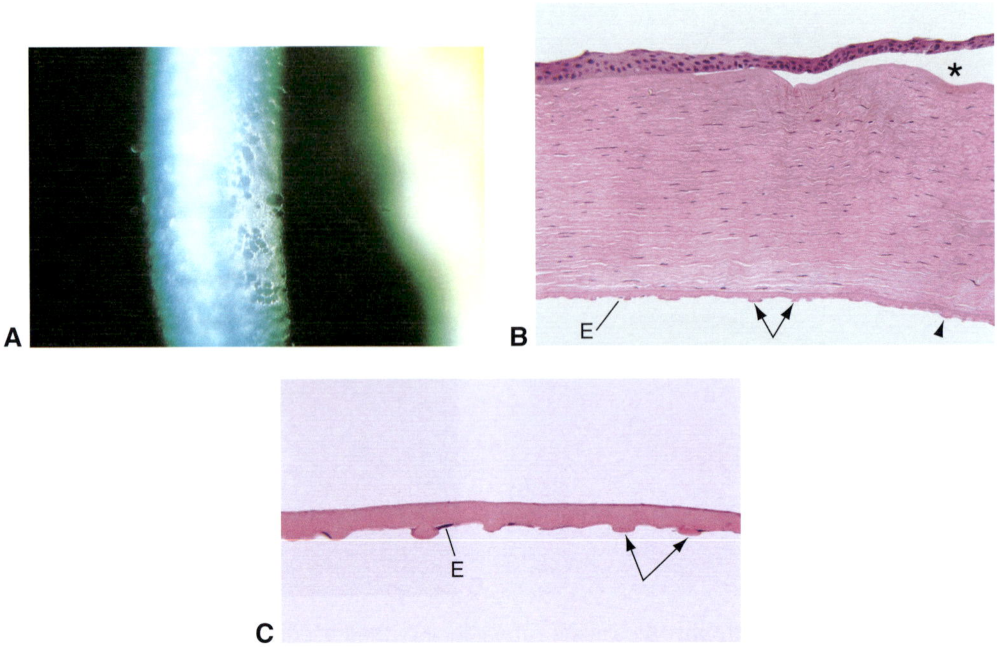

Figure 6-25 Fuchs dystrophy. **A,** Slit-beam illumination of cornea shows "beaten bronze" appearance of Descemet membrane. **B,** Corneal button from penetrating keratoplasty shows endothelial cell loss, with few surviving endothelial cells *(E)*. Numerous guttae are seen in Descemet membrane, either protruding into the anterior chamber *(arrows)* or buried within thickened Descemet membrane *(arrowhead)*. The result of endothelial decompensation is diffuse stromal edema (note loss of interlamellar clefts) and bullous keratopathy *(asterisk)*. **C,** Specimen from Descemet stripping endothelial keratoplasty (DSEK) shows few endothelial cells *(E)* and numerous guttae *(arrows)*. *(Part A reproduced from* External Disease and Cornea: A Multimedia Collection. *San Francisco: American Academy of Ophthalmology; 2000. Parts B and C courtesy of George J. Harocopos, MD.)*

dystrophies (ie, congenital hereditary endothelial dystrophy and posterior polymorphous dystrophy) were discussed previously under Congenital Anomalies.

Neoplasia

Primary conjunctival intraepithelial neoplasia may extend from the limbus and involve the corneal epithelium. This condition is described further in Chapter 5. In rare cases, intraepithelial squamous neoplasia may arise in the cornea.

CHAPTER 7

Anterior Chamber and Trabecular Meshwork

Topography

The anterior chamber is bounded anteriorly by the corneal endothelium, posteriorly by the anterior surface of the iris–ciliary body and pupillary portion of the lens, and peripherally by the trabecular meshwork (Fig 7-1). The depth of the anterior chamber is approximately 3.5 mm. The trabecular meshwork is derived predominantly from the neural crest, while the Schlemm canal is derived from mesoderm.

Histologic features of the anterior chamber angle correlate with gonioscopic landmarks (Fig 7-2). The termination of Descemet membrane is manifested gonioscopically as the Schwalbe line. The scleral spur, a triangular extension of the sclera that appears as a white band gonioscopically, can be identified histologically by tracing the outermost longitudinal ciliary body muscle to its insertion. The trabecular meshwork and the Schlemm

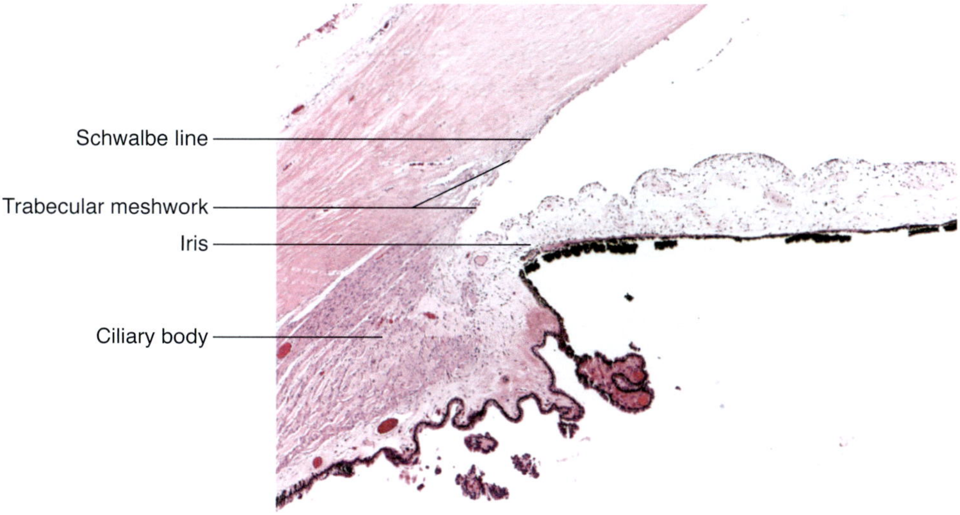

Figure 7-1 The normal anterior chamber angle, the site of drainage for the major portion of the aqueous humor flow, is defined by the anterior border of the iris, the face of the ciliary body, the internal surface of the trabecular meshwork, and the posterior surface of the cornea. *(Courtesy of Nasreen A. Syed, MD.)*

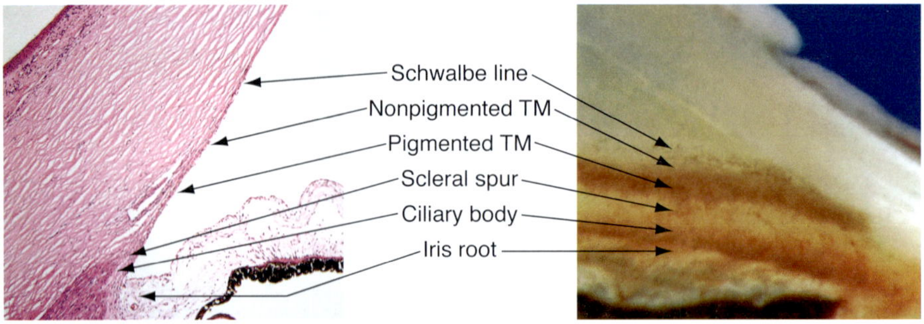

Figure 7-2 Normal anterior chamber angle. Gonioscopic landmarks of the anterior chamber angle with histologic correlation. *TM* = trabecular meshwork. *(Courtesy of Tatyana Milman, MD.)*

canal are nested in the groove formed by the scleral spur and corneoscleral tissue (internal scleral sulcus). See also Figures 2-1B and 2-2 in BCSC Section 10, *Glaucoma.*

Congenital Anomalies

BCSC Section 10, *Glaucoma,* also discusses the conditions described in the following sections.

Primary Congenital Glaucoma

Primary congenital glaucoma, also referred to as *congenital* or *infantile glaucoma,* becomes evident at birth or within the first few years of life. The pathogenesis of primary congenital glaucoma may be related to the arrested development of the anterior chamber angle structures. Histologically, the anterior chamber angle retains an "embryonic" or "fetal" conformation, characterized by anterior insertion of the iris root, a poorly developed scleral spur with insertion of the ciliary body muscle directly into the trabecular meshwork, and mesenchymal tissue in the anterior chamber angle (Fig 7-3). See BCSC Section 6, *Pediatric Ophthalmology and Strabismus,* for detailed discussion.

Anterior Segment Dysgenesis

Anterior segment dysgenesis is the term used for a spectrum of developmental anomalies resulting from abnormalities of neural crest migration and differentiation during embryologic development (Axenfeld-Rieger syndrome, Peters anomaly, posterior keratoconus, and iridoschisis). Maldevelopment of the anterior chamber angle is most prominent in *Axenfeld-Rieger syndrome,* an autosomal dominant disorder, which itself encompasses a spectrum of anomalies, ranging from isolated bilateral ocular defects to a fully manifested systemic disorder. The single most important clinical feature of Axenfeld-Rieger syndrome phenotypes is that they confer at least a 50% risk of developing glaucoma.

Ocular manifestations of Axenfeld-Rieger syndrome include posterior embryotoxon (a thickened and anteriorly displaced Schwalbe line [termination of Descemet membrane]),

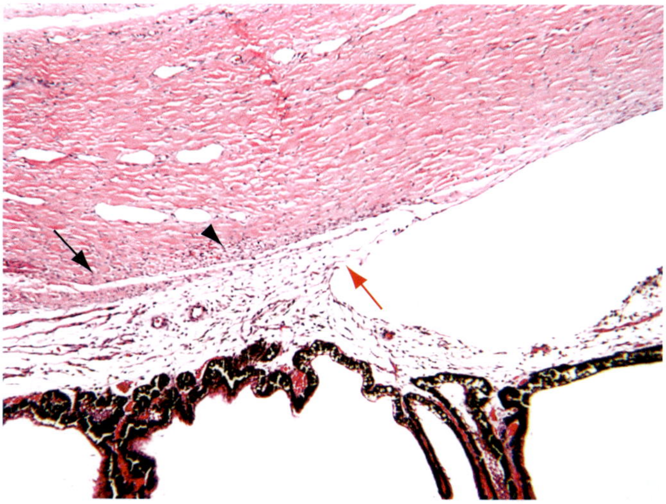

Figure 7-3 Congenital glaucoma. Fetal anterior chamber angle demonstrates anterior insertion of the iris root *(red arrow)*, anteriorly displaced ciliary processes, and a poorly developed scleral spur *(black arrow)* and trabecular meshwork *(arrowhead)*. *(Courtesy of Tatyana Milman, MD.)*

iris strands adherent to the Schwalbe line, iris hypoplasia, corectopia and polycoria, and a maldeveloped or "fetal" anterior chamber angle (discussed earlier) (Figs 7-4, 7-5). See also BCSC Section 8, *External Disease and Cornea.*

Espinoza HM, Cox CJ, Semina EV, Amendt BA. A molecular basis for differential developmental anomalies in Axenfeld-Rieger syndrome. *Hum Mol Genet.* 2002;11(7):743–753.

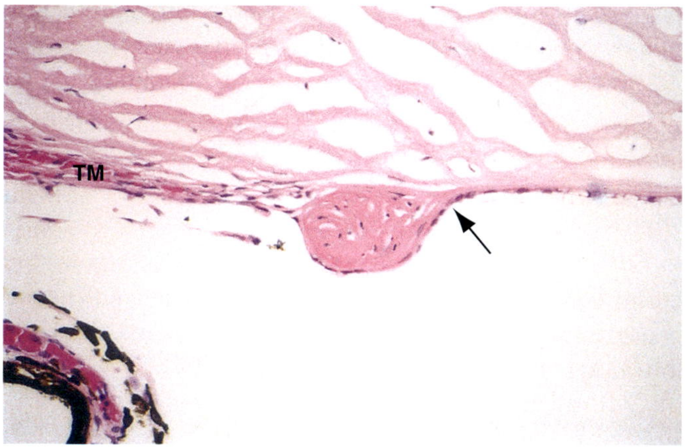

Figure 7-4 Posterior embryotoxon. Light micrograph shows a nodular prominence at the termination of the Descemet membrane *(arrow)*. *TM* = trabecular meshwork. *(Courtesy of Hans E. Grossniklaus, MD.)*

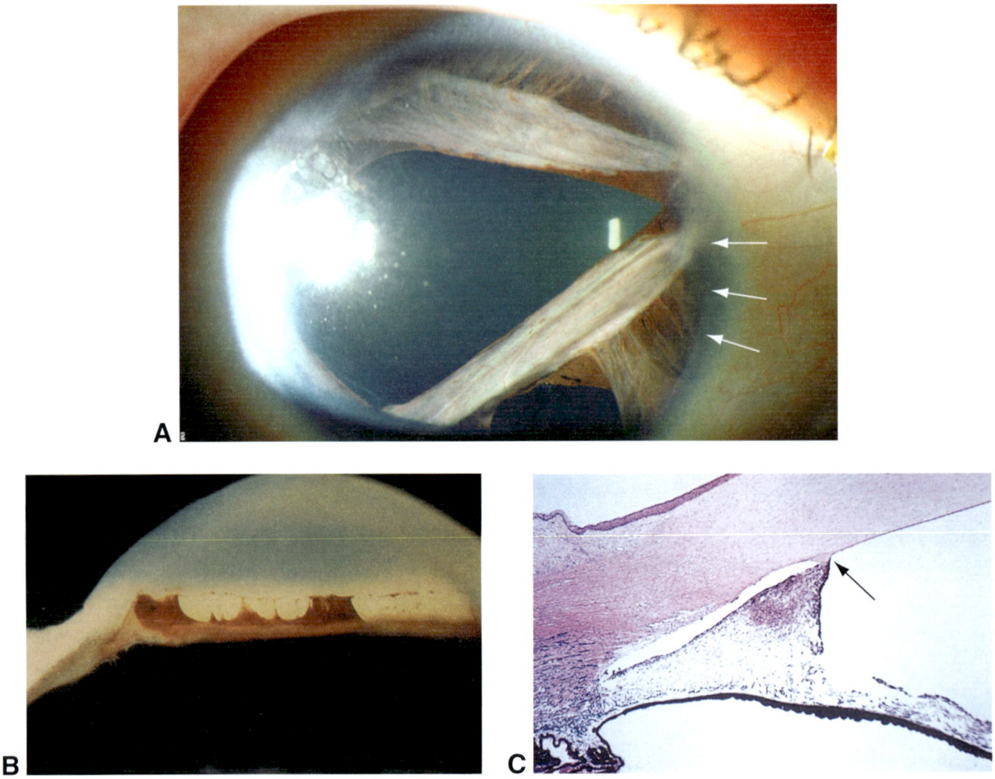

Figure 7-5 **A,** Clinical photograph of the anterior segment in a patient with Axenfeld-Rieger syndrome. Iris atrophy, polycoria, and iris strands in the periphery are present. Posterior embryotoxon can be seen laterally *(arrows).* **B,** Gross photograph shows a prominent Schwalbe line and the anterior insertion of iris strands (Axenfeld anomaly). **C,** Light micrograph shows iris strands that insert anteriorly on the Schwalbe line *(arrow).* *(Part A courtesy of Wallace L.M. Alward, MD. Copyright University of Iowa. Part B courtesy of Robert Y. Foos, MD; part C modified with permission from Yanoff M, Fine BS.* Ocular Pathology: A Color Atlas. *New York: Gower; 1988.)*

Degenerations

Iridocorneal Endothelial Syndrome

Iridocorneal endothelial (ICE) syndrome refers to a spectrum of acquired unilateral abnormalities of the corneal endothelium, anterior chamber angle, and iris typically affecting young to middle-aged adults. Three clinical variants are recognized (the first letter of each type, when combined, forms the mnemonic *ICE*):

- iris nevus (Cogan-Reese) syndrome
- Chandler syndrome
- essential iris atrophy

Epithelial-like metaplasia and abnormal proliferation of the corneal endothelium are constant features of all forms of the ICE syndrome. Abnormal endothelial cells migrate over the anterior chamber angle, leading to peripheral anterior synechiae (PAS) formation and subsequent secondary angle-closure glaucoma in approximately half of the patients with this condition (Fig 7-6). See BCSC Section 8, *External Disease and Cornea,* and Section 10, *Glaucoma,* for further discussion.

Levy SG, McCartney AC, Baghai MH, Barrett MC, Moss J. Pathology of the iridocorneal-endothelial syndrome. The ICE-cell. *Invest Ophthalmol Vis Sci.* 1995;36(13):2592–2601.

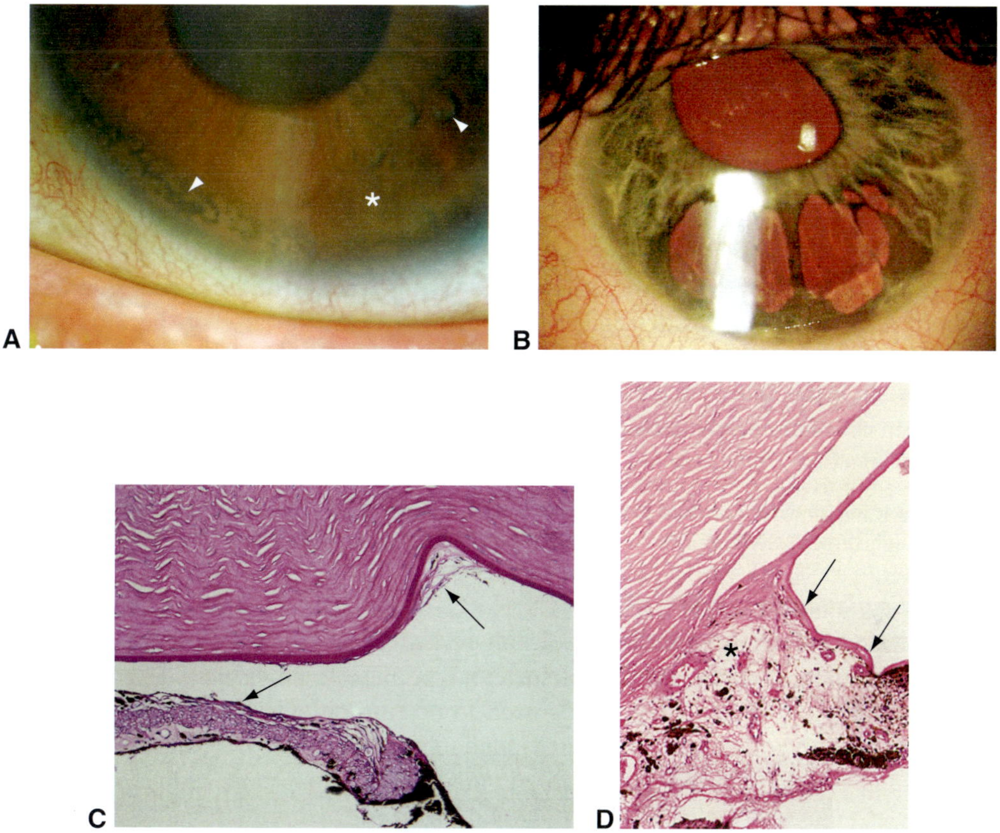

Figure 7-6 ICE syndrome. **A,** Iris nevus syndrome. The normal anterior iris architecture is effaced by a membrane growing on the anterior iris surface *(asterisk).* The membrane pinches off islands of normal iris stroma, resulting in a nodular, nevuslike appearance *(arrowheads).* **B,** Essential iris atrophy. Atrophic holes in the iris and a narrow anterior chamber, consistent with PAS formation. **C,** A membrane composed of spindle cells lines the posterior surface of the cornea and the anterior surface of the atrophic iris *(arrows).* These metaplastic endothelial cells deposit on the iris surface a thin basement membrane that has a positive periodic acid–Schiff reaction and is analogous to the Descemet membrane. **D,** Descemet membrane lines the anterior surface of the iris *(arrows).* The iris is apposed to the cornea (peripheral anterior synechiae, *asterisk*). *(Part A courtesy of Paul A. Sidoti, MD; parts B and C courtesy of Tatyana Milman, MD.)*

Secondary Glaucoma With Material in the Trabecular Meshwork

Exfoliation syndrome

Also known as *pseudoexfoliation,* exfoliation syndrome is a systemic condition that is usually identified in individuals older than 50 years and is characterized by the production and progressive accumulation of a fibrillar material in tissues throughout the anterior segment and in the connective tissue of various visceral organs (Fig 7-7). These deposits distinguish exfoliation syndrome from true exfoliation, which is the splitting of the lens capsule induced by infrared radiation.

Recent data support the pathogenic concept of exfoliation syndrome as a type of stress-induced elastosis associated with the excessive production and abnormal aggregation of elastic fiber components. Mutations in the lysyl oxidase–like 1 gene, *LOXL1,* on chromosome 15 (15q24) were found to be a major genetic risk factor for exfoliation syndrome. Lysyl oxidase is a pivotal enzyme in extracellular matrix formation, catalyzing covalent crosslinking of collagen and elastin.

Exfoliative material is most apparent on the surface of the anterior segment structures, where it exhibits a positive periodic acid–Schiff reaction and presents as delicate, feathery or brushlike fibrils arranged perpendicular to the surfaces of the intraocular structures (Fig 7-8A, B). Exfoliative material also accumulates in the trabecular meshwork and the wall of the Schlemm canal. Associated degenerative changes in the iris pigment epithelium are manifested histologically by a "saw-toothed" configuration (Fig 7-8C). See also BCSC Section 10, *Glaucoma,* and Section 11, *Lens and Cataract.*

Schlötzer-Schrehardt U. Molecular pathology of pseudoexfoliation syndrome/glaucoma—new insights from LOXL1 gene associations. *Exp Eye Res.* 2009;88(4):776–785.

Phacolytic glaucoma

The condition known as *phacolytic glaucoma* occurs when denatured lens protein leaks from a hypermature cataract through an intact but permeable lens capsule. The trabecular

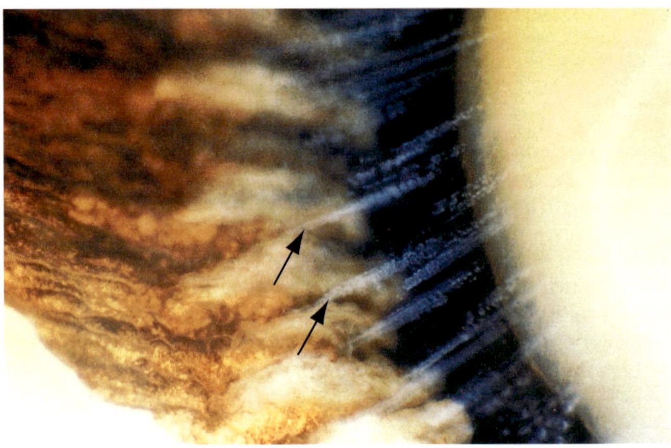

Figure 7-7 Gross photograph shows fibrillar deposits on the lens zonular fibers *(arrows)* in exfoliation syndrome (pseudoexfoliation). *(Courtesy of Hans E. Grossniklaus, MD.)*

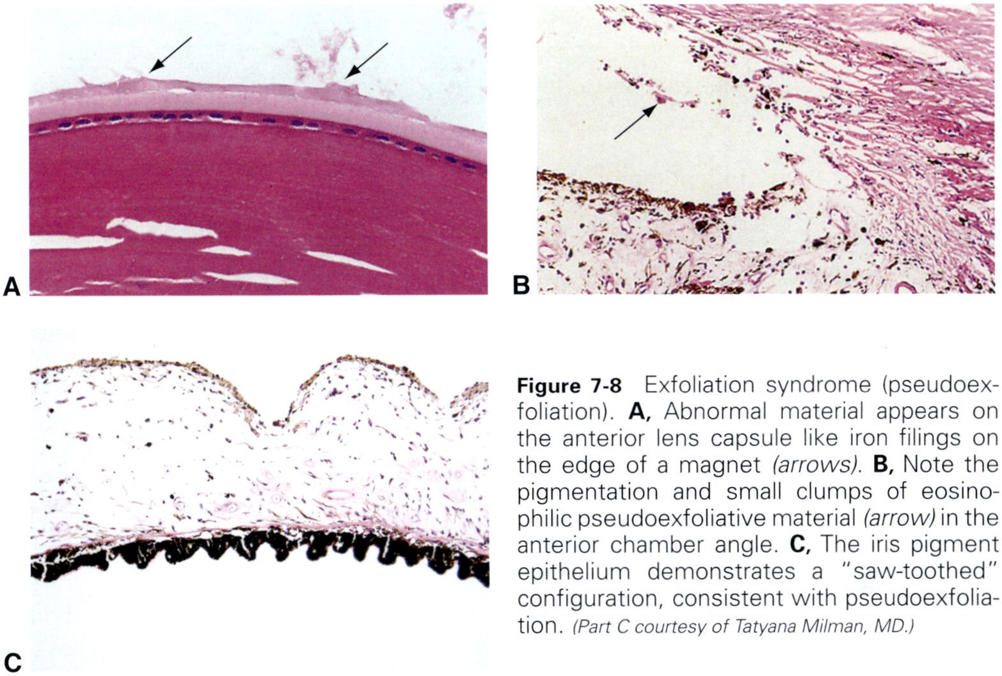

Figure 7-8 Exfoliation syndrome (pseudoexfoliation). **A,** Abnormal material appears on the anterior lens capsule like iron filings on the edge of a magnet *(arrows)*. **B,** Note the pigmentation and small clumps of eosinophilic pseudoexfoliative material *(arrow)* in the anterior chamber angle. **C,** The iris pigment epithelium demonstrates a "saw-toothed" configuration, consistent with pseudoexfoliation. *(Part C courtesy of Tatyana Milman, MD.)*

meshwork becomes occluded by both the lens protein and the macrophages engorged with phagocytosed proteinaceous, eosinophilic lens material (Fig 7-9).

Trauma

Following an intraocular hemorrhage, blood breakdown products may accumulate in the trabecular meshwork. The spherical shape and rigidity of hemolyzed erythrocytes make

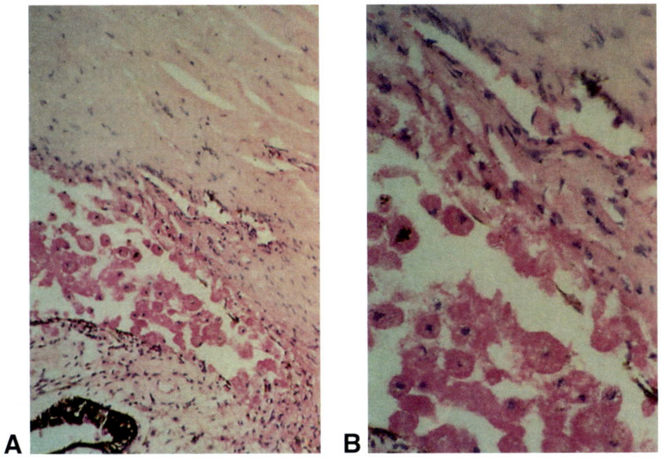

Figure 7-9 Phacolytic glaucoma. **A,** Low magnification of macrophages filled with degenerated lens cortical material in the angle. **B,** Higher magnification.

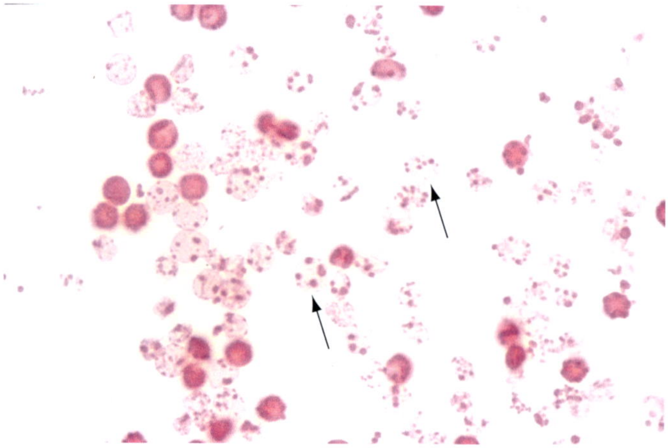

Figure 7-10 Aqueous aspirate demonstrating numerous ghost red blood cells. The degenerating hemoglobin is present as small globules known as Heinz bodies *(arrows)*. (Courtesy of Nasreen A. Syed, MD.)

it difficult for them to escape through the trabecular meshwork, leading to *ghost cell glaucoma* (Fig 7-10).

In *hemolytic glaucoma,* macrophages in the anterior chamber have been noted to phagocytose erythrocytes and their breakdown products. These hemoglobin-laden and hemosiderin-laden macrophages block the trabecular outflow channels (Fig 7-11). It is possible that macrophages are a sign of trabecular obstruction rather than the actual cause of an obstruction.

In other cases of secondary open-angle glaucoma associated with chronic intraocular hemorrhage, histologic examination has revealed hemosiderin within the trabecular endothelium and within many ocular epithelial structures (see Fig 7-11). The presence of hemosiderin may be a sign of damage that occurred during oxidation of hemoglobin. The iron stored in the cells may be an enzyme toxin that damages trabecular function

Figure 7-11 Hemolytic glaucoma. The anterior chamber angle is filled with degenerated red blood cells and macrophages containing rust-colored intracytoplasmic material, hemosiderin *(arrows)*. Hemosiderin is also observed within the trabecular meshwork endothelium *(arrowheads)*. (Courtesy of Tatyana Milman, MD.)

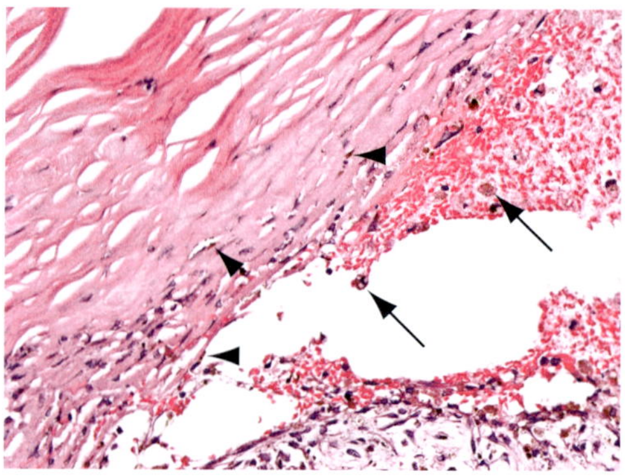

in *hemosiderosis oculi.* Iron deposition in hemosiderosis oculi can be demonstrated by means of the Prussian blue reaction.

Blunt injury to the globe may be associated with *angle recession, cyclodialysis,* and *iridodialysis.* Progressive degenerative changes in the trabecular meshwork can contribute to the pathogenesis of glaucoma after injury. See the section Histologic Sequelae of Ocular Trauma in Chapter 2.

Pigment dispersion associations

Pigment dispersion may be associated with a variety of other conditions in which pigment epithelium or uveal melanocytes are injured, such as uveitis or uveal melanoma. These conditions are characterized by pigment within the trabecular meshwork and in macrophages littering the angle (Fig 7-12).

Secondary open-angle glaucoma can occur as a result of the *pigment dispersion syndrome* (Fig 7-13). This type of glaucoma is characterized by radially oriented defects in the midperipheral iris and pigment in the trabecular meshwork, the corneal endothelium (*Krukenberg spindle;* see Chapter 6, Fig 6-18), and other anterior segment structures, such as the lens capsule. The dispersed pigment is presumed to be from iris pigment epithelium mechanically rubbed off by contact with lens zonular fibers. See also BCSC Section 10, *Glaucoma.*

Neoplasia

Melanocytic nevi and melanomas that arise in the iris or extend to the iris from the ciliary body may obstruct the trabecular meshwork (Fig 7-14). See also Chapter 17. In addition, pigment elaborated from melanomas and melanocytomas may be shed into the trabecular meshwork and produce secondary glaucoma *(melanomalytic glaucoma)* (see Fig 7-12). Occasionally, epibulbar tumors such as conjunctival carcinoma can invade the eye through the limbus, leading to trabecular outflow obstruction and glaucoma. See the section Neoplasia in Chapter 5.

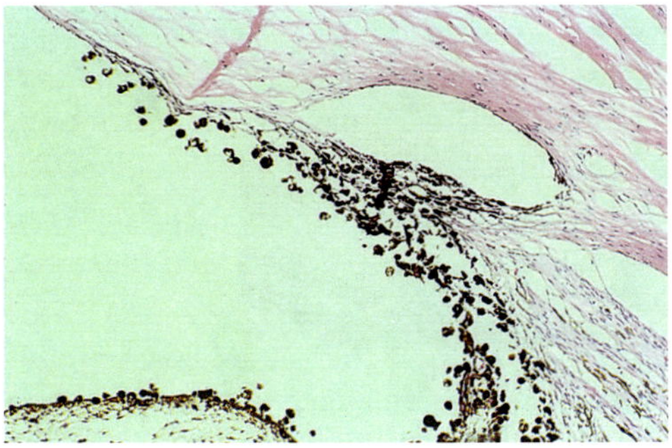

Figure 7-12 Secondary open-angle glaucoma. The trabecular meshwork is obstructed by macrophages that have ingested pigment from a necrotic intraocular melanoma *(melanomalytic glaucoma).*

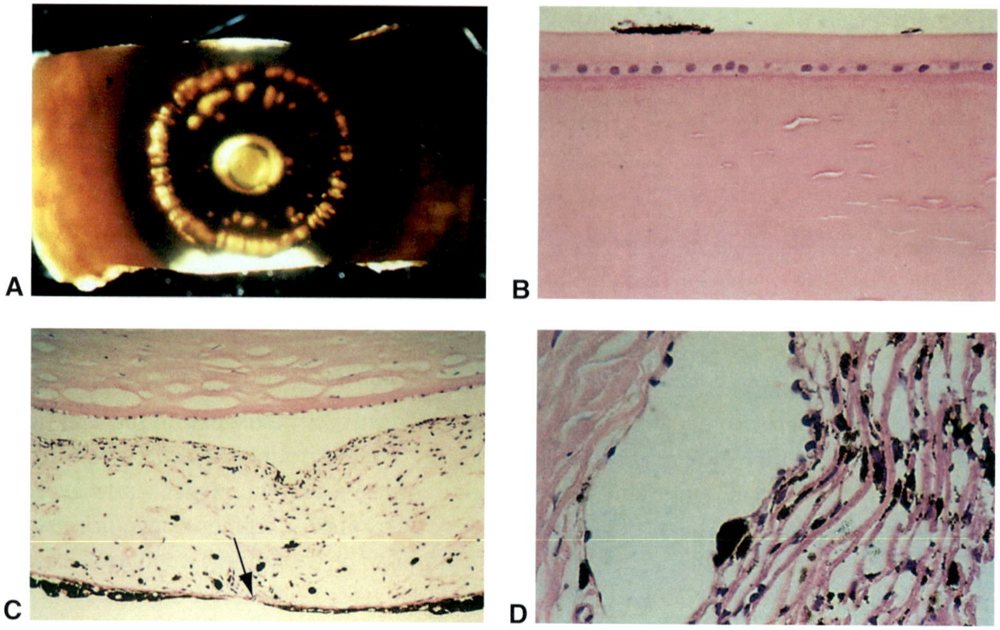

Figure 7-13 Pigment dispersion syndrome. **A,** Gross photograph demonstrating radially oriented transillumination defects in the iris. **B,** Scheie stripe. Melanin is present on the anterior surface of the lens. **C,** Note the focal loss of iris pigment epithelium *(arrow)*. Chafing of the zonules against the epithelium may release the pigment that is dispersed in this condition. **D,** Note the accumulation of pigment in the trabecular meshwork.

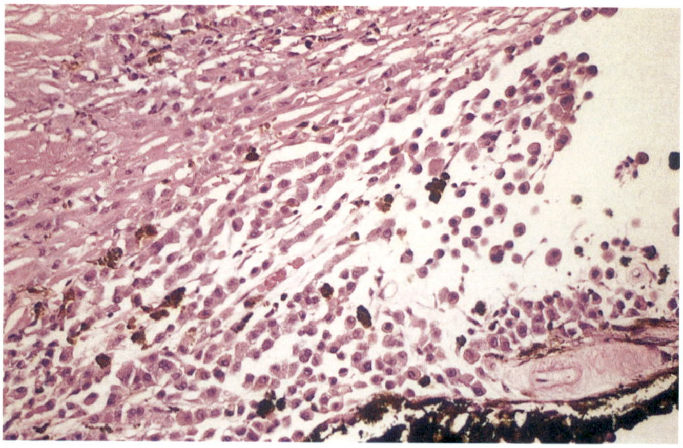

Figure 7-14 Photomicrograph shows melanoma cells filling the anterior chamber angle and obstructing the trabecular meshwork. Note the iris pigment epithelium in the lower right corner of the photomicrograph. *(Courtesy of Hans E. Grossniklaus, MD.)*

CHAPTER 8

Sclera

Topography

The sclera is the white, nearly opaque portion of the outer wall of the eye, covering from four-fifths to five-sixths of the eye's surface area. It is continuous anteriorly at the limbus with the corneal stroma. Posteriorly, the outer two-thirds of the sclera merges with the dura of the optic nerve sheath; the inner one-third continues as the lamina cribrosa, through which pass axonal fibers of the optic nerve (see Chapter 15, Fig 15-1). The diameter of the scleral shell averages 22 mm, and its thickness varies from 1 mm posteriorly to 0.3 mm just posterior to the insertions of the 4 rectus muscles. Histologically, the sclera is divided into 3 layers (from outermost inward): episclera, stroma, and lamina fusca (Fig 8-1). The sclera is derived predominantly from the neural crest.

Episclera

The episclera is a thin, loose fibrovascular tissue that covers the outer surface of the scleral stroma.

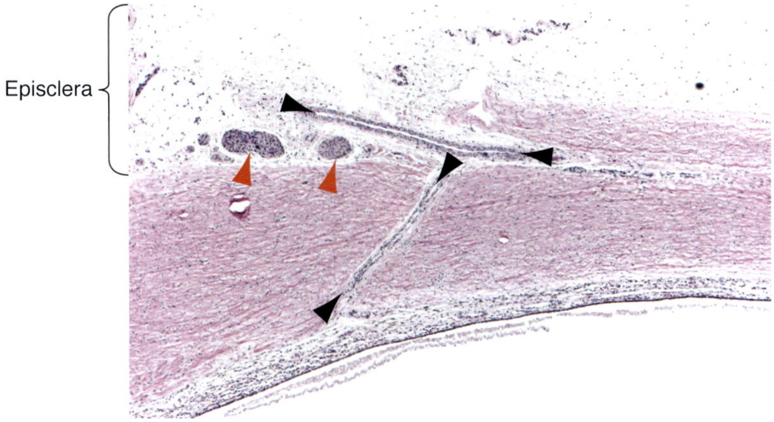

Figure 8-1 Normal sclera demonstrating emissary structures, including ciliary arteries *(black arrowheads)* and nerves *(red arrowheads)* entering and traversing the sclera. *(Courtesy of Nasreen A. Syed, MD.)*

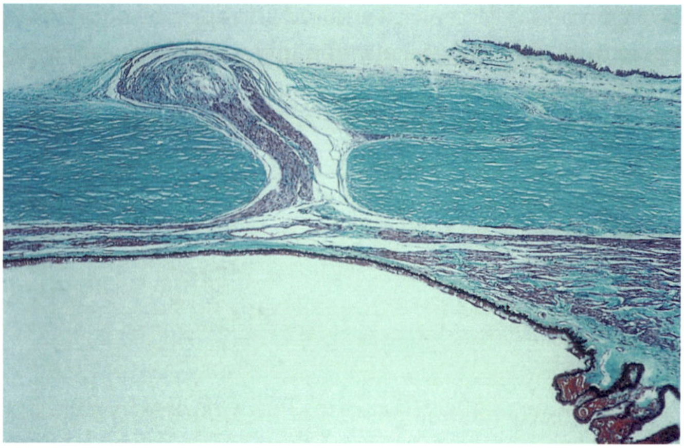

Figure 8-2 An emissary channel through the sclera for the Axenfeld nerve loop is present overlying the pars plana (trichrome stain). *(Courtesy of Harry H. Brown, MD.)*

Stroma

The bulk of the sclera is made up of sparsely vascularized, dense type I collagen fibers whose diameters range from 28 nm to more than 300 nm. In comparison to corneal stroma, scleral collagen fibers are thicker and more variable in thickness and orientation. Transmural emissary channels provide outlets within the stroma as follows (Fig 8-2; see also Fig 8-1):

- in the posterior region, for posterior ciliary arteries and nerves
- in the equatorial region, for vortex veins
- in the anterior regions, for anterior ciliary arteries and veins and long posterior ciliary nerves (Axenfeld nerve loops)

Lamina Fusca

The lamina fusca is a delicate, pigmented fibrovascular tissue that loosely binds the uvea to the sclera. Sclerouveal attachments are strongest along the major emissary channels, the anterior base of the ciliary body, and the juxtapapillary region.

Congenital Anomalies

Choristoma

Epibulbar dermoids and episcleral osseous choristoma are discussed in Chapters 5 and 6.

Nanophthalmos

Nanophthalmos is a rare developmental disorder characterized by an eye with short axial length (15–20 mm), a normal or slightly enlarged lens, thickened sclera, and a predisposition to uveal effusion and glaucoma. The condition is usually bilateral.

In studies, the thick and nonelastic sclera in nanophthalmos was found to demonstrate fraying and splitting of the collagen fibrils and abnormalities in the glycosaminoglycan matrix. These scleral changes may predispose the nanophthalmic eye to uveal effusion due to reduced protein permeability and impaired venous outflow through the vortex veins.

Glaucoma in nanophthalmic eyes may be caused by a variety of mechanisms, including angle closure, pupillary block, and open angle with elevated episcleral venous pressure.

Stewart DH III, Streeten BW, Brockhurst RJ, Anderson DR, Hirose T, Gass DM. Abnormal scleral collagen in nanophthalmos. An ultrastructural study. *Arch Ophthalmol.* 1991;109(7): 1017–1025.

Inflammations

See BCSC Section 8, *External Disease and Cornea,* for additional discussion of episcleritis and scleritis.

Episcleritis

Simple episcleritis is a self-limited, frequently recurrent condition that most commonly presents in the third to fifth decades as a slightly tender, movable, sectorial red area involving the anterior episclera. It affects males and females equally. There is usually no association with antecedent injury or systemic illness. Histologic examination shows vascular congestion; stromal edema; and a chronic nongranulomatous perivascular inflammatory infiltrate, composed primarily of lymphocytes (Fig 8-3).

In contrast to simple episcleritis, *nodular episcleritis* more often affects females and those with systemic illness, such as rheumatoid arthritis. It is characterized by tender, elevated, pink-red nodules on the anterior episclera. Histologically, the nodules are composed of *necrobiotic granulomatous inflammatory infiltrate,* a palisading arrangement of epithelioid histiocytes around a central core of necrotic collagen. This light microscopic pattern is the same as that seen in rheumatoid nodules in subcutaneous tissue.

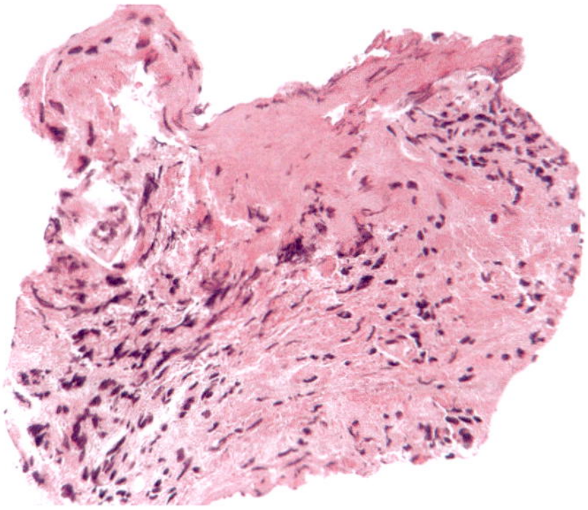

Figure 8-3 Simple episcleritis. Episcleral biopsy specimen from a patient with simple episcleritis demonstrates chronic nongranulomatous inflammatory infiltrate. *(Courtesy of George J. Harocopos, MD.)*

Scleritis

Scleritis is a painful, often progressive ocular disease with potentially serious sequelae. There is a high association with systemic autoimmune vasculitic connective tissue diseases.

Histologic examination of scleritis reveals 2 main categories: necrotizing and nonnecrotizing inflammation. Either type may occur anteriorly or posteriorly. *Necrotizing scleritis* may be nodular or diffuse, so-called brawny scleritis (Figs 8-4, 8-5). Both patterns demonstrate a palisading arrangement of epithelioid histiocytes and multinucleated giant cells surrounding sequestered areas of necrotic collagen (necrobiotic granuloma) (Fig 8-6). Peripheral to the histiocytes is a rim of lymphocytes and plasma cells. Multiple foci may show different stages of evolution. In the course of healing, the necrotic stroma is resorbed, leaving in its wake a thinned scleral remnant prone to staphyloma formation (Fig 8-7). Severe ectasia of the scleral shell predisposes to herniation of uveal tissue through the defect, a condition known as *scleromalacia perforans.*

Nonnecrotizing scleritis is characterized by a perivascular lymphocytic and plasmacytic infiltrate without a granulomatous inflammatory component. Vasculitis may be present in the form of fibrinoid necrosis of vessel walls.

Dubord PJ, Chambers A. Scleritis and episcleritis: diagnosis and management. *Focal Points: Clinical Modules for Ophthalmologists.* San Francisco: American Academy of Ophthalmology; 1995, module 9.

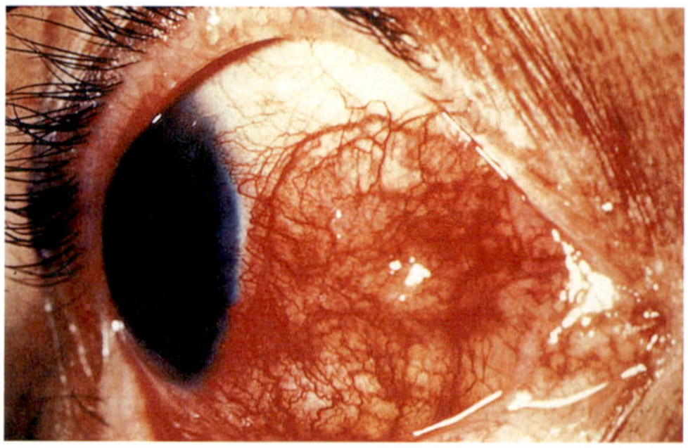

Figure 8-4 This patient has a sectoral nodular anterior scleritis that causes severe ocular pain and photophobia. *(Courtesy of Harry H. Brown, MD.)*

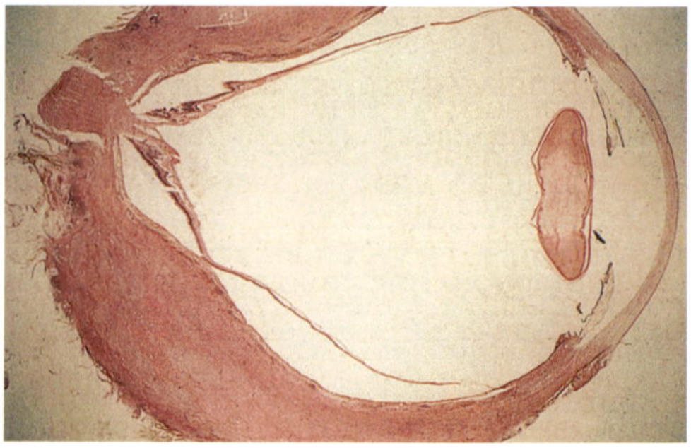

Figure 8-5 Diffuse posterior scleritis (brawny scleritis) demonstrates marked thickening of the posterior sclera. *(Courtesy of Harry H. Brown, MD.)*

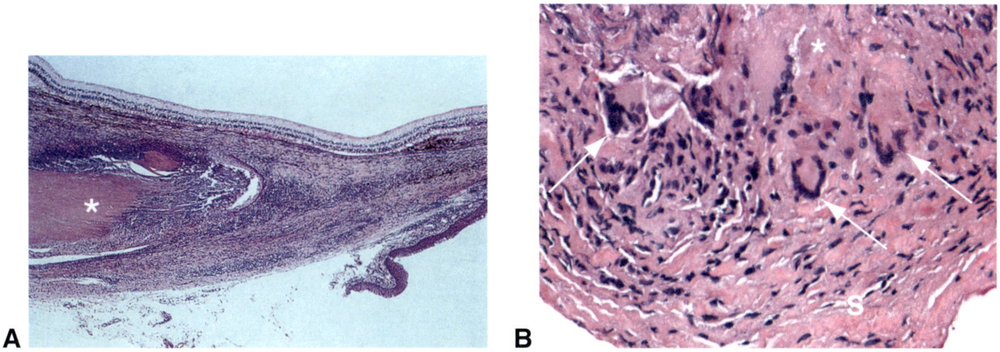

Figure 8-6 Necrotizing granulomatous scleritis. **A,** An area of necrosis *(asterisk)* is sequestered by a zonal inflammatory reaction of histiocytes, lymphocytes, and plasma cells. **B,** High-magnification photomicrograph of scleral *(S)* biopsy illustrates palisading arrangement of histiocytes and multinucleated giant cells *(arrows)* around necrobiotic scleral collagen *(asterisk)*. *(Part A courtesy of Harry H. Brown, MD; part B courtesy of Robert H. Rosa, Jr, MD.)*

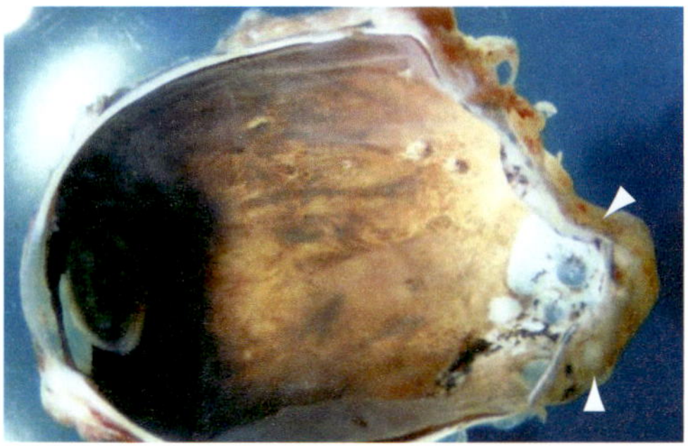

Figure 8-7 A posterior staphyloma *(between arrowheads)* is present in this eye as a sequela of scleritis. *(Courtesy of Hans E. Grossniklaus, MD.)*

Degenerations

Senile Calcific Plaque

Senile calcific plaques occur commonly in elderly individuals as flat, firm, sharply circumscribed, gray rectangular to ovoid patches, measuring 1 cm in greatest dimension. The plaques appear bilaterally and are typically located anterior to the medial and lateral rectus muscle insertions (Fig 8-8A). The etiology is unknown; dehydration, actinic damage, and stress on scleral collagen exerted by rectus muscle insertions have been proposed but not proven.

On histologic sections, the calcium is present within the midportion of the scleral stroma. It initially occurs as a finely granular deposition but may progress to a confluent plaque involving both superficial and deep sclera (Fig 8-8B). Senile plaques may be highlighted by special stains for calcium, such as von Kossa and alizarin red.

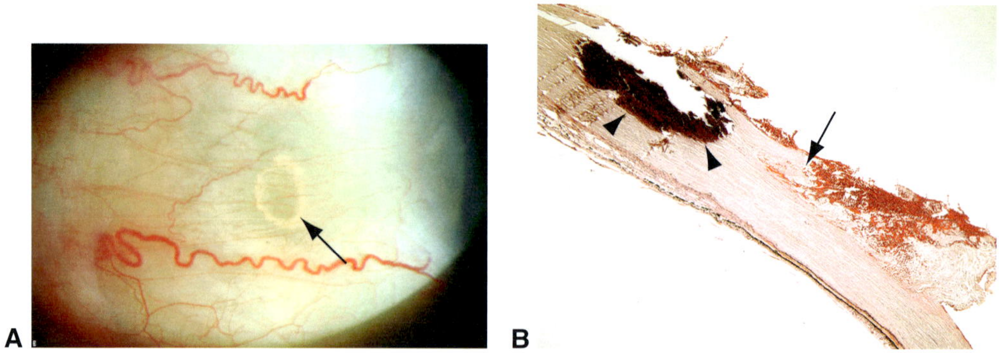

Figure 8-8 A calcific plaque of the sclera. **A,** Calcific plaques *(arrow)* are typically located just anterior to the insertion of the medial and lateral rectus muscles. **B,** Basophilic calcific deposits are noted in the sclera *(arrowheads)* anterior to the rectus muscle insertion *(arrow)*. *(Part A courtesy of Vinay A. Shah, MBBS; part B courtesy of Tatyana Milman, MD.)*

Scleral Staphyloma

Scleral staphylomas are scleral ectasias that are lined internally by uveal tissue and that may occur at points of weakness in the scleral shell, either in inherently thin areas (such as posterior to the rectus muscle insertions; Fig 8-9) or in areas weakened by tissue destruction (as in scleritis; see Fig 8-7). In children, staphylomas may occur as a result of long-standing increased intraocular pressure or axial myopia, owing to the relative distensibility of the sclera in the young. Location and age at onset, therefore, vary according to the underlying etiology. Histologic examination invariably reveals thinned sclera, with or without fibrosis and scarring, again depending on the cause.

Neoplasia

Neoplasms of the sclera are exceedingly rare. Tumors originate predominantly in the episclera or Tenon capsule rather than in the sclera proper.

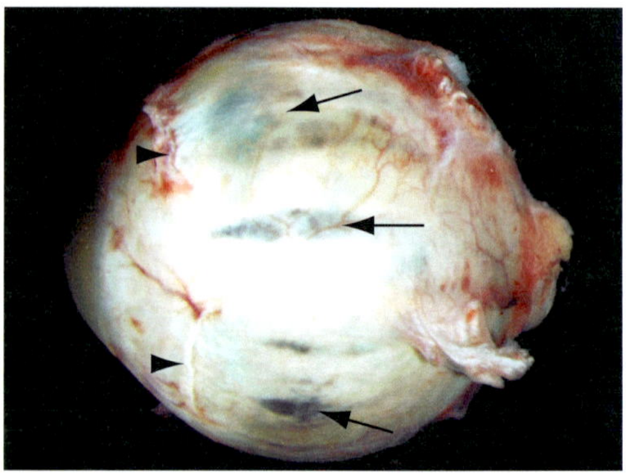

Figure 8-9 Scleral staphylomas. Several regions of scleral thinning *(arrows)*, which appear blue because of the underlying uveal tissue, are present posterior to the rectus muscle insertions *(arrowheads)* and in the equatorial sclera. *(Courtesy of Nasreen A. Syed, MD.)*

Fibrous Histiocytoma

Fibrous histiocytoma, also known as *fibroxanthoma* or *fibrohistiocytic tumor*, is a benign soft-tissue tumor with fibrous differentiation, formed by a proliferation of fibrocytes and histiocytes, characteristically in a whorled (storiform) pattern (see Chapter 14, Fig 14-11). Though more common in the orbit, it may occasionally involve the sclera, particularly the corneoscleral limbus (Fig 8-10). *Malignant fibrous histiocytoma (atypical fibroxanthoma)* of the corneoscleral limbus demonstrates increased mitotic activity, nuclear pleomorphism,

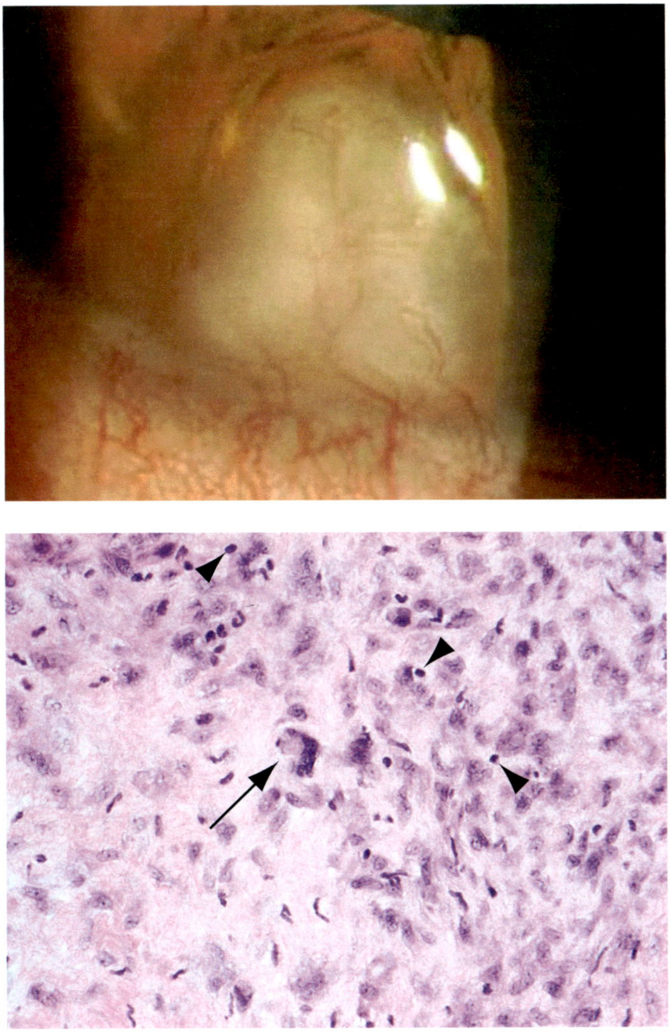

Figure 8-10 Fibrous histiocytoma of the corneoscleral limbus. **A,** A gelatinous, gray, vascularized, dome-shaped nodule extends into the corneal stroma. **B,** Microscopic evaluation reveals a proliferation of spindle fibroblasts, rounded histiocytes, and occasional multinucleated giant cells *(arrow)*; scattered lymphocytes are also seen *(arrowheads)*. *(Part A courtesy of Ira J. Udell; part B courtesy of Tatyana Milman, MD.)*

necrosis, and an invasive growth pattern. Although malignant fibrous histiocytoma of the corneoscleral limbus can be locally aggressive, the tumor generally does not metastasize.

Nodular Fasciitis

Nodular fasciitis is a reactive process that may, in rare instances, cause a tumefaction in the episclera. The disease usually affects young adults as a rapidly growing, round to oval, firm white-gray nodule that measures 0.5–1.5 cm and appears at the limbus or anterior to a rectus muscle insertion. Antecedent trauma has been implicated as an etiologic factor for the development of nodular fasciitis in other body sites, but such an association is infrequent in the sclera. Though self-limited, nodular fasciitis is usually excised because of its rapid growth.

Histologic examination reveals a circumscribed spindle cell proliferation in which the appearance of individual cells resembles that of fibroblasts growing in tissue culture. These spindle cells aggregate in short fascicles, admixed with a chronic inflammatory infiltrate, in a vascular, myxoid stroma (Fig 8-11). Older lesions may show foci of dense collagen deposition. Although mitotic figures may be present, unbalanced (eg, tripolar) mitoses are absent. Because of the cellular nature of these proliferations and the presence of mitotic figures, nodular fasciitis may be misinterpreted histologically as sarcoma (soft-tissue malignancy), a pitfall to avoid.

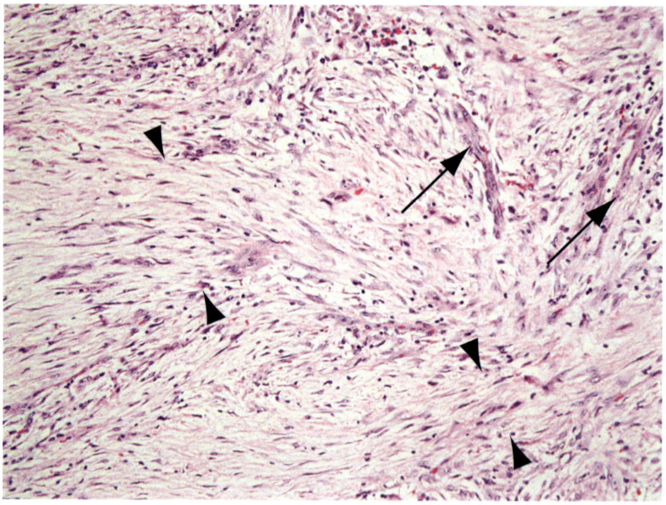

Figure 8-11 Nodular fasciitis. Activated spindled fibroblasts are loosely arranged in short fascicles *(between arrowheads)*. A prominent capillary network *(arrows)* and chronic inflammatory infiltrate are also observed. *(Courtesy of Tatyana Milman, MD.)*

CHAPTER 9

Lens

Topography

The crystalline lens is a soft, elastic, avascular, biconvex structure that in the adult measures approximately 9–10 mm in diameter and 5 mm anteroposteriorly (Fig 9-1). The lens is derived from surface ectoderm. See BCSC Section 11, *Lens and Cataract,* for discussion of the structure, embryology, and pathology of the lens.

Capsule

The lens capsule surrounds the entire lens (Fig 9-2). It is a thick basement membrane elaborated by the lens epithelial cells and composed, in part, of type IV collagen fibers. The lens capsule is thickest anteriorly (12–21 μm) and peripherally near the equator and thinnest posteriorly (2–9 μm). The capsule provides insertions for the zonular fibers and plays an important part in molding the lens shape in accommodation.

Epithelium

The lens epithelium is derived from the cells of the original lens vesicle that did not differentiate into primary lens fibers. The anterior or axial lens epithelium forms a single layer

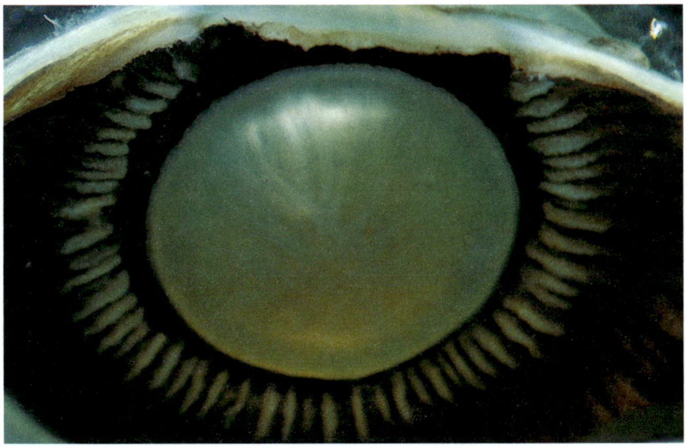

Figure 9-1 Posterior aspect of the crystalline lens, depicting its relationship to the peripheral iris and ciliary body. *(Courtesy of Hans E. Grossniklaus, MD.)*

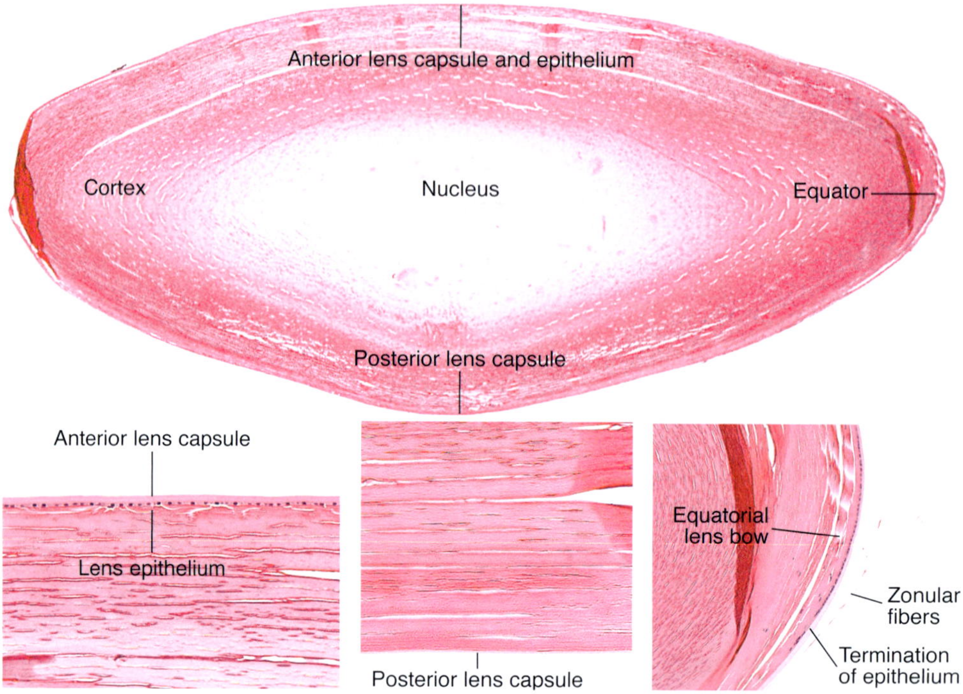

Figure 9-2 Microscopic appearance of the adult lens. *(Courtesy of Tatyana Milman, MD.)*

of cuboidal cells with their basilar surface toward the anterior lens capsule, whereas the equatorial, mitotically active cells appear more elongated as they differentiate into lens fibers. Epithelial cells are not normally observed posterior to the lens equator (see Fig 9-2).

Cortex and Nucleus

The center of the lens contains the oldest lens fibers, the *embryonic and fetal lens nucleus,* while the outer cortical fibers are derived from postnatally differentiated lens epithelial cells. New lens fibers are continuously laid down from the outside as the lens epithelial cells differentiate. Differentiation of lens epithelial cells into cortical lens fibers occurs at the equator. In this region, termed the *equatorial lens bow,* the lens epithelial cells move centrally, elongate, acquire crystallins, lose organelles, and transform into cortical lens fibers. As is the case clinically, the histologic demarcation between the nucleus and cortex is not well defined (see Fig 9-2).

Zonular Fibers

The lens is supported by the zonular fibers that attach to the anterior and posterior lens capsule in the midperiphery (see Fig 9-2 and Chapter 7, Fig 7-7). These fibers hold the lens in place through their attachments to the ciliary body processes.

Congenital Anomalies

See BCSC Section 6, *Pediatric Ophthalmology and Strabismus,* and Section 11, *Lens and Cataract,* for discussion of ectopia lentis and congenital cataract, as well as additional discussion of the following topics.

Congenital Aphakia

Congenital aphakia is a rare anomaly that can be subdivided into 2 forms: primary and secondary. Histologically, the lens is absent in primary congenital aphakia. The histologic findings of secondary congenital aphakia depend on the underlying etiology. Primary congenital aphakia results from failed induction of the surface ectoderm during embryogenesis and has been associated with mutations in the *PAX6* gene and severe ocular and systemic developmental anomalies. In secondary congenital aphakia, the lens has developed but has been resorbed or extruded before or during birth. This form of aphakia is often associated with congenital infections, such as congenital rubella.

Lens Coloboma

A lens coloboma is characterized by a notch in the lens, typically in an inferonasal location. This congenital anomaly is characteristically associated with ciliary body coloboma and likely occurs secondary to the focal absence or abnormal development of zonular fibers.

Anterior Lenticonus (Lentiglobus)

The anterior surface of the lens can assume an abnormal shape, either conical *(lenticonus)* or spherical *(lentiglobus).* Clinically, an "oil droplet" red reflex is present. Anterior lenticonus may be unilateral or bilateral. Bilateral anterior lenticonus is usually associated with *Alport syndrome,* which is typically an autosomal dominant disease and is characterized by hemorrhagic nephritis, deafness, anterior polar cataract, retinal flecks, and retinal and iris neovascularization, in addition to anterior lenticonus. Mutations in type IV collagen genes have been described in some forms of Alport syndrome.

Histology reveals thinning of and dehiscences in the anterior lens capsule, a decrease in the number of anterior lens epithelial cells, and bulging of the anterior cortex. Ultrastructural alterations of lens capsule collagen and immunohistochemical abnormalities in type IV collagen have been observed.

Posterior Lenticonus (Lentiglobus)

Posterior lenticonus is characterized by a spherical deformity of the posterior surface of the lens (Fig 9-3). Clinically, an "oil droplet" red reflex is seen. Posterior lenticonus usually occurs as a sporadic, unilateral anomaly and is associated with congenital cataract. Other, rare ocular associations include microphthalmos, microcornea, persistent anterior hyaloid vasculature, and uveal colobomas. Posterior lenticonus may also occur as a part of Alport syndrome and the oculocerebrorenal syndrome of Lowe. The *oculocerebrorenal syndrome of Lowe* is an X-linked condition characterized by systemic acidosis, renal rickets, hypotonia, and congenital cataracts, which histologically display focal, internally directed excrescences of the lens capsule.

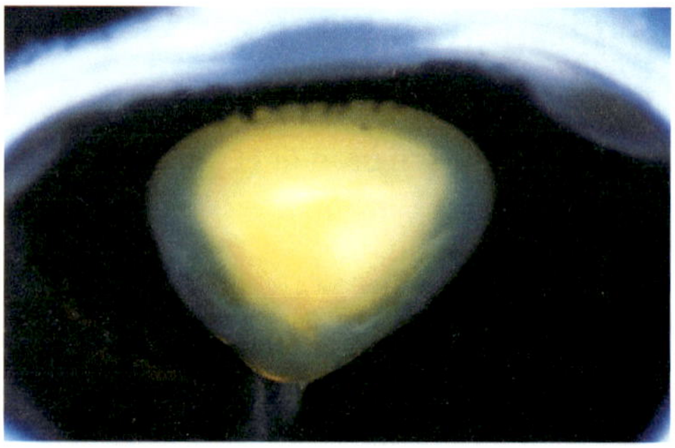

Figure 9-3 Posterior lenticonus. *(Courtesy of Hans E. Grossniklaus, MD.)*

Inflammations

Phacoantigenic Uveitis

Also known as *phacoanaphylactic endophthalmitis* or *lens-induced granulomatous endophthalmitis,* this type of lens-induced intraocular inflammation is mediated by IgG immunoglobulins directed against lens protein. The inflammation may follow accidental or surgical trauma to the lens.

Histologically, lens-induced granulomatous endophthalmitis consists of a central nidus of degenerating lens material surrounded by concentric layers of inflammatory cells (zonal granuloma). Multinucleated giant cells and neutrophils are present within the inner layer adjacent to degenerating lens material. Lymphocytes and plasma cells make up the intermediate mantle of cells. These cells may be surrounded by fibrovascular connective tissue, depending on the duration of the inflammatory response (Figs 9-4, 9-5). See also BCSC Section 9, *Intraocular Inflammation and Uveitis.*

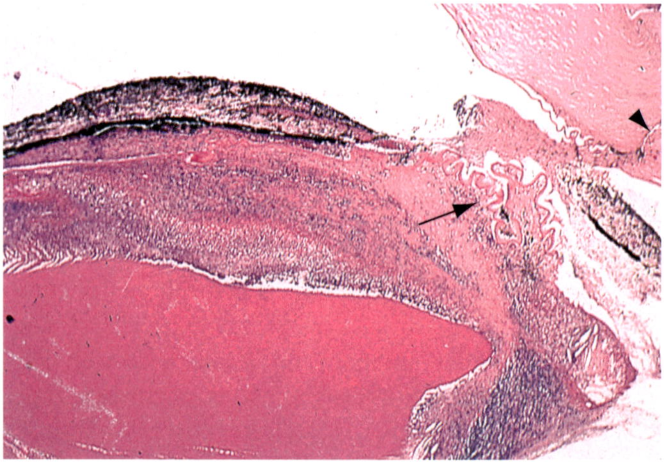

Figure 9-4 Phacoantigenic endophthalmitis, in which inflammatory reaction surrounds the lens *(lower left).* The torn capsule can be observed in the pupillary region *(arrow).* Also note corneal scar *(arrowhead),* representing the site of ocular penetration.

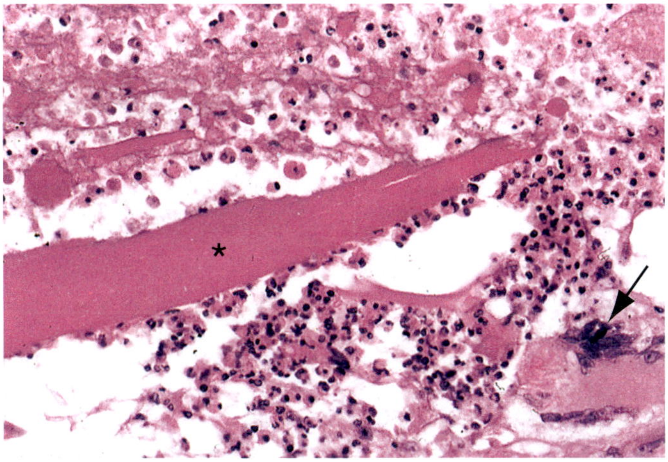

Figure 9-5 Phacoantigenic endophthalmitis. Acute and granulomatous inflammation, including giant cells *(arrow),* surrounds inciting lens fibers *(asterisk).*

Phacolytic Glaucoma

See Chapter 7 for a discussion of this topic.

Propionibacterium acnes Endophthalmitis

Chronic postoperative endophthalmitis secondary to *P acnes* may develop following cataract surgery, usually 2 months to 2 years later. Onset of the inflammation may follow Nd:YAG laser capsulotomy that allows release of the sequestered organisms. *Propionibacterium acnes* endophthalmitis can present with granulomatous keratic precipitates, a small hypopyon, vitritis, and a white plaque containing bacteria and residual lens material sequestered within the capsular bag (Figs 9-6, 9-7).

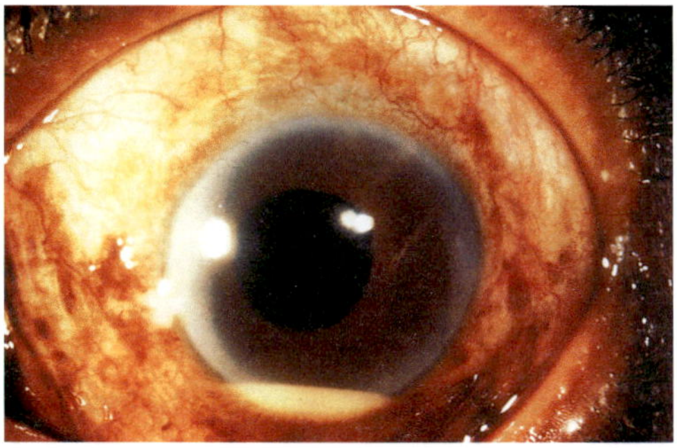

Figure 9-6 Clinical photograph of eye with *P acnes* endophthalmitis. Note injection of the conjunctiva and small hypopyon. *(Courtesy of William C. Lloyd III, MD, and Ralph C. Eagle, Jr, MD.)*

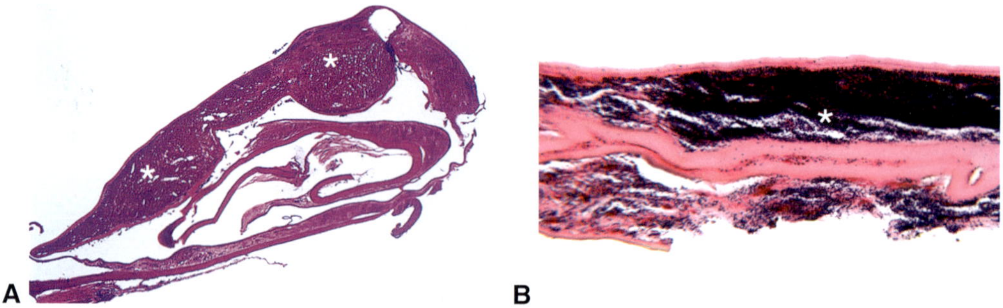

Figure 9-7 Histology of a lens capsule from a case of *P acnes* endophthalmitis. **A,** Colonies of bacteria are sequestered within the PAS-positive capsular bag *(asterisks)*. **B,** Gram-positive coccobacilli *(P acnes)* within the capsular bag *(asterisk)*. *(Part A courtesy of William C. Lloyd III, MD, and Ralph C. Eagle, Jr, MD; part B courtesy of Tatyana Milman, MD.)*

Degenerations

Cataract and Other Abnormalities

Capsule

Mild thickening of the lens capsule can be associated with pathologic proliferation of lens epithelium or with chronic inflammation of the anterior segment. Elements with an affinity for basement membranes, such as copper (chalcosis) and silver (argyrosis), can form pigmented deposits in the anterior lens capsule.

Epithelium

A severe elevation of intraocular pressure causes injury to the lens epithelial cells, leading to degeneration of the cells. Clinically, patches of white flecks *(glaukomflecken)* are seen beneath the lens capsule. Histology shows focal areas of necrotic lens epithelial cells beneath the anterior lens capsule. Associated degenerated subepithelial cortical material is also present. See also BCSC Section 10, *Glaucoma.*

Injury to the lens epithelium can also be caused by inflammation, ischemia, or trauma and can stimulate epithelial hyperplasia and formation of *anterior subcapsular fibrous plaques* (Fig 9-8A). In this situation, the epithelial cells have undergone metaplastic transformation into fibroblast-like cells, which are capable of producing collagen. These functionally transformed epithelial cells arise in response to a variety of stimuli, including inflammation, ischemia, and trauma. Following resolution of the inciting stimulus, the lens epithelium may produce another capsule, thereby completely surrounding the fibrous plaque and producing a *duplication cataract* (Fig 9-8B).

Retention of iron-containing metallic foreign bodies in the lens may lead to lens epithelial degeneration and necrosis, secondary to *siderosis.* The presence of iron within the epithelial cells can be demonstrated by Perls Prussian blue stain.

Posterior subcapsular cataract may be the most common abnormality involving the lens epithelium. There are a number of risk factors for this condition, including chronic

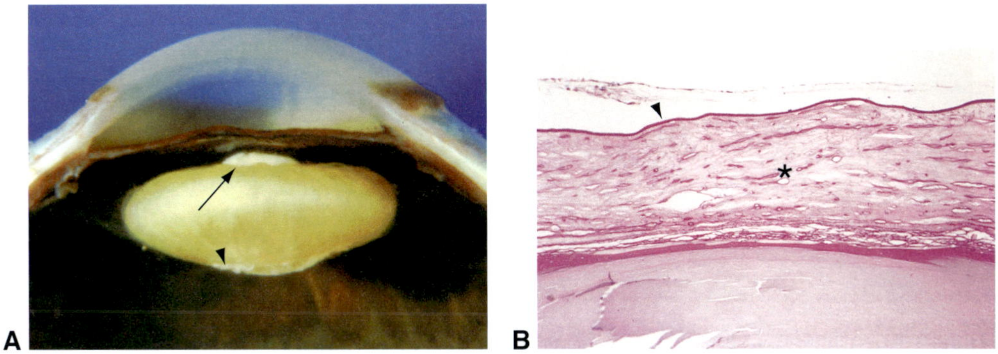

Figure 9-8 Anterior and posterior subcapsular cataracts. **A,** Gross photograph shows white anterior *(arrow)* and posterior *(arrowhead)* subcapsular plaques located centrally. **B,** Fibrous plaque *(asterisk)* is present posterior to the original lens capsule *(arrowhead)*. *(Part A courtesy of Tatyana Milman, MD; part B courtesy of Hans E. Grossniklaus, MD.)*

intraocular inflammation, diabetes mellitus, ionizing radiation exposure, smoking, and prolonged corticosteroid use (Fig 9-9A; see Fig 9-8A). Posterior subcapsular cataract is frequently associated with cortical degeneration and nuclear sclerosis. Histologically, development of this type of cataract begins with epithelial disarray at the equator, followed by posterior migration of the lens epithelium. As the cells migrate posteriorly, they enlarge and swell to 5–6 times their normal size. These swollen cells, referred to as *bladder cells of Wedl,* can cause significant visual impairment if they involve the axial portion of the lens (Fig 9-9B).

Disruption of the lens capsule often results in proliferation of lens epithelial cells. Following extracapsular cataract extraction, for example, remaining epithelial cells can proliferate and cover the inner surface of the posterior lens capsule, producing clinically appreciable posterior capsule opacification. These collections of proliferating epithelial cells may form partially transparent globular masses, called *Elschnig pearls,* which are

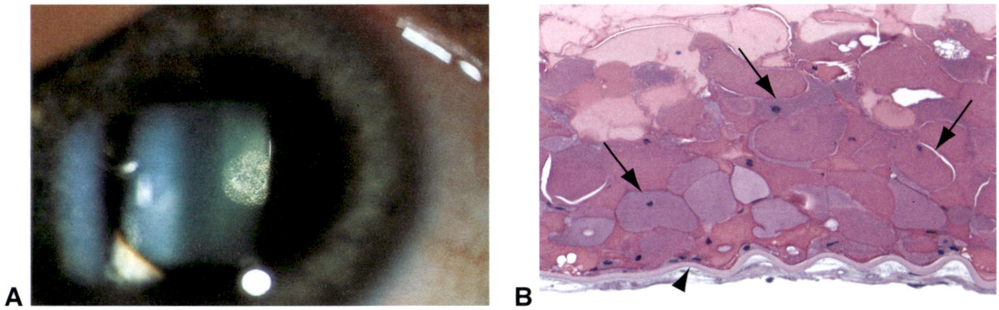

Figure 9-9 Posterior subcapsular cataract. **A,** Viewed at the slit lamp. **B,** Wedl cells. Note the large, round, nucleated bladder or Wedl cells *(arrows)* and the smaller lens epithelial cells lining the posterior lens capsule *(arrowhead)*. *(Part A courtesy of CIBA Pharmaceutical Co., division of CIBA-GEIGY Corp. Reproduced with permission from* Clinical Symposia. *Part B courtesy of Robert H. Rosa, Jr, MD.)*

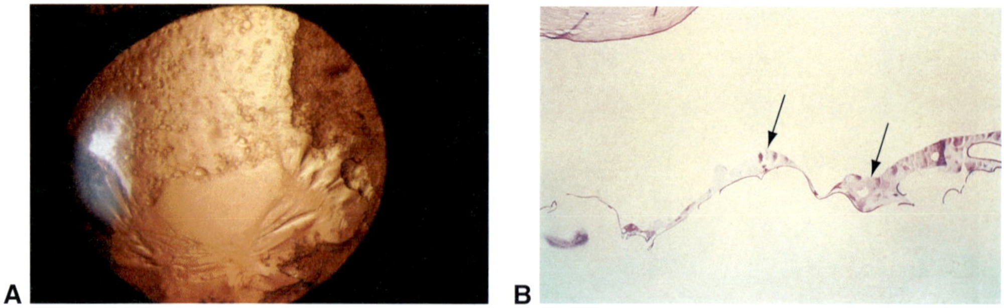

Figure 9-10 Elschnig pearls. **A,** Clinical appearance using retroillumination to demonstrate posterior capsule opacities. **B,** Histology depicting proliferating lens epithelium *(arrows)* on posterior capsule. *(Part A courtesy of Sander Dubovy, MD; part B courtesy of Debra J. Shetlar, MD.)*

histologically identical to bladder cells of Wedl (Fig 9-10). Sequestration of proliferating lens fibers in the equatorial region, often as a result of incomplete cortical removal during cataract surgery, may create a doughnut-shaped configuration referred to as a *Soemmering ring cataract* (Fig 9-11).

Cortex

Opacities of the cortical lens fibers are most often associated with nuclear sclerosis, posterior subcapsular cataracts, and ultraviolet light exposure. Clinically, cortical degenerative changes fall into 2 broad categories: *generalized discolorations with loss of transparency* and *focal opacifications.*

Generalized loss of transparency cannot be diagnosed histologically with reliability, as histologic stains that are used to colorize the lens after it is processed prevent the assessment of lens clarity. The earliest sign of focal cortical degeneration is hydropic swelling of the lens fibers with decreased intensity of the eosinophilic staining. Focal cortical

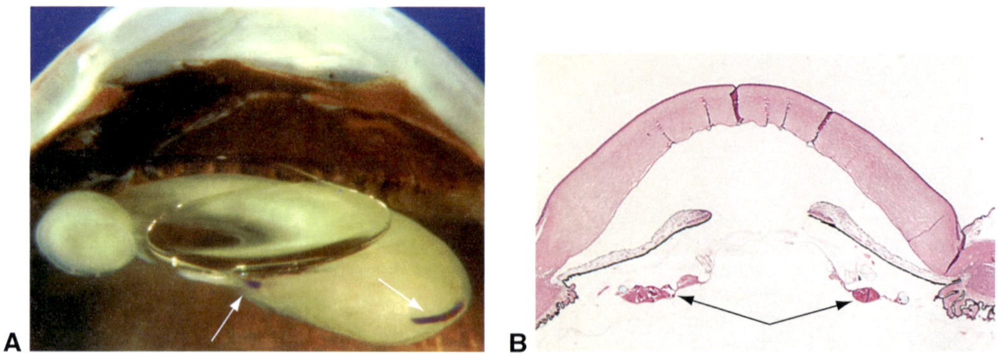

Figure 9-11 Soemmering ring cataract. **A,** Doughnut-shaped white cataractous material is present in the equatorial region of the lens capsule and surrounds one lens haptic *(arrows).* The lens optic and a second haptic are positioned in front of the lens capsular bag, in the sulcus. **B,** Ring cataract, photomicrograph *(arrows).* *(Part A courtesy of Tatyana Milman, MD.)*

opacities become more apparent when fiber degeneration is advanced enough to cause liquefactive change. Light microscopy shows the accumulation of eosinophilic globules *(morgagnian globules)* in slitlike spaces between the lens fibers, which is a reliable histologic sign of cortical degeneration (Fig 9-12; see Fig 9-13C). As focal cortical lesions progress, the slitlike spaces become confluent, forming globular collections of lens protein. Ultimately, the entire cortex can become liquefied, allowing the nucleus to sink downward and the capsule to wrinkle *(morgagnian cataract)* (Fig 9-13).

Denatured lens protein can escape through an intact lens capsule and provoke an anterior chamber macrophagic inflammatory reaction, a condition known as *phacolytic glaucoma* (discussed in Chapter 7).

Nucleus

The continued production of lens fibers subjects the nucleus in the adult lens to the lifelong stress of mechanical compression. This compression causes hardening of the lens nucleus. Aging is also associated with alterations in the chemical composition of the nuclear fibers. The pathogenesis of nuclear discoloration is poorly understood and probably involves more than 1 mechanism, including accumulation of urochrome pigment. Clinically, the lens nucleus may appear yellow, brunescent, or deep brown (Fig 9-14).

Nuclear cataracts are difficult to assess histologically because they take on a subtle homogeneous eosinophilic appearance. The loss of cellular laminations (artifactitious clefts) probably correlates better with firmness of the nucleus than it does with optical opacification clinically (see Fig 9-13C). Occasionally, crystalline deposits, identified as calcium oxalate, may be observed within a nuclear cataract (Fig 9-15). These deposits are birefringent under polarized light.

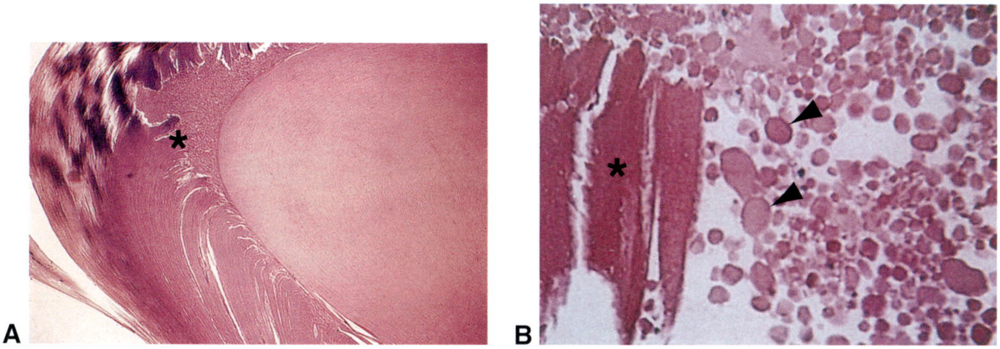

Figure 9-12 Cataract. **A,** Extensive cortical changes are present *(asterisk)*. **B,** Cortical degeneration. Lens cell fibers *(asterisk)* have swollen and fragmented to form morgagnian globules *(arrowheads)*. The lenticular fragments are opaque and will increase osmotic pressure within the capsule. *(Courtesy of Hans E. Grossniklaus, MD.)*

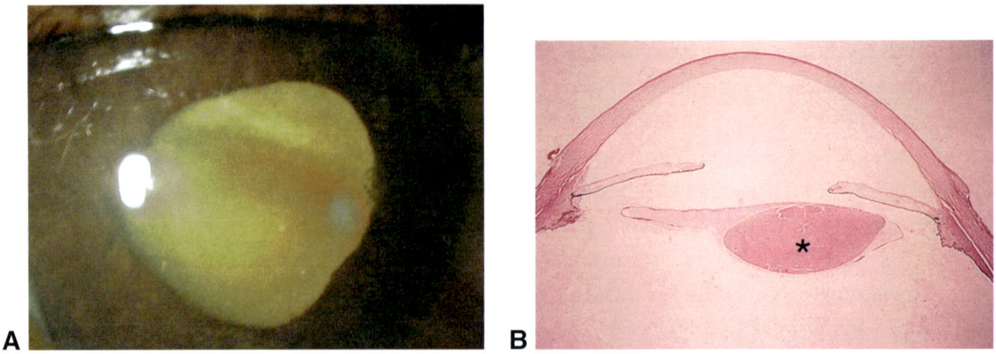

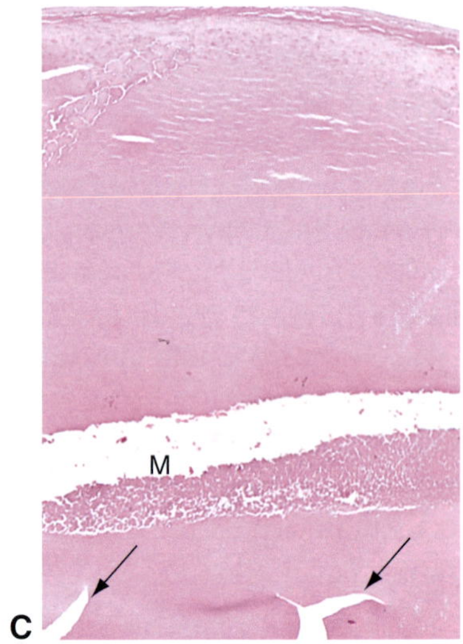

Figure 9-13 Morgagnian cataract. **A,** The brunescent nucleus has sunken inferiorly within the liquefied cortex. **B,** The lens cortex is liquefied, leaving the lens nucleus *(asterisk)* floating free within the capsular bag. **C,** Note the artifactitious, sharply angulated clefts *(arrows)* in this nuclear sclerotic cataract. A zone of morgagnian globules *(M)* is identified. *(Part A courtesy of Bradford Tannen, MD; part B courtesy of Debra J. Shetlar, MD.)*

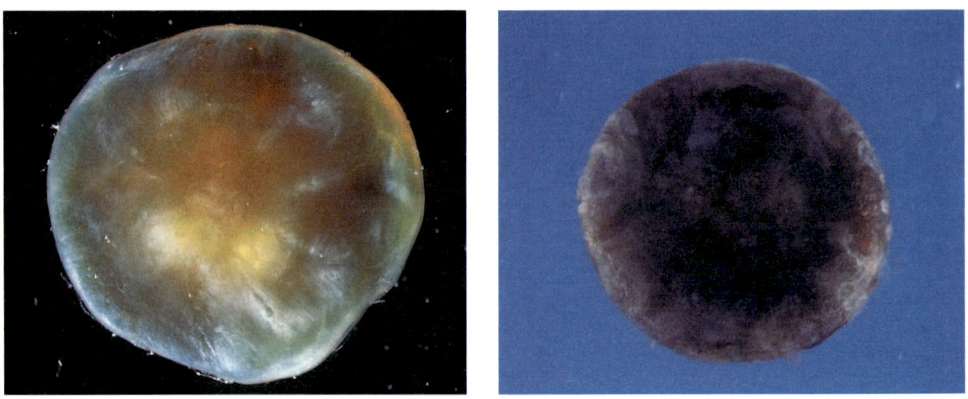

Figure 9-14 Surgically extracted lens nuclei showing varying degrees of brunescence and opacification. *(Courtesy of Hans E. Grossniklaus, MD.)*

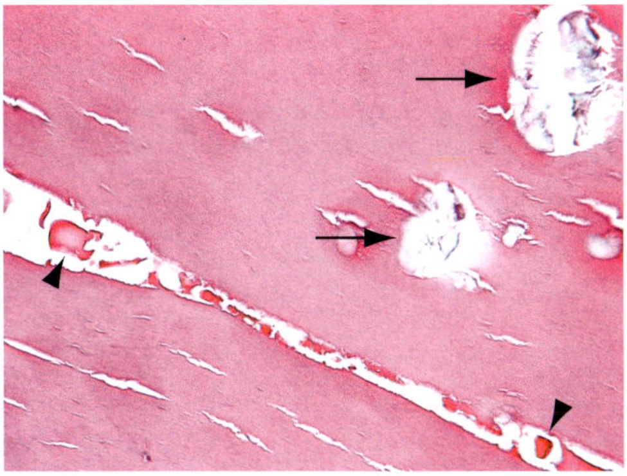

Figure 9-15 Crystalline deposits of calcium oxalate are noted within the lens *(arrows)*. A cortical cleft with morgagnian globules *(arrowheads)* is also seen. *(Courtesy of Tatyana Milman, MD.)*

Neoplasia and Associations With Systemic Disorders

There are no reported examples of neoplasms arising in the human lens. Premature opacification of the lens has been noted in many systemic disorders. See BCSC Section 11, *Lens and Cataract.*

Pathology of Intraocular Lenses

Placement of an intraocular lens following the removal of a cataract has become standard in most cases of cataract surgery. See BCSC Section 11, *Lens and Cataract,* for discussion of this topic.

CHAPTER 10

Vitreous

Topography

The vitreous humor makes up most of the volume of the globe and is important in many diseases that affect the eye. BCSC Section 12, *Retina and Vitreous,* discusses the vitreous in detail.

The average volume of the adult vitreous is 4 mL. The vitreous is composed of 99% water and several macromolecules, including

- types II and IX collagen
- glycosaminoglycans
- soluble proteins
- glycoproteins

The outer portion of the vitreous has a greater number of collagen fibrils and is termed the *vitreous cortex.* The outer surface of the cortex is known as the *hyaloid face.*

The vitreous is bordered anteriorly by the lens, where its attachment to the lens capsule is called the *hyaloideocapsular ligament.* This attachment is firm in young patients and becomes increasingly tenuous with age. The vitreous is attached to the internal limiting membrane (ILM) of the retina by the insertion of the cortical collagen into the basement membrane structure that comprises the basal lamina of the ciliary epithelium and the ILM.

The vitreous attaches most firmly to the vitreous base, a 360° band that straddles the ora serrata and varies in width from 2 to 6 mm. The vitreous base extends more posteriorly with advancing age. Other relatively firm attachments of the vitreous are

- at the margins of the optic nerve head
- along the course of major retinal vessels
- in a circular area around the fovea
- at the edges of areas of vitreoretinal degeneration such as lattice degeneration

The strength of the vitreoretinal attachment is important in the pathogenesis of retinal tears and detachment, macular hole formation, and vitreous hemorrhage from neovascularization.

The embryologic development of the vitreous is generally divided into 3 stages:

1. primary vitreous
2. secondary vitreous
3. tertiary vitreous

The *primary vitreous* consists of fibrillar material; mesenchymal cells; and vascular components: the hyaloid artery, vasa hyaloidea propria, and tunica vasculosa lentis (see Fig 3-3 in BCSC Section 11, *Lens and Cataract*). The *secondary vitreous* begins to form at approximately the ninth week of gestation and is destined to become the main portion of the vitreous in the postnatal and adult eye. The primary vitreous atrophies with formation of the secondary vitreous, leaving only a clear central zone through the vitreous (called the *hyaloid canal,* or the *Cloquet canal*) and, occasionally, the Bergmeister papilla and Mittendorf dot as vestigial remnants (discussed later). The secondary vitreous is relatively acellular and completely avascular. The cells present in the secondary vitreous are called *hyalocytes.* The lens zonular fibers represent the *tertiary vitreous.*

Congenital Anomalies

Persistent Fetal Vasculature

Persistent fetal vasculature (PFV; previously known as *persistent hyperplastic primary vitreous,* or *PHPV*) is characterized by the persistence of variable components of the primary vitreous and is most often unilateral. In most cases of clinically significant PFV, a fibrovascular plaque in the retrolental space extends laterally to involve the ciliary processes, which may be pulled centripetally by traction from the fibrovascular tissue. The clinical and gross appearance of elongated ciliary processes results. The anterior fibrovascular plaque is generally contiguous posteriorly with a remnant of the hyaloid artery that may attach to the optic nerve head (Fig 10-1). Involvement of the posterior structures may be more extensive, with tractional detachment of the peripapillary retina resulting from traction from preretinal membranes. The lens is often cataractous, and nonocular tissues such

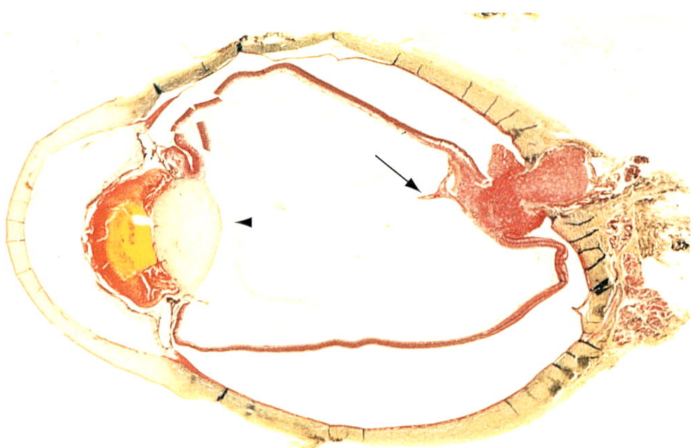

Figure 10-1 Persistent fetal vasculature. Note the prominent anterior fibrovascular plaque *(arrowhead).* The posterior remnant of the persistent hyaloid artery is evident at the optic nerve head *(arrow). (Courtesy of Hans E. Grossniklaus, MD.)*

as adipose tissue and cartilage may be present in the retrolental mass. Eyes affected by PFV are often microphthalmic. See also Chapter 19 in this volume and BCSC Section 6, *Pediatric Ophthalmology and Strabismus.*

Bergmeister Papilla

Persistence of a small part of the posterior portion of the hyaloid artery is referred to as a *Bergmeister papilla.* This anomaly generally takes the form of a veil-like structure or a fingerlike projection extending anteriorly from the surface of the optic nerve head.

Mittendorf Dot

The hyaloid artery attaches to the tunica vasculosa lentis just inferior and nasal to the center of the lens. With regression of these vascular structures, it is not uncommon to see a focal lens opacity at this site, which is referred to as a *Mittendorf dot* (see Fig 2-41 in BCSC Section 2, *Fundamentals and Principles of Ophthalmology*).

Prepapillary Vascular Loops

Retinal vessels may grow into a Bergmeister papilla and then return to the optic nerve head, creating the appearance of a vascular loop. These loops should not be mistaken for neovascularization of the optic nerve head. See Fig 16-5 in BCSC Section 12, *Retina and Vitreous.*

Vitreous Cysts

Vitreous cysts generally occur in eyes with no other pathologic findings, but they have been seen in eyes with retinitis pigmentosa, those with uveitis, and eyes with remnants of the hyaloid system. Histologic studies have suggested the presence of hyaloid remnants in the vitreous cysts. The exact origin of the cysts is not known.

Inflammations

As a relatively acellular and completely avascular structure, the vitreous is not an active participant in inflammatory disorders. It does become involved secondarily in inflammatory conditions of adjacent tissues, however. The term *vitritis* is used to denote the presence of benign or malignant white blood cells in the vitreous. Vitreous inflammation associated with infectious agents, particularly bacteria and fungi, is clinically referred to as *infectious endophthalmitis.* Bacterial endophthalmitis is characterized by neutrophilic infiltration of the vitreous (Fig 10-2). This infiltration leads to liquefaction of the vitreous, with subsequent posterior vitreous detachment. Severe inflammation may be accompanied by formation of fibrocellular membranes, which typically form in the retrolental space and may exert traction on the peripheral retina. The vitreous infiltrate in noninfectious uveitis is typically composed of chronic inflammatory cells, including T and B lymphocytes, macrophages, and histiocytes. See also BCSC Section 9, *Intraocular Inflammation and Uveitis.*

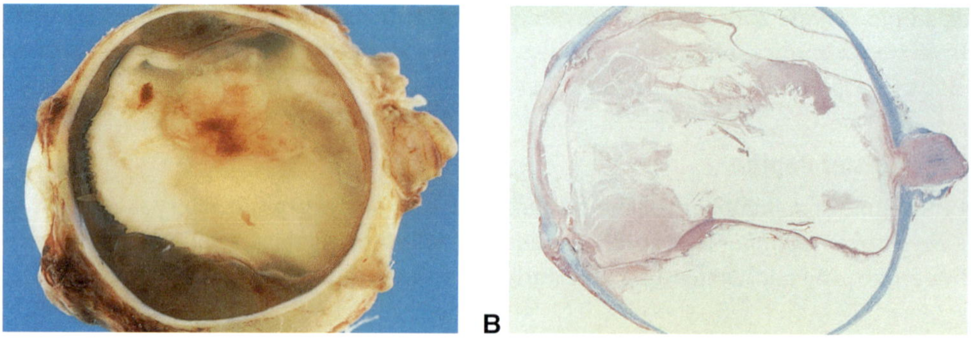

Figure 10-2 **A,** Gross photograph of opacification and infiltration of the vitreous as a result of bacterial endophthalmitis. **B,** Section shows cellular infiltration of vitreous in endophthalmitis (retinal detachment is artifactitious). *(Courtesy of Hans E. Grossniklaus, MD.)*

Degenerations

Syneresis and Aging

Syneresis of the vitreous is defined as liquefaction of the gel. Syneresis of the central vitreous is an almost universal consequence of aging. It also occurs as a consequence of vitreous inflammation and hemorrhage and in the setting of pathologic myopia. The prominent lamellae and strands that develop in aging and following inflammation or hemorrhage are the result of abnormally aggregated collagenous vitreous fibers around syneretic areas (Fig 10-3). Syneresis is one of the contributing factors leading to vitreous detachment.

Posterior Vitreous Detachment

Posterior vitreous detachment (PVD) occurs when a dehiscence in the vitreous cortex allows fluid from a syneretic cavity to gain access to the potential subhyaloid space, causing

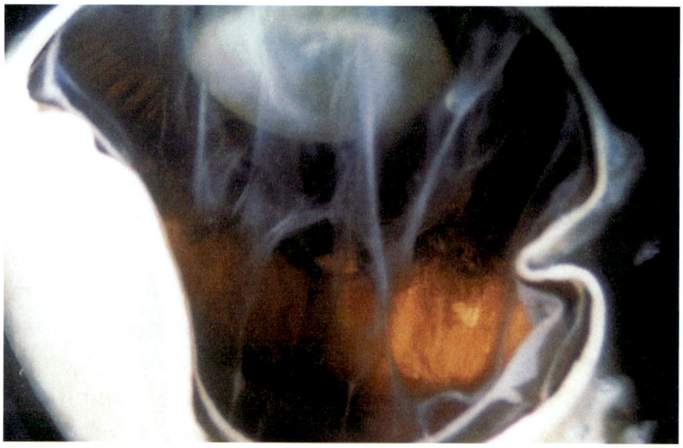

Figure 10-3 Gross photograph of vitreous condensations outlining syneretic cavities. *(Courtesy of Hans E. Grossniklaus, MD.)*

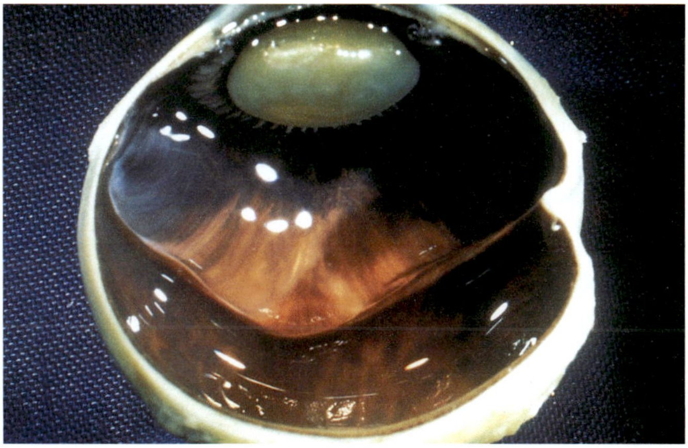

Figure 10-4 Gross photograph of posterior vitreous detachment. *(Courtesy of Hans E. Grossniklaus, MD.)*

the remaining cortex to be stripped from the ILM (Fig 10-4). As fluid drains out of the syneretic cavities under the newly formed posterior hyaloid, the vitreous body collapses anteriorly, remaining attached only at its base. Vitreous detachment generally occurs rapidly over the course of a few hours to days.

A weakening of the adherence of the cortical vitreous to the ILM with age also plays a role in PVDs. The reported incidence of PVD is up to 65% at age 65 and is increased by intraocular inflammation, aphakia or pseudophakia, trauma, and vitreoretinal disease. PVD is important in the pathogenesis of many conditions, including retinal tears and detachment, vitreous hemorrhage, and macular hole formation. See BCSC Section 12, *Retina and Vitreous,* for additional discussion.

Rhegmatogenous Retinal Detachment and Proliferative Vitreoretinopathy

Retinal tears form from vitreous traction on the retina during or after PVD or secondary to ocular trauma. Tears are most likely to occur at sites of greatest vitreoretinal adhesion, such as the vitreous base (Fig 10-5) or the margin of lattice degeneration. The

A 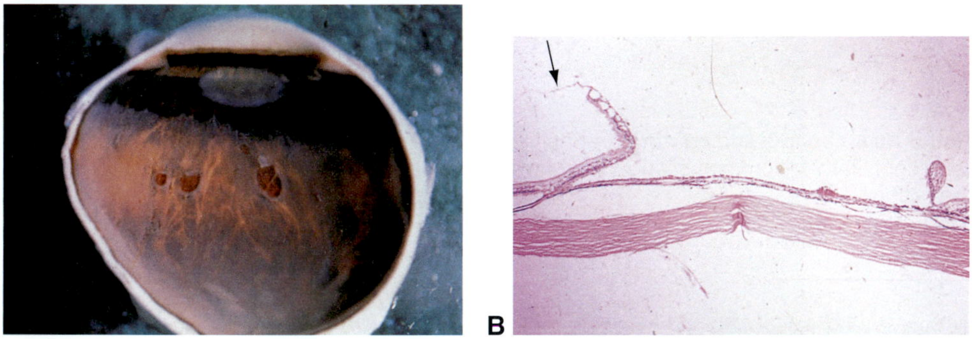 B

Figure 10-5 **A,** Gross photograph of retinal tears at vitreous base. **B,** Photomicrograph shows condensed vitreous *(arrow)* attached to anterior flap of retinal tear. *(Courtesy of W. Richard Green, MD.)*

histopathology of retinal tears reveals that the vitreous is adherent to the retina along the flap of the tear. In the area of retina separated from the underlying retinal pigment epithelium (RPE), there is loss of photoreceptors.

Retinal detachment occurs when vitreous traction and fluid currents resulting from eye movements combine to overcome the forces maintaining retinal adhesion to the RPE. The principal histopathologic findings in retinal detachment consist of the following:

- degeneration of the outer segments of the photoreceptors
- eventual loss of photoreceptor cells
- migration of Müller cells
- proliferation and migration of RPE cells

Small cystic spaces develop in the detached retina, and in chronic detachment, these cysts may coalesce into large macrocysts (Fig 10-6).

With rhegmatogenous retinal detachment, cellular membranes may form on either surface (anterior or posterior) of the retina (Fig 10-7). Clinically, this process is referred to as *proliferative vitreoretinopathy (PVR).* PVR membranes form as a result of proliferation of RPE cells and other cellular elements, including glial cells (Müller cells, fibrous astrocytes), macrophages, fibroblasts, myofibroblasts, and possibly hyalocytes. The cell biology of PVR is complex and involves the interaction of various growth factors, integrins, and cellular proliferation. Studies have shown a significant association between clinical grades of PVR and the expression levels of specific cytokines and/or growth factors in the vitreous fluid.

Harada C, Mitamura Y, Harada T. The role of cytokines and trophic factors in epiretinal membranes: involvement of signal transduction in glial cells. *Prog Retin Eye Res.* 2006;25(2):149–164. Epub 2005 Dec 27.

Macular Holes

Idiopathic macular holes most likely form as the result of degenerative changes in the vitreous. Optical coherence tomography (OCT) has greatly advanced our understanding

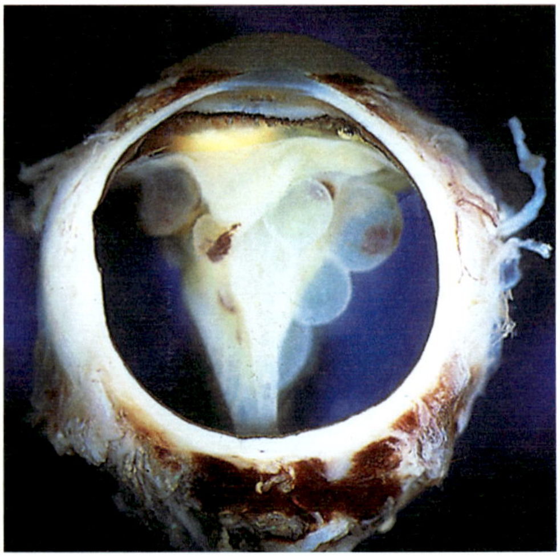

Figure 10-6 Long-standing total retinal detachment with macrocystic degeneration of the retina.

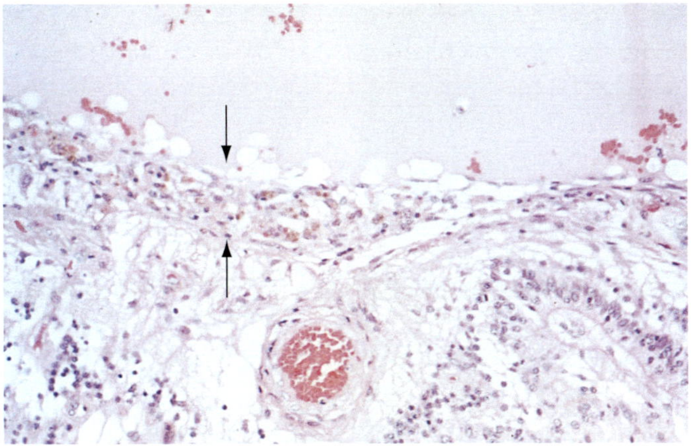

Figure 10-7 Preretinal membrane *(between arrows)* on the surface of the retina, secondary to proliferative vitreoretinopathy. *(Courtesy of David J. Wilson, MD.)*

of the anatomical features of full-thickness macular holes and early macular hole formation. These studies are most consistent with a focal anteroposterior traction mechanism, but some inconsistencies in clinical cases suggest a role for degeneration of the inner retinal layers. Localized perifoveal vitreous detachment (an early stage of age-related PVD) appears to be the primary pathogenetic event in idiopathic macular hole formation (Fig 10-8). Detachment of the posterior hyaloid from the pericentral retina exerts anterior traction on the foveola and localizes the dynamic vitreous traction associated with ocular rotations into the perifoveolar region.

OCT has clarified the pathoanatomy of early macular hole stages, beginning with a foveal pseudocyst (stage 1a), typically followed by disruption of the outer retina (stage 1b), before progressing to a full-thickness dehiscence (stage 2). Histologically, full-thickness macular holes are similar to holes in other locations. A full-thickness retinal defect with rounded tissue margins (stage 3) is accompanied by loss of the photoreceptor outer segments in adjacent retina that is separated from the RPE by subretinal fluid (see Fig 10-8C). An epiretinal membrane composed of Müller cells, fibrous astrocytes, and fibroblasts with myoblastic differentiation is often present on the surface of the retina adjacent to the macular hole. Cystoid macular edema in the parafoveal retina adjacent to the full-thickness macular hole is relatively common. Following surgical repair of macular holes, closer apposition of the remaining photoreceptors and variable glial scarring close the macular defect. See BCSC Section 12, *Retina and Vitreous,* for further discussion.

Gass JD. Reappraisal of biomicroscopic classification of stages of development of a macular hole. *Am J Ophthalmol.* 1995;119(6):752–759.

Smiddy WE, Flynn HW Jr. Pathogenesis of macular holes and therapeutic implications. *Am J Ophthalmol.* 2004;137(3):525–537.

Hemorrhage

A constellation of pathologic features may develop in the vitreous following vitreous hemorrhage. After 3–10 days, red blood cell clots undergo fibrinolysis and red blood cells may

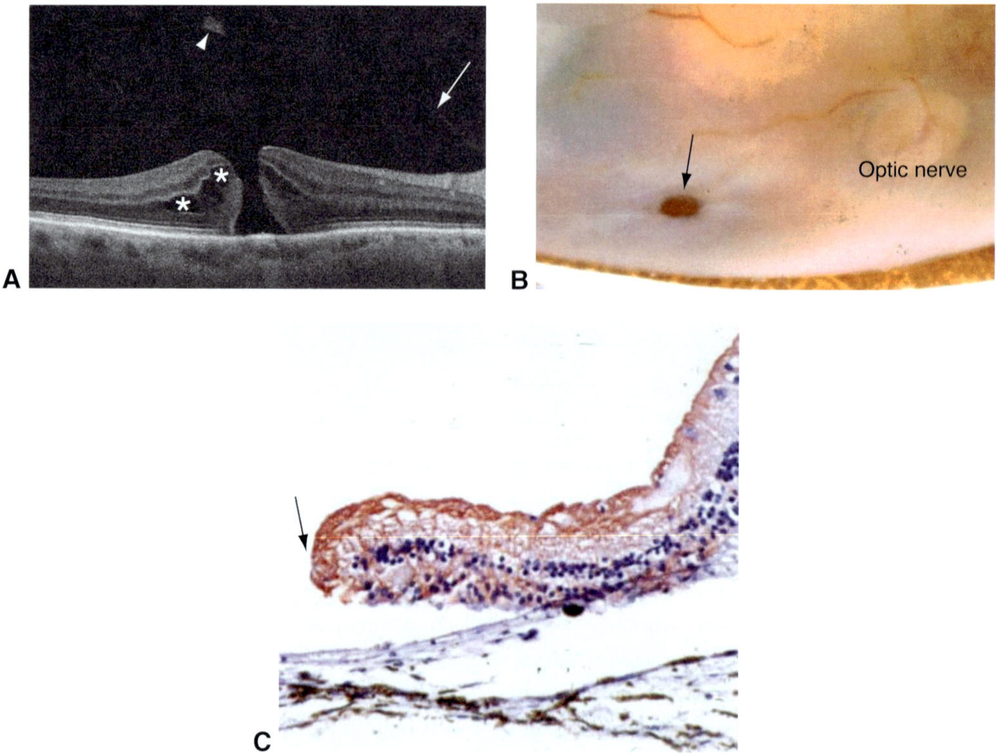

Figure 10-8 Macular holes. **A,** Spectral domain OCT showing stage 3 macular hole with full-thickness retinal defect, rounded margins, cystoid macular edema *(asterisks),* and operculum *(arrowhead).* Note the posterior hyaloid face *(arrow)* tethered to the peripapillary retina near the optic disc. **B,** Gross photograph of full-thickness macular hole *(arrow).* **C,** Histology of full-thickness macular hole showing rounded gliotic margin *(arrow)* with positive staining for glial fibrillary acidic protein (GFAP), highlighting the Müller cells and fibrous astrocytes. *(Parts A and B courtesy of Robert H. Rosa, Jr, MD, and Terry Hanke, CRA; part C courtesy of Patricia Chévez-Barrios, MD.)*

diffuse throughout the vitreous cavity. At this time, breakdown of the red blood cells also occurs. Loss of hemoglobin from the red blood cells produces ghost cells (see Chapter 7, Fig 7-10) and hemoglobin spherules (Fig 10-9). Obstruction of the trabecular meshwork by these cells may lead to *ghost cell glaucoma.* See also BCSC Section 10, *Glaucoma.*

The process of red blood cell dissolution attracts macrophages, which phagocytose the effete red blood cells. The hemoglobin is broken down to hemosiderin and then removed from the eye. In massive hemorrhages, cholesterol crystals caused by the breakdown of red blood cell membranes may be present, often surrounded by a foreign body giant cell reaction. Cholesterol appears clinically as refractile intravitreal crystals (synchesis scintillans). Syneresis of the vitreous and PVD are common after vitreous hemorrhage.

Asteroid Hyalosis

Asteroid hyalosis is a condition with a spectacular clinical appearance (see Fig 16-8 in BCSC Section 12, *Retina and Vitreous*) but little clinical significance. Histologically, asteroid bodies are rounded structures measuring 10–100 nm that stain positively with alcian

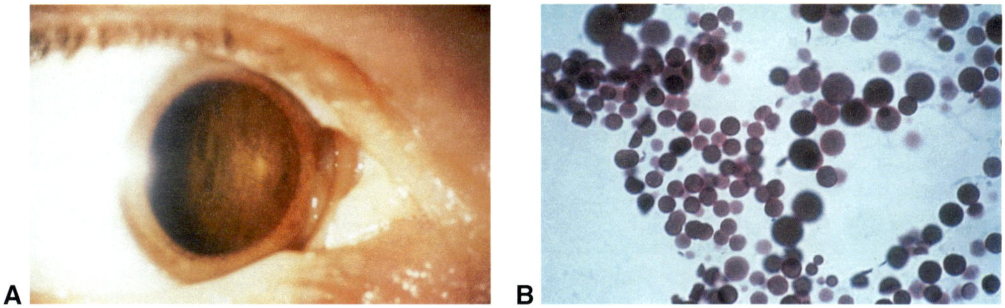

Figure 10-9 **A,** Clinical photograph of retrolental hemoglobin spherules. **B,** Cytologic preparation of hemoglobin spherules removed from the vitreous cavity. *(Reproduced with permission from Spraul CW, Grossniklaus HE. Vitreous hemorrhage.* Surv Ophthalmol. *1997;42(1):3–39.)*

blue and positively with stains for neutral fats, phospholipids, and calcium (Fig 10-10). The bodies stain metachromatically and exhibit birefringence. Occasionally, asteroid bodies will be surrounded by a foreign body giant cell, but the condition is not generally associated with vitreous inflammation.

The exact mechanism of formation of asteroid bodies is not known; however, element mapping by electron spectroscopic imaging has revealed a homogeneous distribution of calcium, phosphorus, and oxygen. The electron energy loss spectra of these elements show details similar to those found for hydroxyapatite. Immunofluorescence microscopy has revealed the presence of chondroitin-6-sulfate at the periphery of asteroid bodies; and carbohydrates specific for hyaluronic acid were observed by lectin-gold labeling to be part of the inner matrix of asteroid bodies. Thus, asteroid bodies exhibit structural and elemental similarity to hydroxyapatite, and proteoglycans and their glycosaminoglycan side chains appear to play a role in regulating the biomineralization process.

Winkler J, Lünsdorf H. Ultrastructure and composition of asteroid bodies. *Invest Ophthalmol Vis Sci.* 2001;42(5):902–907.

Vitreous Amyloidosis

The term *amyloidosis* refers to a group of diseases that lead to extracellular deposition of amyloid. Amyloid is composed of various proteins that have a characteristic ultrastructural

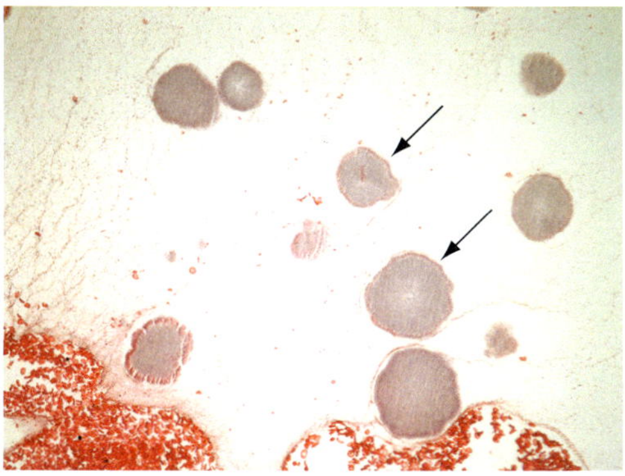

Figure 10-10 Asteroid bodies *(arrows)* and erythrocytic debris within the vitreous. *(Courtesy of Tatyana Milman, MD.)*

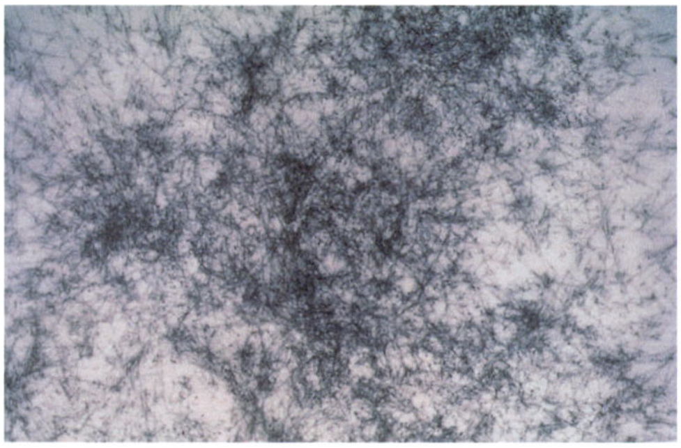

Figure 10-11 Electron photomicrograph shows characteristic amyloid fibrils. *(Courtesy of David J. Wilson, MD.)*

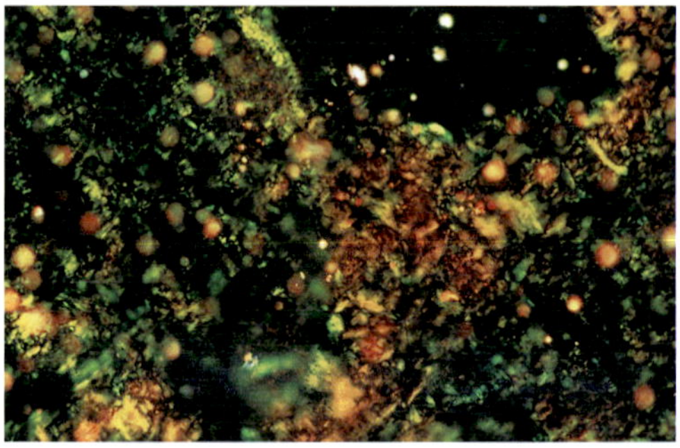

Figure 10-12 Polarized light photomicrograph of the Congo red–stained vitreous from a patient with familial amyloid polyneuropathy. *(Courtesy of David J. Wilson, MD.)*

appearance of nonbranching fibrils with variable length and a diameter of 75–100 Å (Fig 10-11). The proteins forming amyloid also have in common the ability to form a tertiary structure characterized as a β-pleated sheet, which then enables the proteins to bind Congo red stain and show birefringence in polarized light (Fig 10-12).

Amyloid may be derived from various types of protein, and the protein of origin is characteristic for different forms of amyloidosis. Amyloid deposits occur in the vitreous when the protein forming the amyloid is *transthyretin,* previously known as *prealbumin.* Multiple genetic mutations have been described that result in various amino acid substitutions in the transthyretin protein. The most common mutations were originally described in *familial amyloid polyneuropathy (FAP)* types I and II. Systemic manifestations in patients with FAP include vitreous opacities and perivascular infiltrates (Fig 10-13), peripheral neuropathy, cardiomyopathy, and carpal tunnel syndrome.

The mechanism by which the vitreous becomes involved is not known with certainty. Because amyloid deposits are found within the walls of retinal vessels and in the RPE, amyloid may gain access to the vitreous through these tissues. In addition, because transthyretin is a blood protein, it may gain access to the vitreous by crossing the blood–aqueous or blood–retina barrier.

Neoplasia

Intraocular Lymphoma

Primary neoplastic involvement of the vitreous is uncommon because of the relatively acellular nature of the vitreous. However, the vitreous can be the site of primary involvement

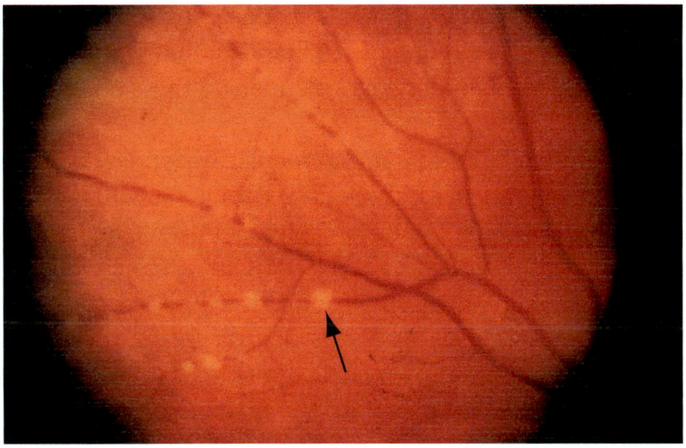

Figure 10-13 Perivascular sheathing *(arrow)* associated with vitreous amyloidosis. *(Courtesy of Hans E. Grossniklaus, MD.)*

in cases of B-cell lymphoma. This type of lymphoma has been referred to as *primary intraocular/central nervous system lymphoma, large cell lymphoma,* and *vitreoretinal/ retinal lymphoma.* Immunohistochemical and molecular genetic studies have confirmed that this entity is typically a B-cell lymphoma; however, T-cell lymphomas may occur in rare instances.

Clinically, *primary intraocular lymphoma (PIOL)* presents most commonly as a vitritis. Some patients have sub-RPE infiltrates (Fig 10-14) with a very characteristic speckled pigmentation overlying tumor detachments of the RPE. The sub-RPE infiltrates are present in a minority of patients with intraocular lymphoma. Recent evidence suggests that the lymphoma cells may be attracted to the RPE by B-cell chemokines and subsequently migrate from the sub-RPE space into the vitreous. More than half of patients presenting with ocular findings have or will develop involvement of the central nervous system.

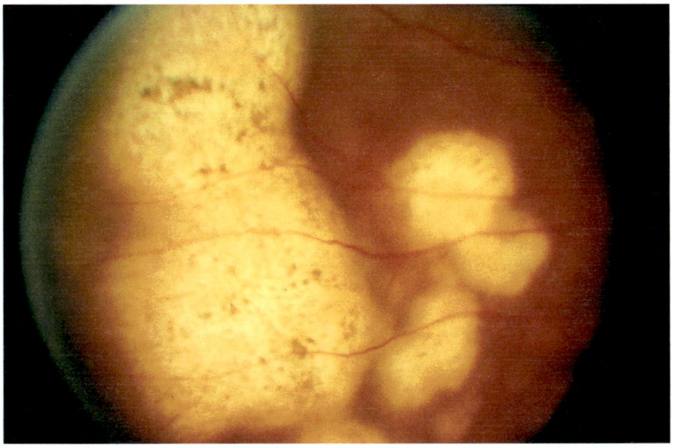

Figure 10-14 Sub-RPE infiltrates in a patient with primary intraocular lymphoma. Note the characteristic speckled pigmentation over the tumor detachments of the RPE. *(Courtesy of Robert H. Rosa, Jr, MD.)*

The diagnosis of intraocular lymphoma is made by cytologic analysis of vitrectomy specimens. Immunohistochemical study of cell markers, flow cytometry, or gene amplification studies can be performed on vitreous specimens, although the standard method of diagnosis is cytology.

Cytologically, the vitreous infiltrate in intraocular lymphoma is heterogeneous. The atypical cells are large lymphoid cells, frequently with a convoluted nuclear membrane and multiple, conspicuous nucleoli. An accompanying infiltrate of small lymphocytes almost always appears, and the normal cells may obscure the neoplastic cell population. These small round lymphocytes are mostly reactive T cells. Numerous cell ghosts are usually present, and this feature is very suggestive of a diagnosis of intraocular lymphoma (Fig 10-15). Immunohistochemically, the viable tumor cells can be labeled as a monoclonal population of B cells. Flow cytometry is helpful in demonstrating a monoclonal population. Other laboratory tests that may be useful in the diagnosis and follow-up of patients with intraocular lymphoma are determination of the interleukin-10 to interleukin-6 ratio and the use of microdissection and polymerase chain reaction (PCR) for the detection of immunoglobulin gene rearrangement and translocation.

The subretinal/sub-RPE infiltrates are composed of neoplastic lymphoid cells (Fig 10-16). With or without treatment, the subretinal infiltrates may resolve, leaving a focal area of RPE atrophy. Optic nerve and retinal infiltration may also be present. Infiltrates in these locations tend to be perivascular and may lead to ischemic retinal or optic nerve damage. The choroid is most often free of lymphoma cells; however, secondary chronic inflammation may be present in the choroid. In the setting of systemic lymphoma with ocular involvement, the choroid (rather than the vitreous, retina, or subretinal space) is the primary site of involvement.

Coupland SE, Hummel M, Müller HH, Stein H. Molecular analysis of immunoglobulin genes in primary intraocular lymphoma. *Invest Ophthalmol Vis Sci.* 2005;46(10):3507–3514.

Levy-Clarke GA, Chan CC, Nussenblatt RB. Diagnosis and management of primary intraocular lymphoma. *Hematol Oncol Clin North Am.* 2005;19(4):739–749.

Read RW, Zamir E, Rao NA. Neoplastic masquerade syndromes. *Surv Ophthalmol.* 2002;47(2): 81–124.

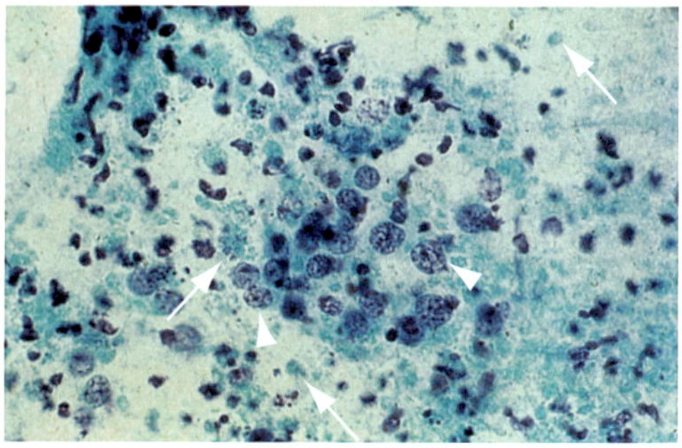

Figure 10-15 Cytologic preparation of vitreous lymphoma. Note the atypical cells *(arrowheads)* with large nuclei and multiple nucleoli. Cell ghosts *(arrows)* are also present. *(Courtesy of David J. Wilson, MD.)*

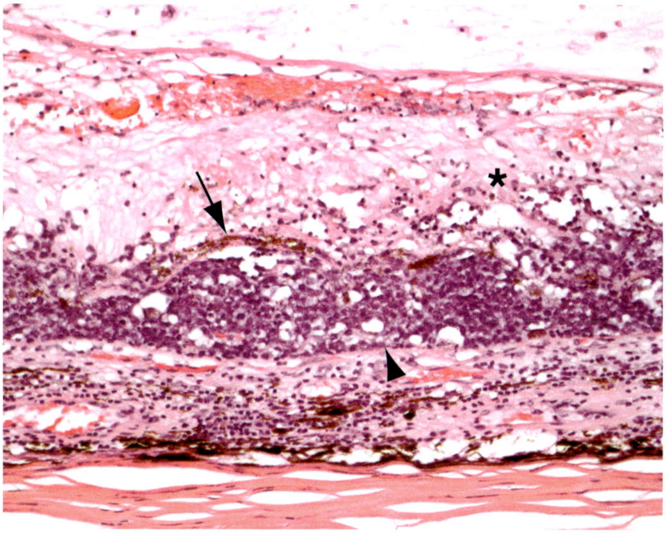

Figure 10-16 Primary intraocular lymphoma. Note the detachment of the RPE by tumor *(arrow)* overlying retinal gliosis *(asterisk)*, and intact Bruch membrane *(arrowhead)*. Secondary chronic inflammation is present in the choroid. *(Courtesy of Robert H. Rosa, Jr, MD.)*

CHAPTER **11**

Retina and Retinal Pigment Epithelium

Topography

The retina and the retinal pigment epithelium (RPE) make up 2 distinct layers that together line the inner two-thirds of the globe:

1. The RPE is a pigmented layer derived from the outer layer of the optic cup.
2. The neurosensory retina is a delicate, transparent layer derived from the inner layer of the optic cup.

Anteriorly, the RPE becomes continuous with the pigmented epithelium of the ciliary body, and the retina becomes continuous with the nonpigmented ciliary body epithelium. Posteriorly, the RPE terminates at the optic nerve, just prior to the termination of the Bruch membrane. The nuclear, photoreceptor, and synaptic layers of the retina gradually taper at the optic nerve head, and only the nerve fiber layer (NFL) continues on to form the optic nerve. See BCSC Section 12, *Retina and Vitreous*, for additional discussion.

Neurosensory Retina

The topographic variation in the structures of the retina is striking, with regional variation in the neural structures as well as the retinal vasculature. The neurosensory retina has 9 layers (Fig 11-1). Beginning on the vitreous side and progressing to the choroidal side, they are

1. internal limiting membrane (ILM; a true basement membrane synthesized by Müller cells)
2. nerve fiber layer
3. ganglion cell layer
4. inner plexiform layer
5. inner nuclear layer
6. outer plexiform layer
7. outer nuclear layer (nuclei of the photoreceptors)
8. external limiting membrane (ELM; not a true membrane but rather an apparent membrane formed by a series of desmosomes between Müller cells and photoreceptors)
9. photoreceptors (inner and outer segments) of the rods and cones

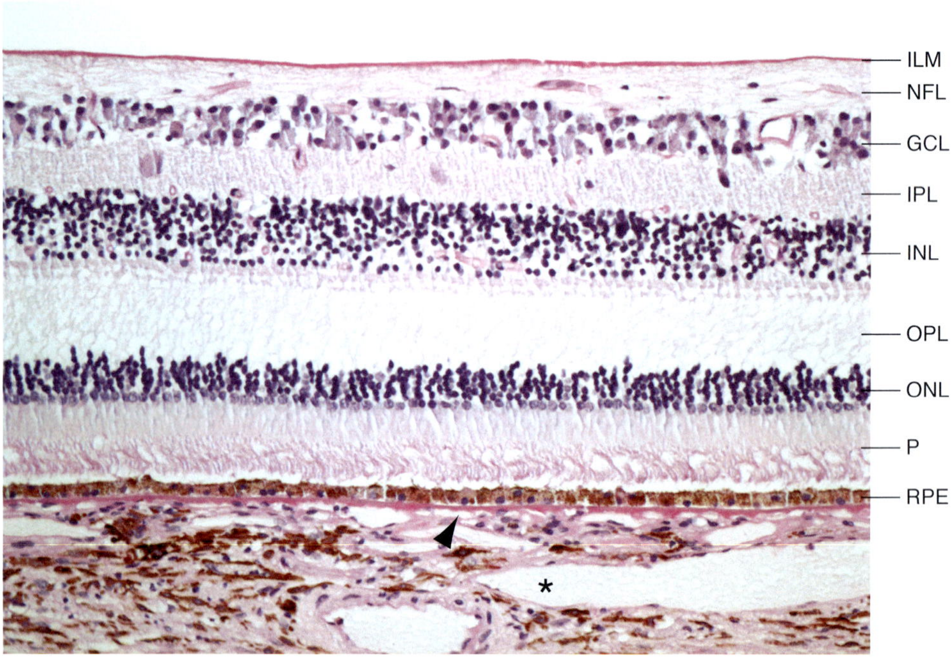

Figure 11-1 Normal retinal layers. From vitreous to choroid: *ILM* = internal limiting membrane, *NFL* = nerve fiber layer, *GCL* = ganglion cell layer, *IPL* = inner plexiform layer, *INL* = inner nuclear layer, *OPL* = outer plexiform layer, *ONL* = outer nuclear layer, *P* = photoreceptors (inner/outer segments) of rods and cones. *RPE* = retinal pigment epithelium. Bruch membrane, *arrowhead;* choroid, *asterisk.* The external limiting membrane (ELM) is not shown in this figure. *(Courtesy of Robert H. Rosa, Jr, MD.)*

The arrangement of the retina (in tissue sections oriented perpendicular to the retinal surface) is vertical from outer to inner layers, except for the NFL, where the axons run horizontally toward the optic nerve head. Consequently, deposits and hemorrhages in the deep retinal layers have a round appearance clinically when viewed on edge, whereas those in the NFL have a feathery appearance.

The blood supply of the retina comes from 2 sources, with a watershed zone inside the inner nuclear layer. The *retinal blood vessels* supply the NFL, ganglion cell layer, inner plexiform layer, and inner two-thirds of the inner nuclear layer. The *choroidal vasculature* supplies the outer one-third of the inner nuclear layer, outer plexiform layer, outer nuclear layer, photoreceptors, and RPE. Because of this division of the blood supply to the retina, ischemic choroidal vascular lesions and ischemic lesions attributed to the retinal vasculature produce different histologic pictures. Ischemic retinal injury produces inner ischemic atrophy of the retina (see Fig 11-13), and choroidal ischemia produces outer ischemic retinal atrophy (see Fig 11-12).

Histologically, the term *macula* refers to that area of the retina where the ganglion cell layer is thicker than a single cell (Fig 11-2). Clinically, this area corresponds approximately with the area of the retina bound by the inferior and superior vascular arcades. The macula is subdivided into the *foveola,* the *fovea,* the *parafovea,* and the *perifovea.* Only

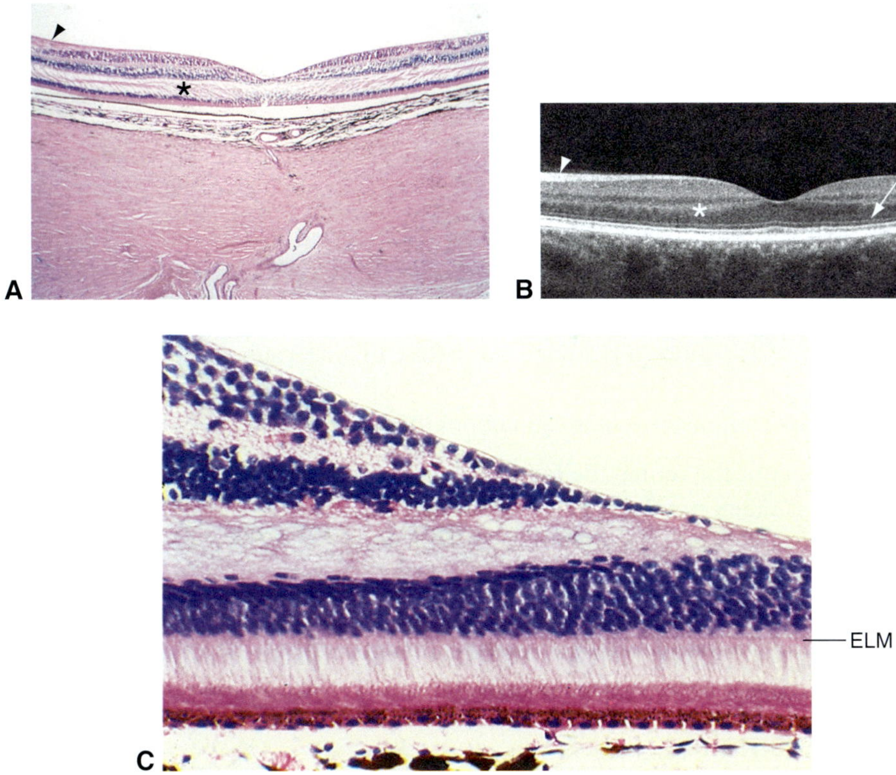

Figure 11-2 **A,** The normal macula is identified histologically by a multicellular, thick ganglion cell layer and an area of focal thinning, the foveola. Note the nerve fiber layer *(arrowhead)* in the nasal macular region and the oblique orientation of the nerve fiber layer of Henle (outer plexiform layer, *asterisk*). Clinically, the macula lies between the inferior and superior vascular arcades. **B,** Spectral domain optical coherence tomography (SD-OCT) of the macula showing in vivo histologic assessment with tremendous details of the lamellar architecture of the retina. Note the nerve fiber layer *(arrowhead)* in the nasal macular region, the nerve fiber layer of Henle (outer plexiform layer, *asterisk*), and the external limiting membrane *(arrow)*. **C,** In the region of the foveola, the inner cellular layers are absent, with an increased density of pigment in the RPE. Note the external limiting membrane *(ELM)*. The incident light falls directly on the photoreceptor outer segments, reducing the potential for distortion of light by overlying tissue elements. *(Part B courtesy of Robert H. Rosa, Jr, MD.)*

photoreceptor cells appear in the central foveola; the ganglion cells, other nucleated cells (including Müller cells), and blood vessels are not present. The concentration of cones is greater in the macula than in the peripheral retina, and only cones are present in the fovea.

Nerve fibers in the outer plexiform layer (nerve fiber layer of Henle) of the macula run obliquely (see Fig 11-2A). This morphologic feature results in the flower-petal appearance of cystoid macular edema (CME) observed on fluorescein angiography and the star-shaped configuration of hard exudates observed ophthalmoscopically in conditions that cause macular edema. Xanthophyll pigment gives the macula its yellow appearance clinically and grossly (macula lutea), but the xanthophyll dissolves during tissue processing and is not present in histologic sections.

Retinal Pigment Epithelium

The RPE consists of a monolayer of hexagonal cells with apical microvilli and a basement membrane at the base of the cells. This monolayer has the following specialized functions:

- vitamin A metabolism
- maintenance of the outer blood–retina barrier
- phagocytosis of the photoreceptor outer segments
- absorption of light
- heat exchange
- formation of the basal lamina of the inner portion of the Bruch membrane
- production of the mucopolysaccharide matrix that surrounds the photoreceptor outer segments
- active transport of materials into and out of the subretinal space

Compared with that of the retina, the topographic variation of the RPE is subtle. In the macula, the RPE is taller, narrower, and more heavily pigmented, and it forms a regular hexagonal array. In the equatorial and midperipheral area, the RPE cells are larger in diameter and thinner. Variability in the diameter of the RPE cells increases in the peripheral retina. The amount of cytoplasmic pigment, primarily lipofuscin, increases with age, particularly within the RPE in the macular region.

Congenital Anomalies

Albinism

Albinism is a general term that refers to a congenital dilution of the pigment of the skin, the eyes and the skin, or just the eyes. The condition results from genetic mutations that cause abnormalities in the biosynthesis of melanin pigment. True albinism has been subdivided into *oculocutaneous* and *ocular albinism*. This distinction is somewhat helpful clinically, but in reality all cases of ocular albinism have some degree of mild cutaneous involvement. There is a pathophysiologic difference between the 2 types of albinism. In oculocutaneous albinism, transmission is commonly autosomal recessive, and the amount of melanin in each melanosome is reduced, whereas in ocular albinism, transmission is commonly X-linked recessive, and the number of melanosomes is reduced (Fig 11-3). See BCSC Section 6, *Pediatric Ophthalmology and Strabismus,* and Section 12, *Retina and Vitreous,* for further discussion.

Myelinated Nerve Fibers

Generally, myelination of the nerve fibers in the optic pathways terminates at the lamina cribrosa. However, myelination produced by oligodendroglial cells in the NFL can occur (see Fig 26-7 in BCSC Section 6, *Pediatric Ophthalmology and Strabismus*). Though usually contiguous with the optic nerve head, myelination may also occur in isolation away from the optic nerve head and, if large, can produce a clinically significant scotoma. Myelinated nerve fibers have been associated with myopia, amblyopia, strabismus, and nystagmus.

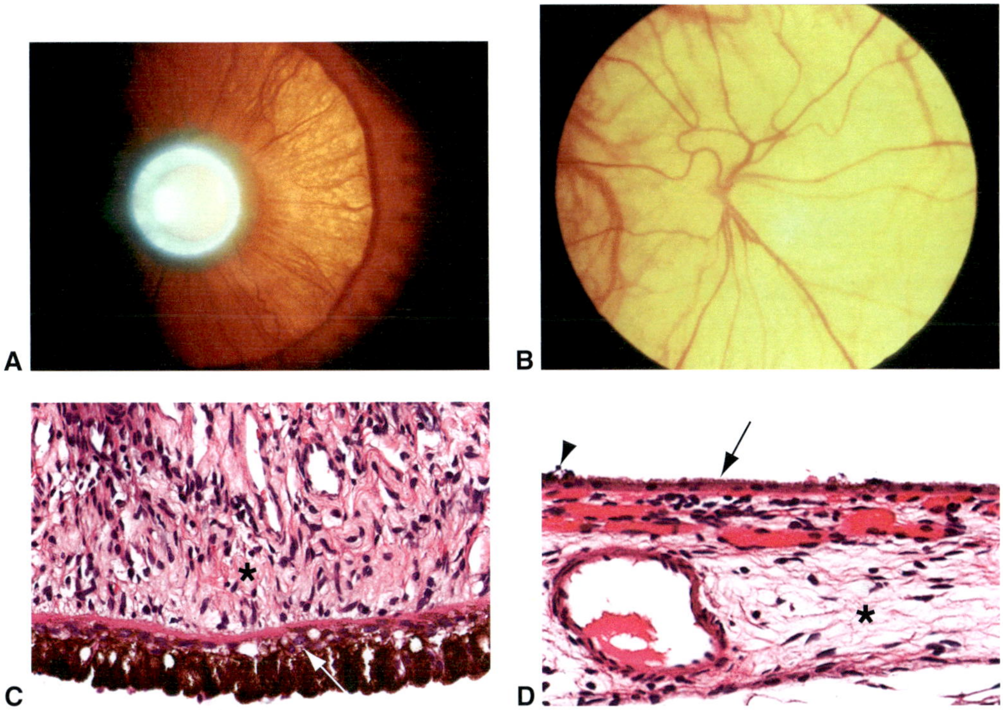

Figure 11-3 Albinisim. **A,** Iris transillumination. **B,** Fundus hypopigmentation. **C,** Photomicrograph illustrates decreased pigmentation in the iris pigment epithelium (smaller melanosomes) allowing visualization of the nuclei *(arrow).* No appreciable pigmentation is present in the iris stroma *(asterisk).* **D,** Photomicrograph shows RPE and choroid in an albino eye. Note the apical distribution of melanin granules and overall decreased pigmentation in the RPE *(arrow),* rare giant melanosomes *(arrowhead)* in the RPE, and lack of appreciable pigmentation in the choroidal stroma *(asterisk).* *(Parts A and B courtesy of Robert H. Rosa, Jr, MD; parts C and D courtesy of Tatyana Milman, MD, and Ralph C. Eagle, Jr, MD.)*

Vascular Anomalies

There are numerous congenital anomalies of the retinal vasculature, including capillary hemangioma and cavernous hemangioma, parafoveal telangiectasia, and Coats disease. Many of these anomalies and their clinical features are covered in BCSC Section 12, *Retina and Vitreous.* In Coats disease, exudative retinal detachment occurs as a result of leakage from abnormalities in the peripheral retina, including telangiectatic vessels, microaneurysms, and saccular dilations of retinal vessels (Fig 11-4). Histologically, retinal detachments secondary to Coats disease are characterized by the presence of "foamy" macrophages and cholesterol crystals in the subretinal space.

Congenital Hypertrophy of the RPE

Congenital hypertrophy of the RPE (CHRPE), a relatively common congenital lesion, is characterized clinically by a flat, dark black lesion varying in size from a few to 10 mm in diameter (see Chapter 17, Fig 17-10). Frequently, central lacunae and a peripheral zone of less dense pigmentation appear within the lesion. This lesion is histologically characterized

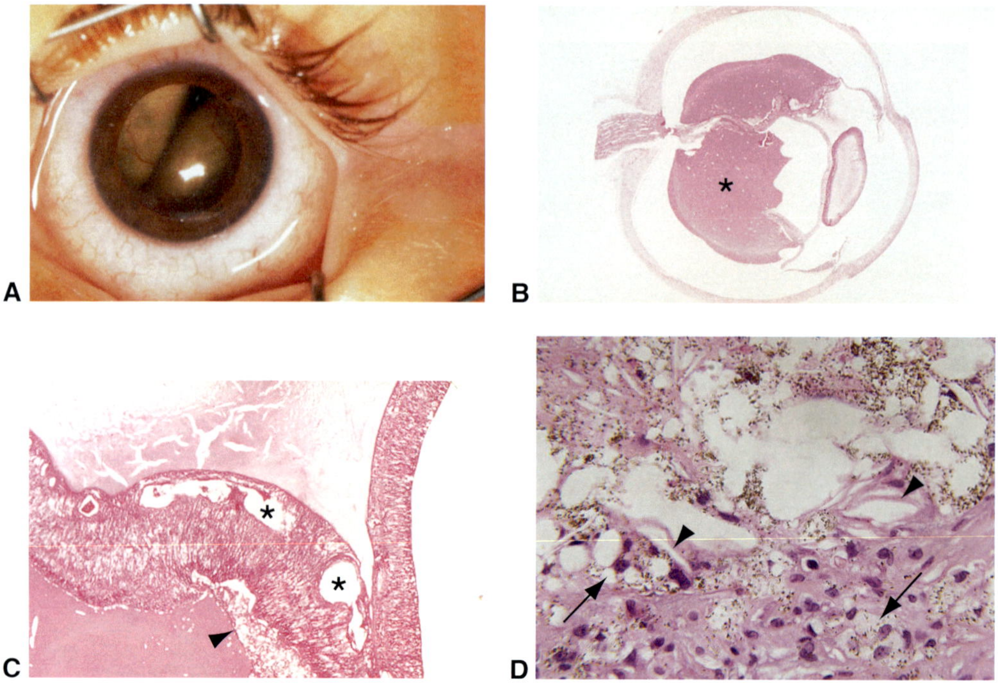

Figure 11-4 **A,** Leukocoria as a result of Coats disease. **B,** Total exudative retinal detachment in Coats disease. Note the dense subretinal proteinaceous fluid *(asterisk)*. **C,** Telangiectatic vessels *(asterisks)* and "foamy" macrophages *(arrowhead)* typical of Coats disease. **D,** High magnification of subretinal exudate showing lipid- and pigment-laden macrophages *(arrows)* and cholesterol clefts *(arrowheads)*. *(Parts A–C courtesy of Hans E. Grossniklaus, MD; part D courtesy of George J. Harocopos, MD.)*

by enlarged RPE cells with densely packed and larger-than-normal, spherical melanin granules (Fig 11-5). This benign congenital condition can generally be distinguished from choroidal nevi and melanoma on the basis of ophthalmoscopic features. Adenoma and adenocarcinoma of the RPE may develop, in rare instances, in an area of CHRPE. RPE lesions mimicking CHRPE may be present in Gardner syndrome, or familial adenomatous polyposis. Histologic study of the RPE changes in Gardner syndrome reveals that they are more consistent with hyperplasia of the RPE than with hypertrophy. The RPE changes in

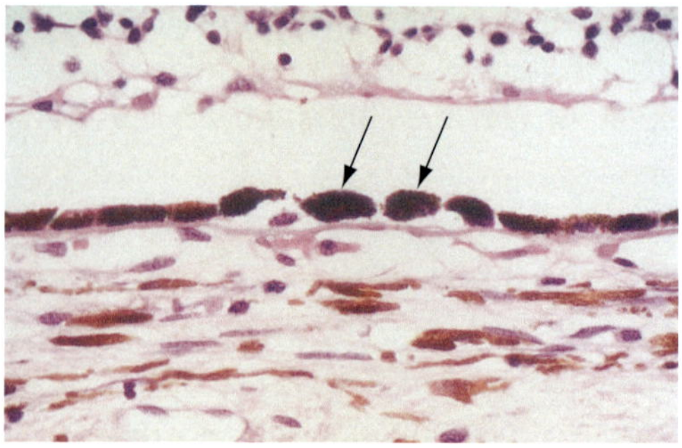

Figure 11-5 In CHRPE, the RPE cells are larger than normal and contain more densely packed melanin granules *(arrows)*. For clinical images of CHRPE, see Chapter 17, Figure 17-10. *(Courtesy of Hans E. Grossniklaus, MD.)*

Gardner syndrome are probably more appropriately termed *hamartomas,* consistent with the loss of regulatory control of cell growth that gives rise to the other soft-tissue changes in this syndrome.

Traboulsi EI. Ocular manifestations of familial adenomatous polyposis (Gardner syndrome). *Ophthalmol Clin North Am.* 2005;18(1):163–166.

Inflammations

Infectious

Viral

Multiple viruses may cause retinal infections, including rubella, measles, human immunodeficiency virus (HIV), herpes simplex virus (HSV), varicella-zoster virus (VZV, or herpes zoster), and cytomegalovirus (CMV). Two of the most frequent clinical presentations of retinal viral infection, acute retinal necrosis (ARN) and CMV retinitis, are discussed here.

Acute retinal necrosis is a rapidly progressive, necrotizing retinitis caused by infection with HSV types 1 and 2, VZV, and, in rare instances, CMV. ARN can occur in healthy or immunocompromised persons. The histologic findings include inflammation in the vitreous and anterior chamber, with a prominent obliterative retinal vasculitis and retinal necrosis (Fig 11-6A). Electron microscopy has demonstrated viral inclusions in retinal cells (Fig 11-6B). Polymerase chain reaction (PCR) analysis of aqueous or vitreous biopsy specimens can be used to rapidly demonstrate the viral cause of ARN, reducing the need for other diagnostic techniques such as viral culture, intraocular antibody analysis, or immunohistochemistry.

CMV retinitis is an opportunistic infection that may occur in immunosuppressed patients, especially AIDS patients (Fig 11-7). This infection is histologically characterized by retinal necrosis, which leads to a thin fibroglial scar with healing. Acute lesions show large neurons (20–30 μm) that contain large eosinophilic intranuclear or intracytoplasmic inclusion bodies. At the cellular level, CMV may infect vascular endothelial cells, retinal neurons, and macrophages.

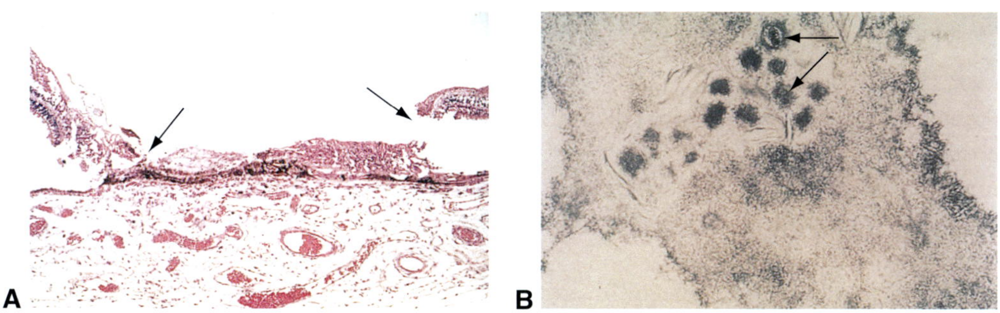

Figure 11-6 **A,** Acute retinal necrosis (ARN) is characterized by full-thickness necrosis of the retina *(between arrows).* **B,** Electron microscopy demonstrates viral particles *(arrows)* within retinal cells. *(Courtesy of Hans E. Grossniklaus, MD.)*

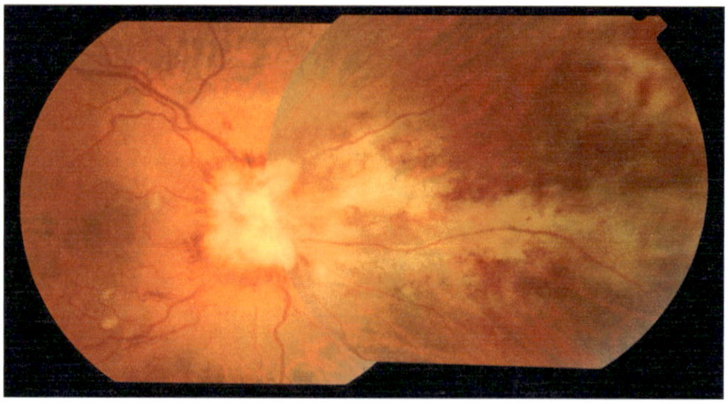

A

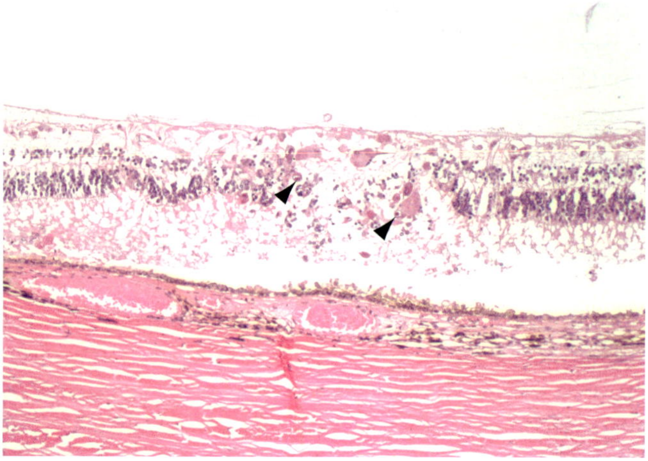

B

Figure 11-7 **A,** CMV retinitis/papillitis. Intraretinal hemorrhages and areas of opaque retina are present nasal to the optic disc. Note the marked optic disc and peripapillary retinal swelling and cotton-wool spots temporal to the optic disc. **B,** Histologically, full-thickness retinal necrosis, cytomegalo cells, and intranuclear *(arrowheads)* and/or intracytoplasmic inclusions are present. *(Part A courtesy of R. Doug Davis, MD; part B courtesy of Robert H. Rosa, Jr, MD.)*

Bacterial

See the discussion of endophthalmitis in Chapter 10 and in BCSC Section 9, *Intraocular Inflammation and Uveitis.*

Fungal

Fungal infections of the retina are uncommon, occurring almost exclusively in immunosuppressed patients as a result of fungemia. These infections usually begin as single or multiple foci of choroidal and retinal infection (Fig 11-8). The most common causative fungi are *Candida* species. Less common agents include *Aspergillus* species and *Cryptococcus neoformans.*

Histologically, fungal infections are typified by necrotizing granulomatous inflammation. A central zone of necrosis is typically surrounded by granulomatous inflammation, and a surrounding infiltrate of lymphocytes is common. With treatment, the lesions

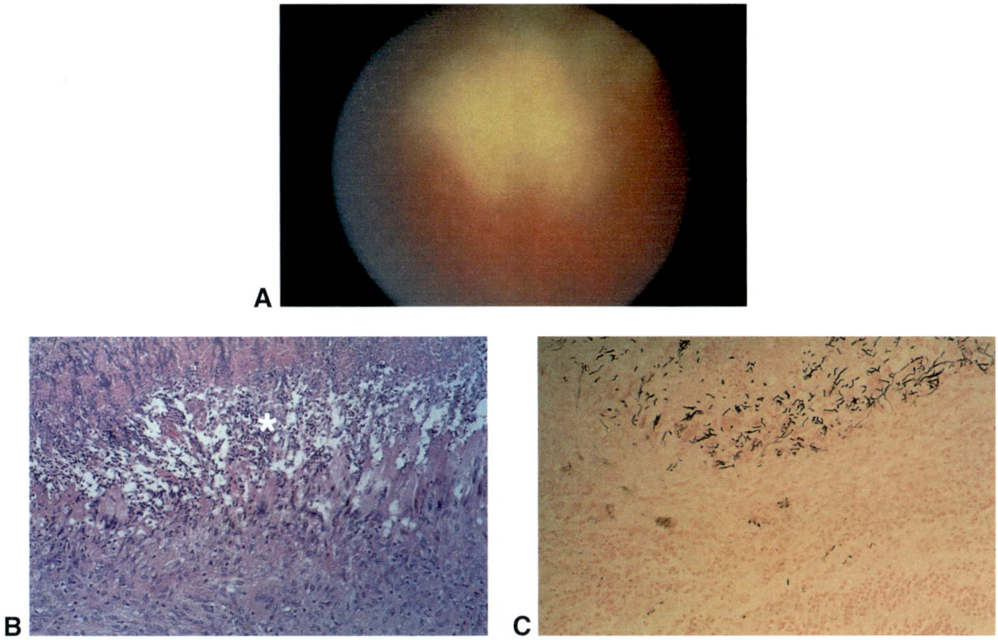

Figure 11-8 **A,** Vitreous, retinal, and choroidal infiltrate in a patient with fungal chorioretinitis. **B,** Granulomatous infiltration surrounding central area of necrosis *(asterisk).* **C,** Gomori methenamine–silver nitrate stain of section parallel to **B** shows numerous fungal hyphae (black staining). *(Courtesy of David J. Wilson, MD.)*

heal with a fibrous scar. The causative agent can usually be identified by culture or by the specific features of the fungal hyphae in histopathologic material.

Toxoplasmosis

Ocular toxoplasmosis, the most common infectious retinitis, may occur because of reactivation of congenitally acquired disease or as the result of an acquired *Toxoplasma* infection in healthy or immunocompromised persons. In patients with reactivated disease, ocular toxoplasmosis typically presents as a posterior uveitis or panuveitis with marked vitritis and focal retinochoroiditis adjacent to a pigmented chorioretinal scar. The absence of prior chorioretinal scarring suggests newly acquired disease. Microscopic examination of active toxoplasmic retinitis reveals necrosis of the retina, a prominent infiltrate of neutrophils and lymphocytes, and *Toxoplasma* organisms in the form of cysts and tachyzoites (Fig 11-9). There is generally a prominent lymphocytic infiltrate of the vitreous and the anterior segment and, not uncommonly, granulomatous inflammation in the inner choroid. Healing brings resolution of the inflammatory cell infiltrate with encystment of the organisms in the retina adjacent to the chorioretinal scar.

Noninfectious

Noninfectious (autoimmune) inflammatory conditions involving the retina are discussed in BCSC Section 9, *Intraocular Inflammation and Uveitis,* and Section 12, *Retina and Vitreous.*

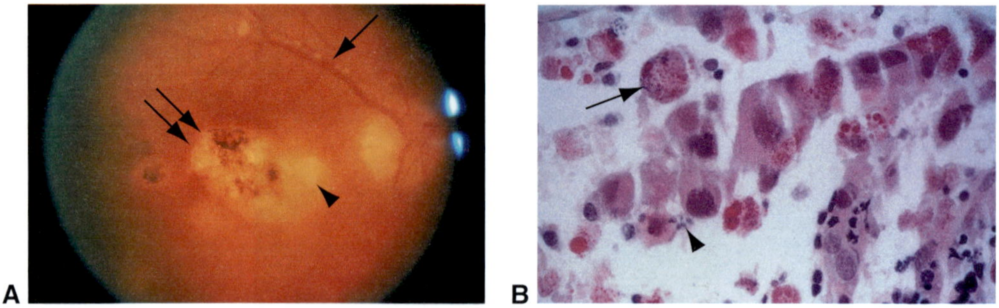

Figure 11-9 **A,** Chorioretinal scars with pigmentation *(double arrow)* typical of prior infection with toxoplasmosis. Active retinitis *(arrowhead)* and perivascular sheathing *(arrow)* are present. **B,** Cysts *(arrow)* and released organisms (tachyzoites, *arrowhead*) in active toxoplasmosis. *(Courtesy of Hans E. Grossniklaus, MD.)*

Degenerations

Typical and Reticular Peripheral Cystoid Degeneration and Retinoschisis

Typical peripheral cystoid degeneration (TPCD) is a universal finding in the eyes of persons older than 20 years. In TPCD, cystic spaces develop in the outer plexiform layer of the retina. *Reticular peripheral cystoid degeneration (RPCD)* is less common. In RPCD, the cystic spaces are present in the NFL. When present, RPCD occurs posterior to areas of TPCD (Fig 11-10). Coalescence of the cystic spaces of TPCD forms *typical degenerative retinoschisis,* which is usually inferotemporal in location. In *reticular degenerative retinoschisis,* the splitting of retinal layers occurs in the NFL.

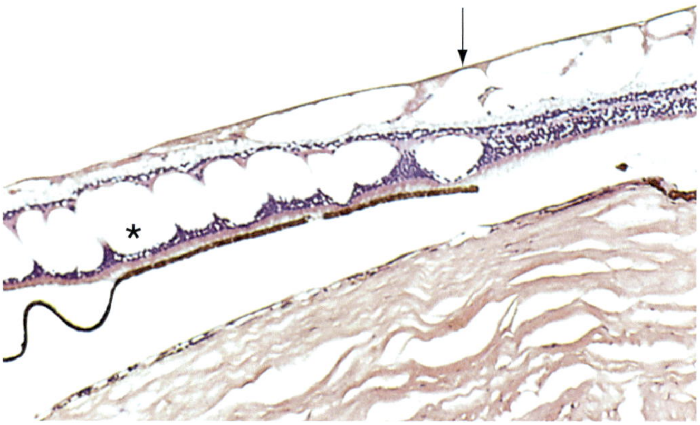

Figure 11-10 Retinal degeneration. Typical peripheral cystoid degeneration consists of cystoid spaces in the outer plexiform layer *(asterisk)* on the lower left (anterior retina). In the upper right (posterior retina), reticular peripheral cystoid degeneration *(arrow)* is present.

Lattice Degeneration

Lattice degeneration may be a familial condition (Fig 11-11). It is found in up to 10% of the general population, but only a small number of affected persons develop retinal detachment. In contrast, lattice degeneration is seen in up to 40% of all rhegmatogenous detachments. The most important histopathologic features of lattice degeneration include

- discontinuity of the ILM of the retina
- an overlying pocket of liquefied vitreous
- sclerosis of the retinal vessels, which remain physiologically patent
- condensation and adherence of vitreous at the margins of the lesion
- variable degrees of atrophy of the inner layers of the retina

Although atrophic holes often develop in the center of the lattice lesion, they are rarely the cause of retinal detachment because the vitreous is liquefied over the surface of the lattice, and thus no vitreous traction occurs. Retinal detachment associated with lattice degeneration is generally the result of vitreous adhesion at the margin of lattice degeneration, leading to retinal tears in this location with vitreous detachment. *Radial perivascular*

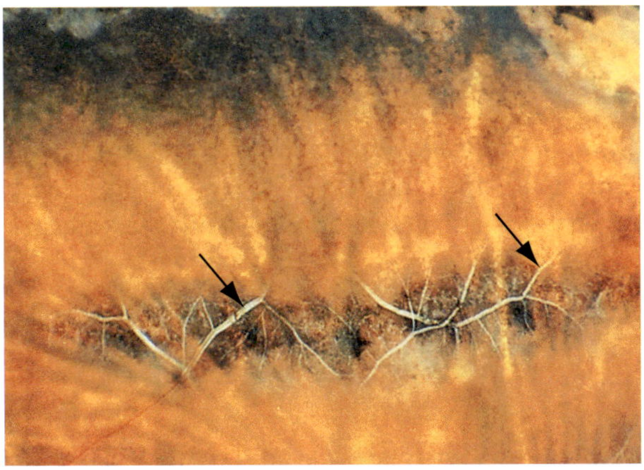
A

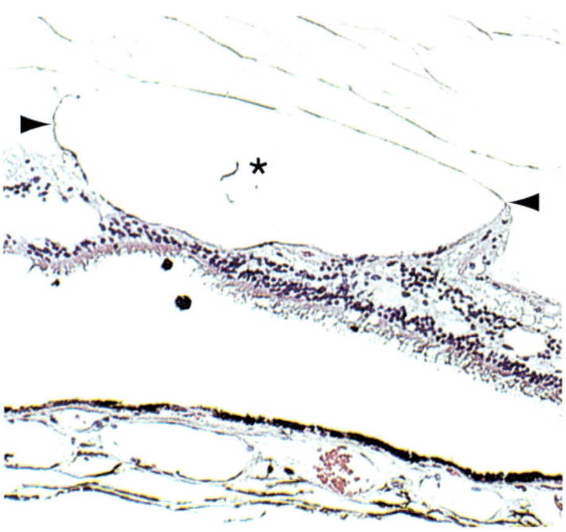
B

Figure 11-11 Retinal lattice degeneration. **A,** Lattice degeneration may present as prominent sclerotic vessels *(arrows)* in a wicker or lattice pattern. The clinical presentation has many variations. **B,** The vitreous directly over lattice degeneration is liquefied *(asterisk),* but formed vitreous remains adherent at the margins *(arrowheads)* of the degenerated area. The internal limiting membrane is discontinuous, and the inner retinal layers are atrophic.

lattice degeneration has the same histopathologic features as typical lattice degeneration but occurs more posteriorly along the course of retinal vessels.

Paving-Stone Degeneration

In contrast to retinal vascular occlusion, which leads to inner retinal ischemia, occlusion of the choriocapillaris can lead to loss of the outer retinal layers and RPE. This type of atrophy, called *cobblestone* or *paving-stone degeneration,* is very common in the retinal periphery. The well-demarcated, flat, pale lesions seen clinically correspond to circumscribed areas of outer retinal and RPE atrophy with adherence of the inner nuclear layer to the Bruch membrane (Fig 11-12).

Ischemia

There are many causes of retinal ischemia, including diabetes mellitus, retinal artery and vein occlusion, radiation retinopathy, retinopathy of prematurity, sickle cell retinopathy, vasculitis, and carotid occlusive disease. The specific aspects of some of these diseases are discussed later in the chapter. However, certain histopathologic findings are common to all the disorders that result in retinal ischemia. The retinal changes that occur with ischemia can be grouped into cellular responses and vascular responses.

Cellular responses

The neurons in the retina are highly active metabolically, requiring, on a per gram of tissue basis, large amounts of oxygen for production of adenosine triphosphate (ATP) (see also BCSC Section 2, *Fundamentals and Principles of Ophthalmology,* Part IV, Biochemistry and Metabolism). This makes them highly sensitive to interruption of their blood supply. With prolonged oxygen deprivation (greater than 90 minutes in experimental studies), the

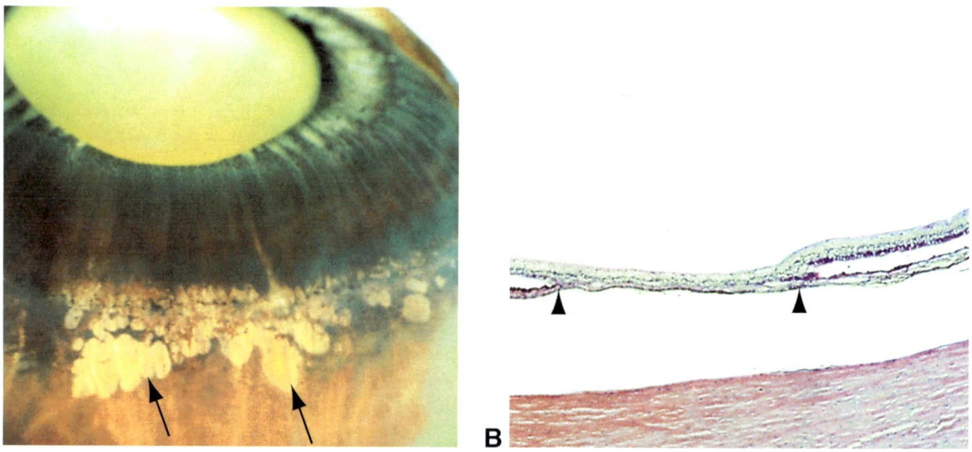

A B

Figure 11-12 **A,** Paving-stone degeneration appears as areas of depigmentation *(arrows)* in the periphery of the retina near the ora serrata. **B,** Histologically, paving-stone degeneration consists of atrophy of the outer retinal elements and chorioretinal adhesion to the remaining inner retinal elements. A sharp boundary *(arrowheads)* exists between normal and atrophic retina, corresponding to the clinical appearance of paving-stone degeneration.

neuronal cells become pyknotic; they are subsequently phagocytosed, and they disappear. The extent and the location of the area of atrophic retina resulting from ischemia depend on the size of the occluded vessel and on whether it is a retinal or a choroidal blood vessel. As described earlier, the retinal circulation supplies the inner retina, and the choroidal circulation supplies the outer retina and RPE. Infarctions of the retinal circulation lead to *inner ischemic retinal atrophy* (Fig 11-13), and infarctions of the choroidal circulation lead to *outer ischemic retinal atrophy* (Fig 11-14).

The neuronal cells of the retina have no capacity for regeneration after ischemic damage. Following ischemic damage to the nerve fibers of the ganglion cells, *cytoid bodies* (swollen axons) become apparent histologically (Fig 11-15). These are localized accumulations of axoplasmic material that are present in ischemic infarcts of the NFL. *Cotton-wool spots* are the clinical correlate of ischemic infarcts of the NFL that resolve over 4–12 weeks, leaving an area of inner ischemic atrophy.

Glial cells, like axons, degenerate in areas of infarction. Proliferation of the glial cells may occur adjacent to local areas of infarction or in areas of ischemia without infarction, resulting in a glial scar.

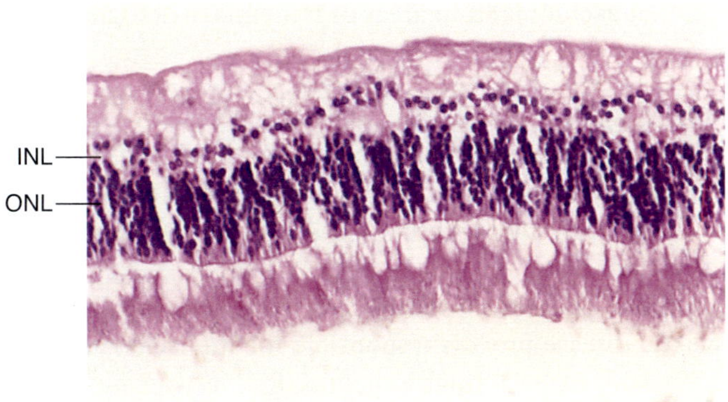

Figure 11-13 Inner retinal ischemia. The photoreceptor nuclei (outer nuclear layer, *ONL*) and the outer portion of the inner nuclear layer *(INL)* are identifiable. The inner portion of the inner nuclear layer is absent. There are no ganglion cells, and the NFL is absent. This pattern of ischemia corresponds to the supply of the retinal arteriolar circulation and may be observed in arterial and venular occlusions.

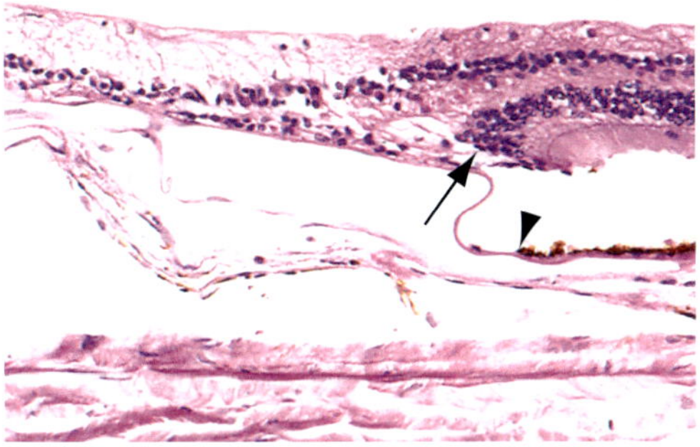

Figure 11-14 Begin at the right edge of the photograph and trace the ganglion cell and the inner nuclear layer toward the left. In this case, there is loss of the nuclei of the photoreceptor layer (outer nuclear layer, *arrow*), the photoreceptor inner and outer segments, and the RPE *(arrowhead)*. This is the pattern of outer retinal atrophy, secondary to interruption in the choroidal vascular blood supply. Compare with Figure 11-13.

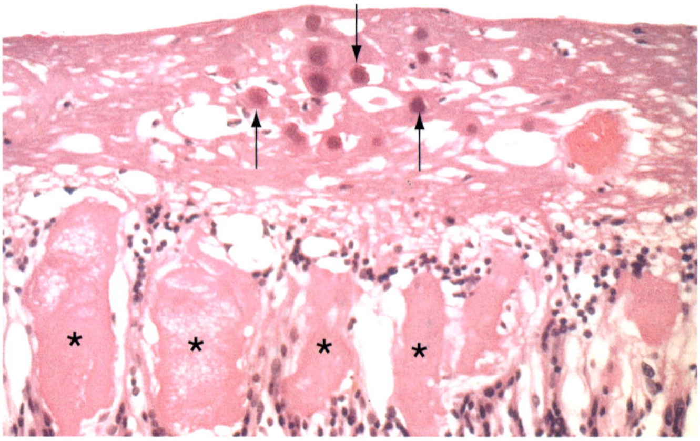

Figure 11-15 Cytoid bodies *(arrows)* within the NFL. Cystoid spaces *(asterisks)* are filled with proteinaceous fluid. *(Courtesy of W. Richard Green, MD.)*

Microglial cells are actually tissue macrophages rather than true glial cells. These cells are involved in the phagocytosis of necrotic cells as well as of extracellular material, such as lipid and blood, that accumulates in areas of ischemia. Microglial cells are fairly resistant to ischemia.

Vascular responses

Many of the vascular changes in retinal ischemia are mediated by vascular endothelial growth factor (VEGF). This growth factor is a potent mediator of vascular permeability and angiogenesis. It has been shown to play a role in numerous ocular conditions associated with vascularization.

In addition to those changes secondary to ischemia itself, vascular changes may be caused by the specific disease process responsible for the ischemia. Edema and hemorrhages are common with acute retinal ischemia. Retinal capillary closure, microaneurysms, lipid exudates, and neovascularization may develop with chronic retinal ischemia.

Edema, one of the earliest manifestations of retinal ischemia, is a result of transudation across the inner blood–retina barrier (Fig 11-16). Fluid and serum components accumulate in the extracellular space, and the fluid pockets are delimited by the surrounding neurons and glial cells. Exudate accumulating in the outer plexiform layer of the macula (Henle layer) produces a star figure because of the orientation of the nerve fibers in this layer (Fig 11-17). In cases of chronic edema, the extracellular deposits will become richer in protein and lipids, as the water component of the exudate is more efficiently removed, resulting in so-called *hard exudates.* Histologically, retinal exudates appear as eosinophilic, sharply circumscribed spaces within the retina (Fig 11-18). Chronic edema may result in intraretinal lipid deposits that are contained within the microglial cells.

Intravitreally administered triamcinolone acetonide (IVTA) and recently developed biologic agents inhibiting VEGF (pegaptanib, ranibizumab, and bevacizumab) are now being employed in the treatment of various retinal diseases associated with macular

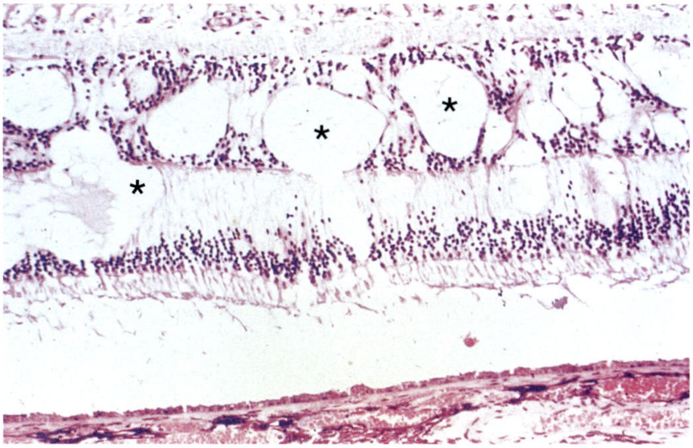

Figure 11-16 Cystoid spaces in inner nuclear and outer plexiform layers *(asterisks). (Courtesy of W. Richard Green, MD.)*

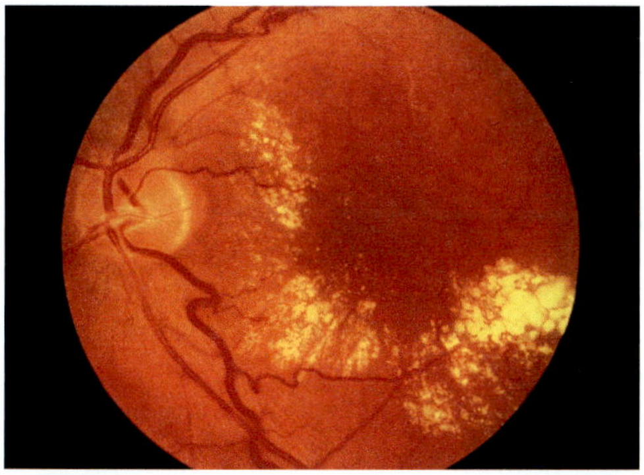

Figure 11-17 Intraretinal lipid deposits, or hard exudates. *(Courtesy of David J. Wilson, MD.)*

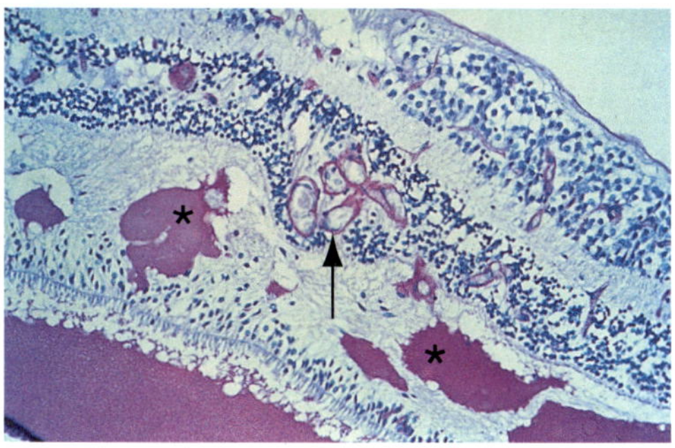

Figure 11-18 Intraretinal exudates *(asterisks)* surrounding intraretinal microvascular abnormalities *(arrow). (Courtesy of W. Richard Green, MD.)*

edema and choroidal neovascularization. Gain in visual acuity, which is mostly secondary to a decrease in macular edema, has been demonstrated in studies in which these treatments were used for such conditions as diabetic macular edema, central and branch retinal vein occlusions, uveitic macular edema, and retinal and choroidal neovascularization (Fig 11-19). Hypotheses regarding the mechanism of action of IVTA include an anti-inflammatory effect, inhibition of VEGF, improvement in diffusion, and reestablishment

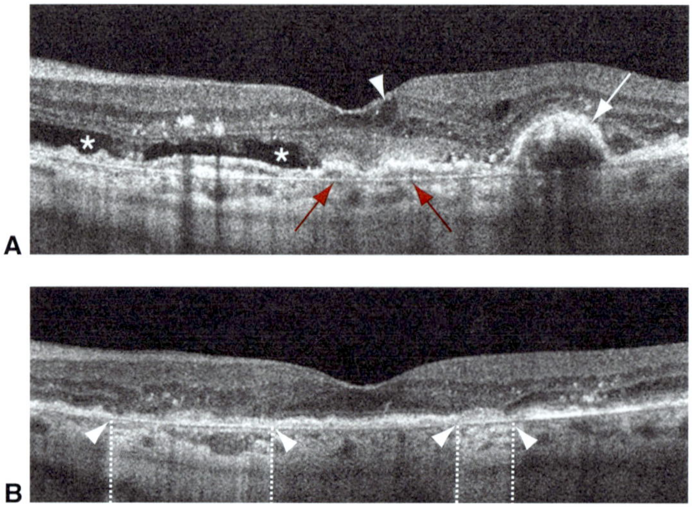

Figure 11-19 **A,** SD-OCT shows cystoid macular edema *(arrowhead),* subretinal fluid *(asterisks),* and irregular elevation and detachment of the RPE *(white arrow)* secondary to exudative age-related macular degeneration. Note the outer aspect of Bruch membrane *(red arrows).* **B,** SD-OCT after anti-vascular endothelial growth factor therapy shows resolution of the cystoid macular edema and detachment of the RPE. Focal areas of geographic atrophy of the RPE with attenuation of the photoreceptor cell layer are more apparent *(between arrowheads).* Note the hyperreflectivity *(between dashed lines)* in the choroid corresponding to the areas of geographic atrophy. *(Courtesy of Robert H. Rosa, Jr, MD.)*

of the blood–retina barrier through a reduction in permeability. VEGF inhibition in the eye arrests angiogenesis and reduces vascular permeability. Pegaptanib is an RNA aptamer (an oligonucleotide ligand) that binds specifically to the $VEGF_{165}$ isoform, thereby preventing receptor binding of the VEGF isoform. Ranibizumab is a recombinant humanized monoclonal antibody fragment, whereas bevacizumab is a full-length monoclonal antibody. Both ranibizumab and bevacizumab inhibit receptor binding of all isoforms of VEGF-A, which may explain the enhanced anatomical and visual effects that have been observed clinically with use of these agents.

Retinal hemorrhages also develop as a result of ischemic damage to the inner blood–retina barrier. As with edema and exudates, the shape of the hemorrhage conforms to the surrounding retinal tissue. Consequently, hemorrhages in the nerve fiber are flame-shaped, whereas those in the nuclear or inner plexiform layer are circular, or "dot and blot" (Fig 11-20). Subhyaloid and sub-ILM hemorrhages have a boat-shaped configuration. White-centered hemorrhages *(Roth spots)* may be present in a number of conditions. The white centers of the hemorrhages can have a number of causes, including aggregates of white blood cells, platelets, and fibrin; or they may be due to retinal light reflexes. Hemorrhages clear over a period of time ranging from days to months.

Chronic retinal ischemia leads to architectural changes in the retinal vessels. The capillary bed becomes acellular in an area of vascular occlusion. Adjacent to acellular areas, dilated irregular vascular channels known as *intraretinal microvascular abnormalities (IRMA)* and microaneurysms often appear (Figs 11-21, 11-22). *Microaneurysms* are

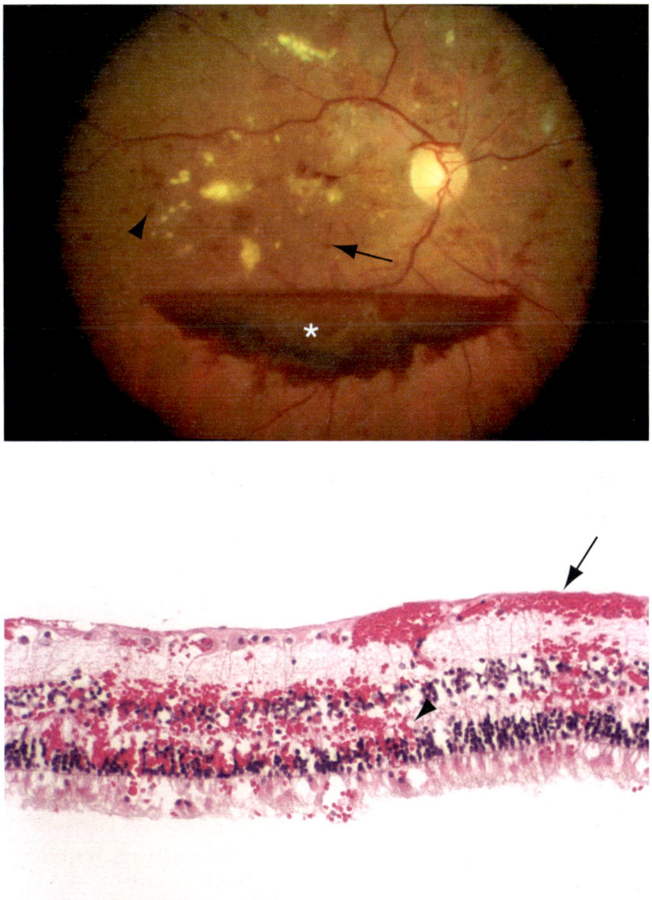

A

B

Figure 11-20 Intraretinal hemorrhage. **A,** Fundus photograph showing dot-and-blot *(arrowhead),* flame-shaped *(arrow),* and boat-shaped *(asterisk)* hemorrhages in diabetic retinopathy. **B,** Histologically, the dot-and-blot hemorrhage corresponds to blood in the middle layers (inner nuclear and outer plexiform layers) of the retina *(arrowhead).* The flame-shaped hemorrhage corresponds to blood in the NFL *(arrow),* and the boat-shaped hemorrhage corresponds to subhyaloid blood. *(Courtesy of Robert H. Rosa, Jr, MD.)*

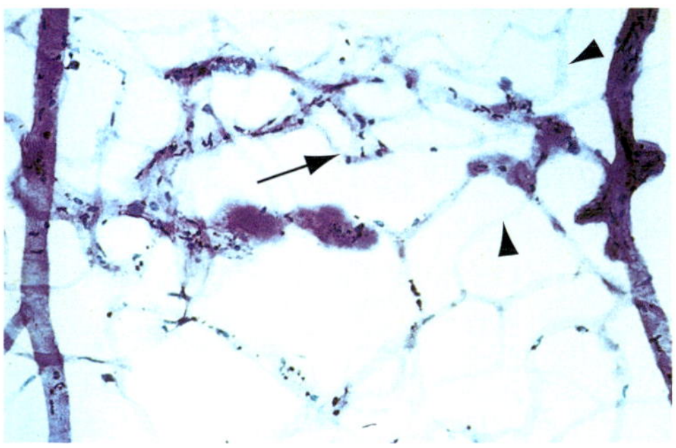

Figure 11-21 Trypsin digest preparation, illustrating acellular capillaries *(arrowheads)* adjacent to intraretinal microvascular abnormalities (IRMA, *arrow*). *(Courtesy of W. Richard Green, MD.)*

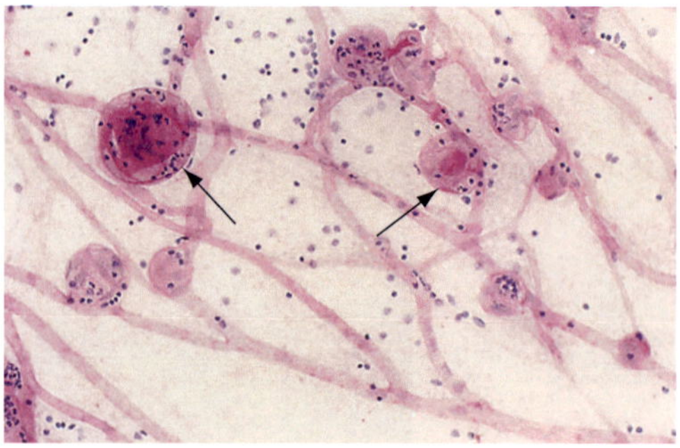

Figure 11-22 Retinal trypsin digest preparation, showing diabetic microaneurysms *(arrows).*

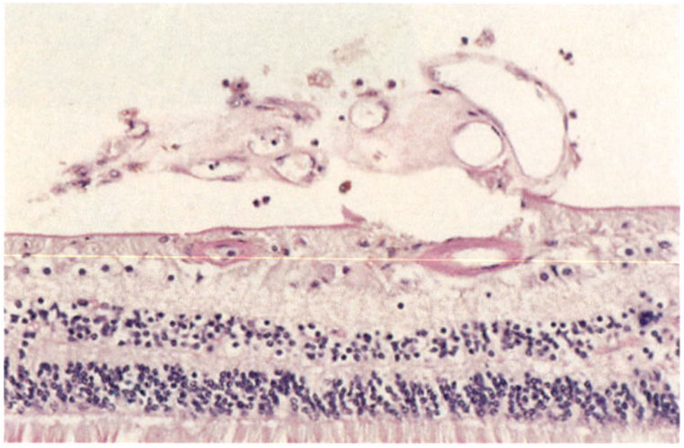

Figure 11-23 Retinal neovascularization. The new blood vessels have broken through the internal limiting membrane.

fusiform or saccular outpouchings of the retinal capillaries best seen clinically with fluorescein angiography and histologically with PAS-stained trypsin digest preparations (see Fig 11-22). The density of the endothelial cells lining the microaneurysms and IRMA is frequently variable. Microaneurysms evolve from thin-walled hypercellular microaneurysms to hyalinized, hypocellular microaneurysms.

In some cases of retinal ischemia, neovascularization of the retina and the vitreous may occur, most commonly in diabetes and central retinal vein occlusion. Retinal neovascularization generally consists of the growth of new vessels on the vitreous side of the ILM (Fig 11-23); only rarely does neovascularization occur within the retina itself. Hemorrhage may develop from retinal neovascularization as the associated vitreous exerts traction on the fragile new vessels. Retinal neovascularization should be distinguished from retinal collaterals and arteriovenous shunts, which represent dilation and increased flow in existing retinal vessels.

Specific Ischemic Retinal Disorders

Central and branch retinal artery and vein occlusions

Central retinal artery occlusions (CRAO) result from localized arteriosclerotic changes, an embolic event, and, in rare instances, vasculitis (as in temporal arteritis). As the retina becomes ischemic, it swells and loses its transparency. This swelling is best appreciated clinically and histologically in the posterior pole, where the NFL and the ganglion cell

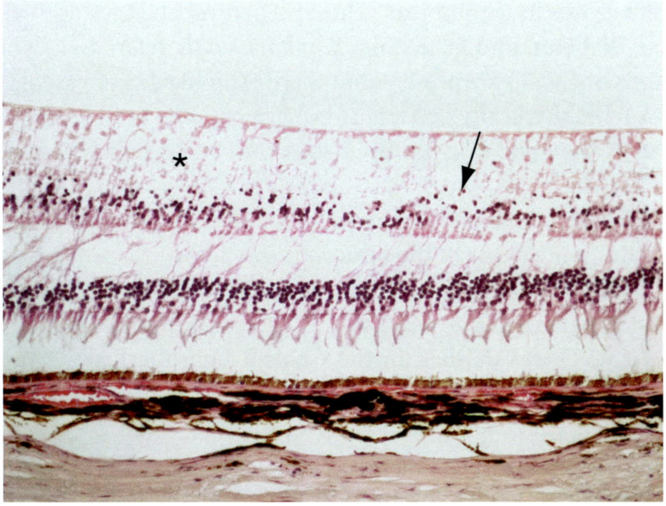

Figure 11-24 Acute central retinal artery occlusion. Histologically, necrosis occurs in the inner retina *(asterisk)* corresponding to the retinal whitening observed by ophthalmoscopic examination. Note the pyknotic nuclei *(arrow)* in the inner aspect of the inner nuclear layer. *(Courtesy of Robert H. Rosa, Jr, MD.)*

layer are the thickest (Fig 11-24). Because the ganglion cell layer and the NFL are thickest in the macula but absent in the fovea, the normal color of the choroid shows through in the fovea and produces a cherry-red spot, ophthalmoscopically suggesting CRAO. The retinal swelling eventually clears and leaves the classic histologic picture of inner ischemic atrophy (see Fig 11-13). Scarring and neovascularization following CRAO are rare.

Branch retinal artery occlusion (BRAO) is usually the result of emboli that lodge at the bifurcation of a retinal arteriole. *Hollenhorst plaques,* which are cholesterol emboli within retinal arterioles, seldom occlude the vessel. Emboli may be the first or most important clue to a significant systemic disorder such as carotid vascular disease (Hollenhorst plaques), cardiac valvular disease (calcific emboli), or thromboembolism (platelet-fibrin emboli).

The histology of the acute phase of BRAO is characterized by swelling of the inner retinal layers with the death of all nuclei. As the edema resolves, a classic picture emerges of inner ischemic atrophy in the distribution of the retina supplied by the occluded arteriole. The NFL, the ganglion cell layer, the inner plexiform layer, and the inner nuclear layer are affected (see Fig 11-13). Arteriolar occlusions result in infarcts with complete postnecrotic atrophy of the affected layers.

Central retinal vein occlusion (CRVO) occurs at the level of the lamina cribrosa. The pathophysiology of CRVO is the same as that of hemiretinal vein occlusion but different from that of branch retinal vein occlusion (see the following discussion). CRVOs develop as a result of structural changes in the central retinal artery and the lamina cribrosa that lead to compression of the central retinal vein. This compression creates turbulent flow in the vein and predisposes to thrombosis. These structural changes occur in arteriosclerosis, hypertension, diabetes, and glaucoma. *Papillophlebitis* refers to a condition in which the clinical features of CRVO are present, but there is no history of vascular disease. In this variant of CRVO, which typically occurs in younger patients (<50 years), inflammation of the retinal vessels at the optic disc has been shown to be a causative factor in retinal vein occlusion.

CRVO is recognized clinically by the presence of retinal hemorrhages in all 4 quadrants. Usually, prominent edema of the optic nerve head occurs, along with dilation of the retinal veins, variable numbers of cotton-wool spots, and macular edema. CRVO occurs in 2 forms: a milder, perfused type and a more severe, nonperfused type.

Nonperfused CRVO was defined in the Central Vein Occlusion Study (CVOS) as a CRVO in which greater than 10 disc areas showed nonperfusion on fluorescein angiography. Nonperfused CRVOs typically have extensive retinal edema and hemorrhage. Marked venular dilation and a variable number of cotton-wool spots are found.

Acute ischemic CRVO is characterized histologically by marked retinal edema; focal retinal necrosis; and subretinal, intraretinal, and preretinal hemorrhage. With long-standing CRVO, glial cells respond to the insult by replication and intracellular deposition of filaments *(gliosis).* The hemorrhage, hemosiderosis, disorganization of the retinal architecture, and gliosis seen in vein occlusions distinguish the final histologic picture from that seen in CRAO (Fig 11-25). Numerous microaneurysms are present in the retinal capillaries following CRVO, and acellular capillary beds are present to a variable degree. With time, dilated collateral vessels develop at the optic nerve head. Neovascularization of the iris is common following ischemic CRVO.

Branch retinal vein occlusion (BRVO) is a disorder in which occlusion of a tributary retinal vein occurs at the site of an arteriovenous crossing. At the crossing of a branch retinal artery and vein, the 2 vessels share a common adventitial sheath. With arteriosclerotic changes in the arteriole, the retinal venule may become compressed, leading to turbulent flow, which predisposes to thrombosis. This condition is more common in patients with arteriosclerosis and hypertension.

BRVO leads to retinal hemorrhages and cotton-wool spots. Because BRVO does not always result in total inner retinal ischemia and death of all tissue, neovascularization is unlikely unless the ischemia is extensive (>5 disc diameters). Findings in eyes with permanent vision loss from BRVO include CME, retinal nonperfusion, pigmentary macular disturbance, macular edema with hard lipid exudates, subretinal fibrosis, and epiretinal membrane formation.

The histologic picture of BRVO resembles that seen in CRVO but is localized to the area of the retina in the distribution of the occluded vein. Inner ischemic retinal atrophy is a characteristic late histologic finding in both retinal arterial and venous occlusions (see Fig 11-13). Numerous microaneurysms and dilated collateral vessels may be present. Acellular retinal capillaries are present to a variable degree, correlating with retinal capillary nonperfusion on fluorescein angiography.

Baseline and early natural history report. The Central Vein Occlusion Study. *Arch Ophthalmol.* 1993;111(8):1087–1095.

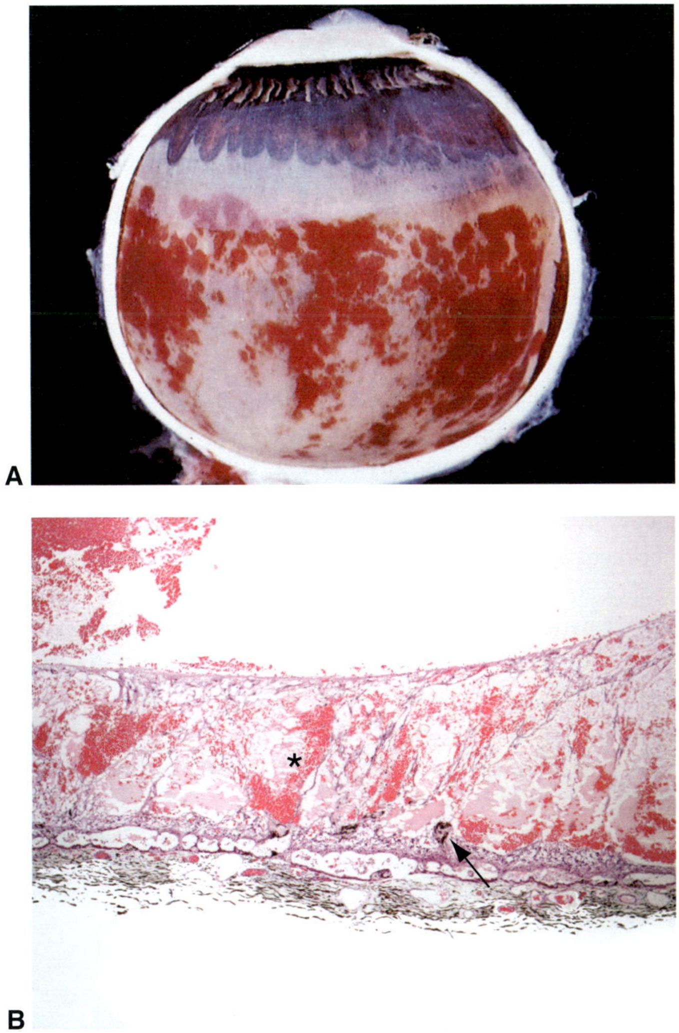

Figure 11-25 **A,** Diffuse retinal hemorrhage following CRVO. The damaged retina will be replaced by gliosis. **B,** Histology of long-standing CRVO shows loss of the normal lamellar architecture of the retina, marked edema with cystic spaces *(asterisk)* containing blood and proteinaceous exudate, vitreous hemorrhage, and nodular hyperplasia of the RPE *(arrow).* *(Part B courtesy of Robert H. Rosa, Jr, MD.)*

Diabetic Retinopathy

Diabetic retinopathy is 1 of the 4 most frequent causes of new blindness in the United States and the leading cause among 20- to 60-year-olds. Early in the course of diabetic retinopathy, certain physiologic abnormalities occur:

- impaired autoregulation of the retinal vasculature
- alterations in retinal blood flow
- breakdown of the blood–retina barrier

Histologically, the primary changes occur in the retinal microcirculation. These changes include

- thickening of the retinal capillary basement membrane
- selective loss of pericytes compared with retinal capillary endothelial cells
- microaneurysm formation (see Fig 11-22)
- retinal capillary closure (see Fig 11-21) (histologically recognized as acellular capillary beds)

Dilated intraretinal telangiectatic vessels, or intraretinal microvascular abnormalities (IRMA), may develop, as shown in Figure 11-21, and neovascularization may follow (see Fig 11-23). Intraretinal edema, hemorrhages, exudates, and microinfarcts of the inner retina may develop secondary to the primary retinal vascular changes. Acutely, microinfarcts of the inner retina (see Fig 11-15) are characterized clinically as cotton-wool spots. Subsequently, focal inner ischemic atrophy appears (see Fig 11-13).

Other histologic changes in diabetes

In diabetes, the corneal epithelial basement membrane is thickened. This change is associated with inadequate adherence of the epithelium to the underlying Bowman layer, predisposing diabetic patients to corneal abrasions and poor corneal epithelial healing. Lacy vacuolation of the iris pigment epithelium (Fig 11-26) occurs in association with hyperglycemia; histologically, the intraepithelial vacuoles contain glycogen (PAS-positive and diastase-sensitive). Histopathologically, thickening of the pigmented ciliary epithelial basement membrane (see Fig 11-26) is almost universally present in diabetic eyes. The incidence of cataract formation is increased.

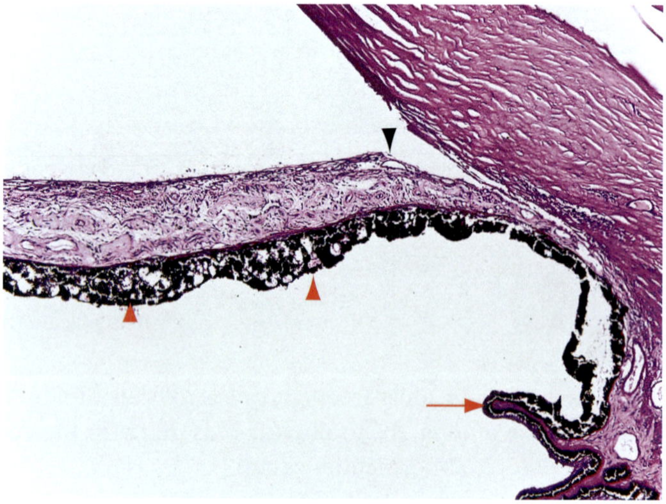

Figure 11-26 Photomicrograph showing iris neovascularization *(black arrowhead),* lacy vacuolation of the iris pigment epithelium *(red arrowheads),* and thickening of the basement membrane of the pigmented ciliary epithelium *(red arrow).* These histologic findings are typically found in the eyes of patients with diabetes. *(Courtesy of Tatyana Milman, MD.)*

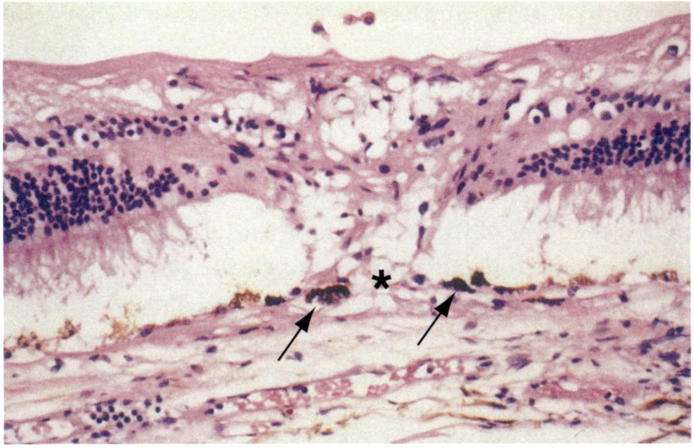

Figure 11-27 Laser photocoagulation scar characterized by absence of the RPE centrally *(asterisk)* with peripheral RPE hyperplasia *(arrows)* and loss of the photoreceptors, the outer nuclear layer, and a portion of the inner nuclear layer. *(Courtesy of David J. Wilson, MD.)*

Argon laser photocoagulation, used in diabetic retinopathy, results in variable destruction of the outer retina, destruction of the RPE, and occlusion of the choriocapillaris (Fig 11-27). These lesions heal by proliferation of the adjacent RPE and glial scarring.

Retinopathy of Prematurity

Retinal ischemia also plays a role in retinopathy of prematurity (ROP). This ischemia develops not because of the occlusion of existing vessels but rather because of the absence of retinal vessels in the incompletely developed retinal periphery. A decrease in retinal blood flow from oxygen-induced vasoconstriction may also be a contributing factor.

The clinical and histologic features of ROP are somewhat different from those present in other retinal ischemic states. Retinal edema and exudates do not develop. Retinal hemorrhages and retinal vascular dilation develop only in the most severe cases *(plus* or *rush disease)*. Neovascularization of the retina and vitreous may develop as a result of proliferation of new vessels at the border between the vascularized and avascular peripheral retina. Fibrovascular proliferation into the vitreous at this site may lead to tractional retinal detachment, macular heterotopia, and high myopia. See BCSC Section 6, *Pediatric Ophthalmology and Strabismus,* and Section 12, *Retina and Vitreous,* for a more detailed discussion.

Age-Related Macular Degeneration

Age-related macular degeneration (AMD) is the leading cause of new blindness in the United States. Although the etiology of AMD remains unknown, evidence suggests that both genes and environmental factors play a role in the disease pathogenesis. Genome-wide and candidate association studies have identified risk loci for AMD and implicated certain genes, including *CFH, C3, C2-CFB, CFI, HTRA1/LOC387715/ARMS2, CTEP, TIMP3, LIPC, VEGFA, COL10A1, TNFRSF10A,* and *APOE.* Increasing age, cigarette smoking, positive family history, and cardiovascular disease increase the risk of developing AMD. In addition, randomized clinical trials showing the benefit of antioxidant supplementation in AMD provide support for the role of oxidative stress in progression of the disease. See BCSC Section 12, *Retina and Vitreous,* for additional discussion.

Several characteristic changes in the retina, RPE, Bruch membrane, and choroid occur in AMD. Perhaps the first detectable pathologic change is the appearance of deposits between the basement membrane of the RPE and the elastic portion of the Bruch membrane (basal linear deposits) and similar deposits between the plasma membrane of the RPE and the basement membrane of the RPE (basal laminar deposits). These deposits are not clinically visible and may require electron microscopy to be distinguished. In advanced cases, these deposits may become confluent and can be seen at the light microscopic level (Fig 11-28). This appearance has been described as *diffuse drusen.*

The first clinically detectable feature of AMD is the appearance of drusen. The clinical term *drusen* has been correlated pathologically to large PAS-positive deposits between the RPE and Bruch membrane. Many eyes with clinically apparent drusen (especially soft drusen) are found to have basal laminar and/or basal linear deposits and diffuse drusen on histologic analysis. Drusen, which may be transient, have been classified clinically as follows:

- *hard (hyaline) drusen:* the typical discrete, yellowish lesions that are PAS-positive nodules composed of hyaline material between the RPE and Bruch membrane (Fig 11-29)

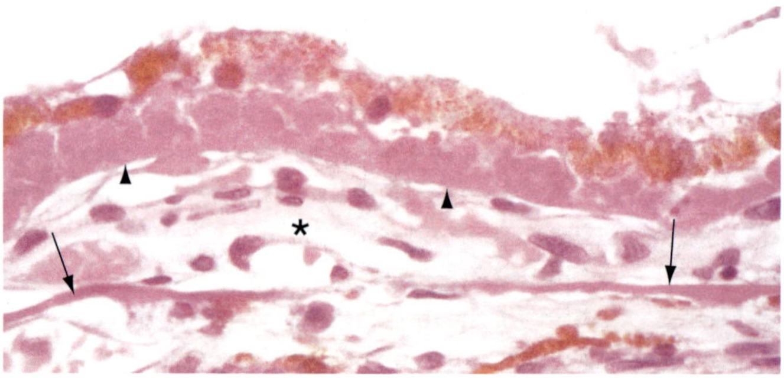

Figure 11-28 Diffuse drusen. There is diffuse deposition of eosinophilic material *(arrowheads)* beneath the RPE. Choroidal neovascularization *(asterisk)* is present between the diffuse drusen and the elastic portion of the Bruch membrane *(arrows). (Courtesy of Hans E. Grossniklaus, MD.)*

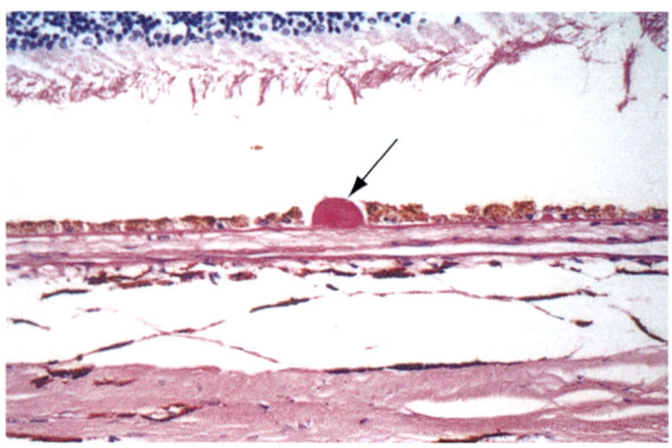

Figure 11-29 Hard drusen *(arrow).* Note the periodic acid–Schiff staining of the dome-shaped, nodular, hard druse. *(Reproduced with permission from Spraul CW, Grossniklaus HE. Characteristics of drusen and Bruch's membrane in postmortem eyes with age-related macular degeneration.* Arch Ophthalmol. *1997;115(2):267–273. © 1997, American Medical Association.)*

- *soft drusen:* drusen with amorphous, poorly demarcated boundaries, usually >63 µm in size; histologically, they represent cleavage of the RPE and basal laminar or linear deposits from the Bruch membrane (Fig 11-30)
- *basal laminar or cuticular drusen:* diffuse, small, regular, and nodular deposits of drusenlike material in the macula
- *calcific drusen:* sharply demarcated, glistening, refractile lesions usually associated with RPE atrophy

Photoreceptor atrophy occurs to a variable degree in macular degeneration. It is not clear whether this atrophy is a primary abnormality of the photoreceptors or is secondary to the underlying changes in the RPE and Bruch membrane. In addition to photoreceptor atrophy, large zones of RPE atrophy may appear (Fig 11-31). When this occurs centrally, it is termed *geographic atrophy* (formerly, *central areolar atrophy of the RPE*). Drusen, photoreceptor atrophy, and RPE atrophy may all be present to varying degrees in *dry,* or *non-exudative, AMD.*

Eyes with choroidal neovascularization *(neovascular, wet,* or *exudative AMD)* have fibrovascular tissue present between the inner and outer layers of the Bruch membrane, beneath the RPE, or in the subretinal space (Fig 11-32). The new blood vessels leak fluid and may rupture easily, producing the exudative consequences of neovascular AMD, including macular edema, serous retinal detachment, and subretinal and intraretinal hemorrhages. VEGF inhibition achieved with intravitreally administered anti-VEGF agents (pegaptanib, ranibizumab, or bevacizumab) has been shown to reduce the macular edema, slow the progression of the choroidal neovascularization, and improve the visual outcomes of patients with neovascular AMD (also see the section "Vascular responses").

Subretinal choroidal neovascular membranes have been classified as type 1 or type 2, based on their pathologic and clinical features. *Type 1 neovascularization* (Fig 11-32A) is typically associated with the presence of basal laminar deposits and diffuse drusen and characterized by neovascularization within the Bruch membrane in the sub-RPE space. In this type of neovascularization, the RPE is often abnormally oriented or absent across a broad expanse of the inner portion of Bruch membrane. *Type 2 neovascularization* (Fig 11-32B) occurs in the subretinal space and generally features only a small defect in

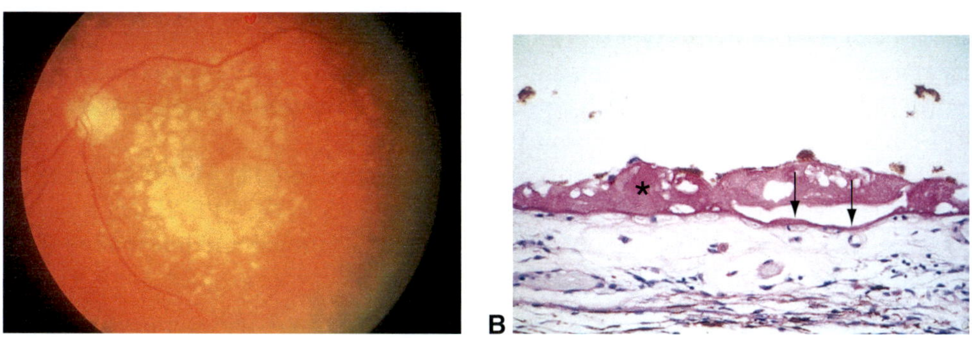

A B

Figure 11-30 **A,** Clinical photograph of multiple confluent drusen. **B,** Thick eosinophilic deposits *(asterisk)* between the RPE and the elastic portion *(arrows)* of Bruch membrane. *(Reproduced with permission from Spraul CW, Grossniklaus HE. Characteristics of drusen and Bruch's membrane in postmortem eyes with age-related macular degeneration.* Arch Ophthalmol. *1997;115(2):267–273. © 1997, American Medical Association.)*

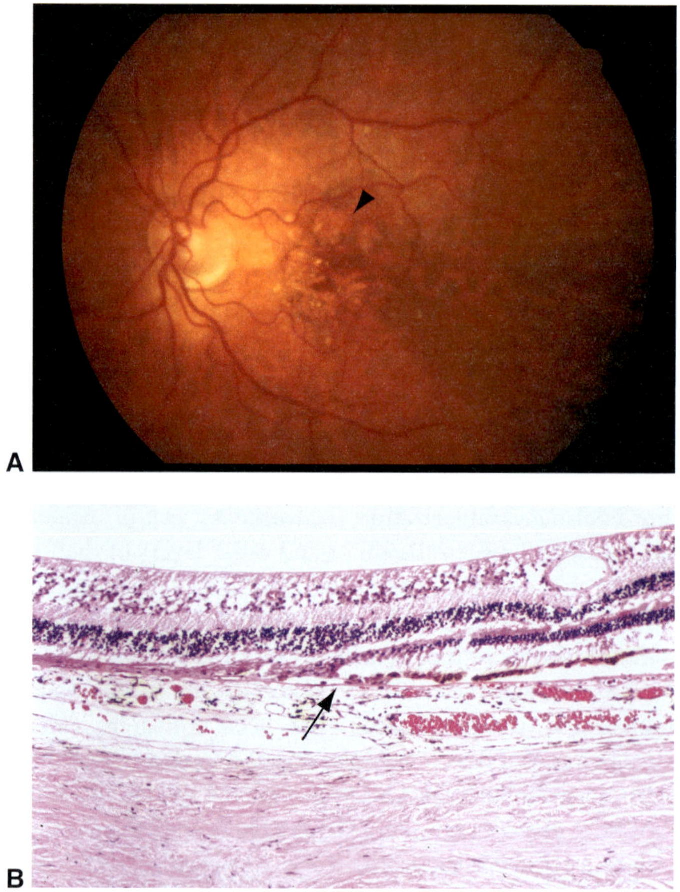

Figure 11-31 Geographic atrophy of the RPE. **A,** Fundus photograph shows focal geographic atrophy of the RPE *(arrowhead)* and drusen in nonexudative AMD. **B,** Histologically, there is loss of the photoreceptor cell layer, RPE, and choriocapillaris *(left of arrow)* with an abrupt transition zone *(arrow)* to a more normal-appearing retina/RPE *(right of arrow)*. Note the thickened ganglion cell layer identifying the macular region. *(Courtesy of Robert H. Rosa, Jr, MD.)*

which the RPE is abnormally oriented or absent. Type 1 neovascularization is more characteristic of AMD, whereas type 2 is more characteristic of ocular histoplasmosis. Type 2 membranes are more amenable to surgical removal than are type 1 membranes because native RPE would be excised with a type 1 membrane, leaving an atrophic lesion (without RPE) in the area of membrane excision.

Surgically excised choroidal neovascular membranes (see Fig 11-32) are composed of vascular channels, RPE, and various other components of the RPE–Bruch membrane complex, including photoreceptor outer segments, basal laminar and linear deposits, hyperplastic RPE, and inflammatory cells.

Grossniklaus HE, Gass JD. Clinicopathologic correlations of surgically excised type 1 and type 2 submacular choroidal neovascular membranes. *Am J Ophthalmol.* 1998;126(1):59–69.

Grossniklaus HE, Miskala PH, Green WR, et al. Histopathologic and ultrastructural features of surgically excised subfoveal choroidal neovascular lesions: submacular surgery trials report no. 7. *Arch Ophthalmol.* 2005;123(7):914–921.

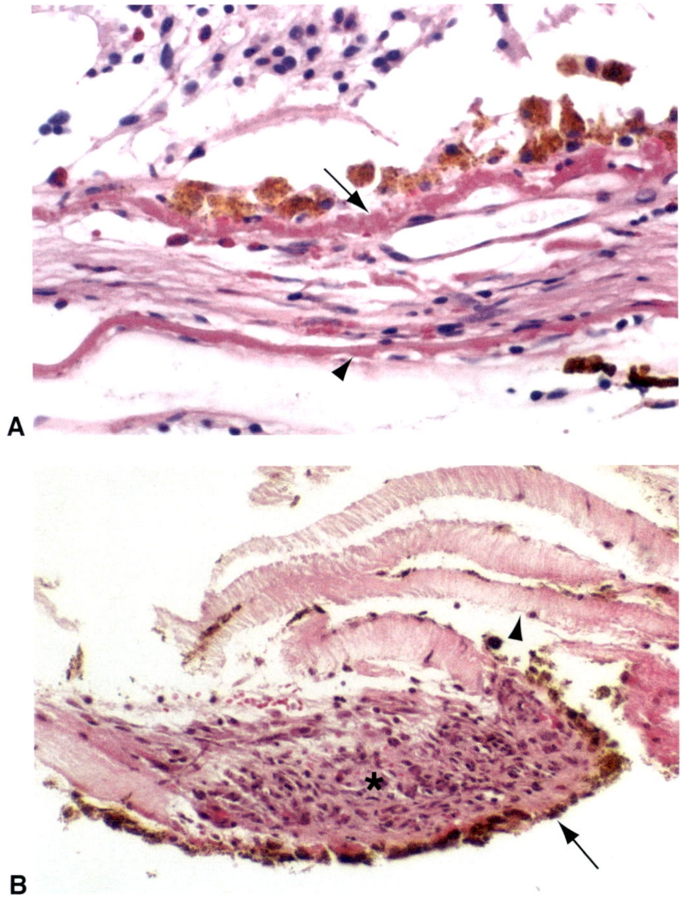

Figure 11-32 **A,** Choroidal neovascularization (CNV) located between the inner *(arrow)* and outer *(arrowhead)* layers of Bruch membrane (sub-RPE, type 1 CNV). Note loss of the overlying photoreceptor inner and outer segments, RPE hyperplasia, and the PAS-positive basal laminar deposit *(arrow).* **B,** Surgically excised CNV (subretinal, type 2 CNV) composed of fibrovascular tissue *(asterisk)* lined externally by RPE *(arrow)* with adherent photoreceptor outer segments *(arrowhead). (Courtesy of Robert H. Rosa, Jr, MD.)*

Ratnapriya R, Chew EY. Age-related macular degeneration—clinical review and genetics update. *Clin Genet.* 2013;84(2):160–166.

Polypoidal Choroidal Vasculopathy

Polypoidal choroidal vasculopathy (PCV), previously described as *posterior uveal bleeding syndrome* and *multiple recurrent serosanguineous RPE detachments,* is a disorder in which dilated, thin-walled vascular channels (Figs 11-33, 11-34), apparently arising from the short posterior ciliary arteries, penetrate into the Bruch membrane. Associated choroidal neovascularization is often present in these lesions, as observed in several histologic specimens.

Rosa RH Jr, Davis JL, Eifrig CW. Clinicopathologic reports, case reports, and small case series: clinicopathologic correlation of idiopathic polypoidal choroidal vasculopathy. *Arch Ophthalmol.* 2002;120(4):502–508.

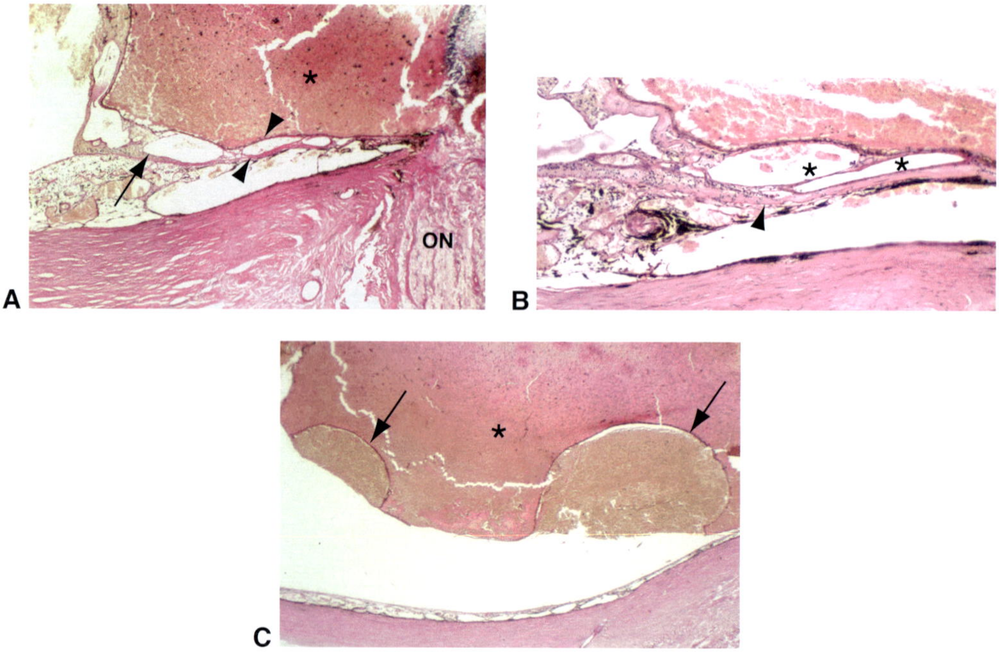

Figure 11-33 Polypoidal choroidal vasculopathy (PCV). **A,** Peripapillary dilated vascular channels *(arrow)* between the RPE and outer aspect of Bruch membrane *(arrowheads).* Note the dense subretinal hemorrhage *(asterisk). ON* = optic nerve. **B,** Higher-power view of thin-walled vascular channels *(asterisks)* interposed between the RPE and Bruch membrane *(arrowhead).* **C,** Hemorrhagic RPE detachments *(arrows)* and serosanguineous subretinal fluid *(asterisk).* *(Courtesy of Robert H. Rosa, Jr, MD.)*

Macular Dystrophies

See BCSC Section 12, *Retina and Vitreous,* for additional discussion of the following topics.

Fundus flavimaculatus and Stargardt disease

Fundus flavimaculatus and Stargardt disease are thought to represent 2 ends of the spectrum of a disease process characterized by yellowish flecks at the level of the RPE, a generalized vermilion (reddish) color to the fundus on clinical examination, a dark choroid on fluorescein angiography (Fig 11-35A, B; see also Figs 12-7 and 12-8 in BCSC Section 12, *Retina and Vitreous*), and gradually decreasing visual acuity. The inheritance pattern is generally autosomal recessive, but autosomal dominant forms have been reported as well. Several genetic mutations have been observed in patients with a Stargardt-like phenotype, including the *ABCA4, STGD4, ELOV4,* and *RDS/peripherin* genes. Mutations in *ABCA4* are responsible for most cases of Stargardt disease. The *ABCA4* gene encodes a protein called RIM protein, which is a member of the adenosine triphosphate (ATP)-binding cassette transporter family. It is expressed in the rims of rod and cone photoreceptor disc membranes and is involved in the transport of vitamin A derivatives to the RPE. The most striking feature of Stargardt disease on light and electron microscopy is the marked engorgement of RPE cells (Fig 11-35C, D; see also Fig 12-9 in BCSC Section 12, *Retina and Vitreous*) with lipofuscin-like, PAS-positive material, with apical displacement of the normal RPE melanin granules.

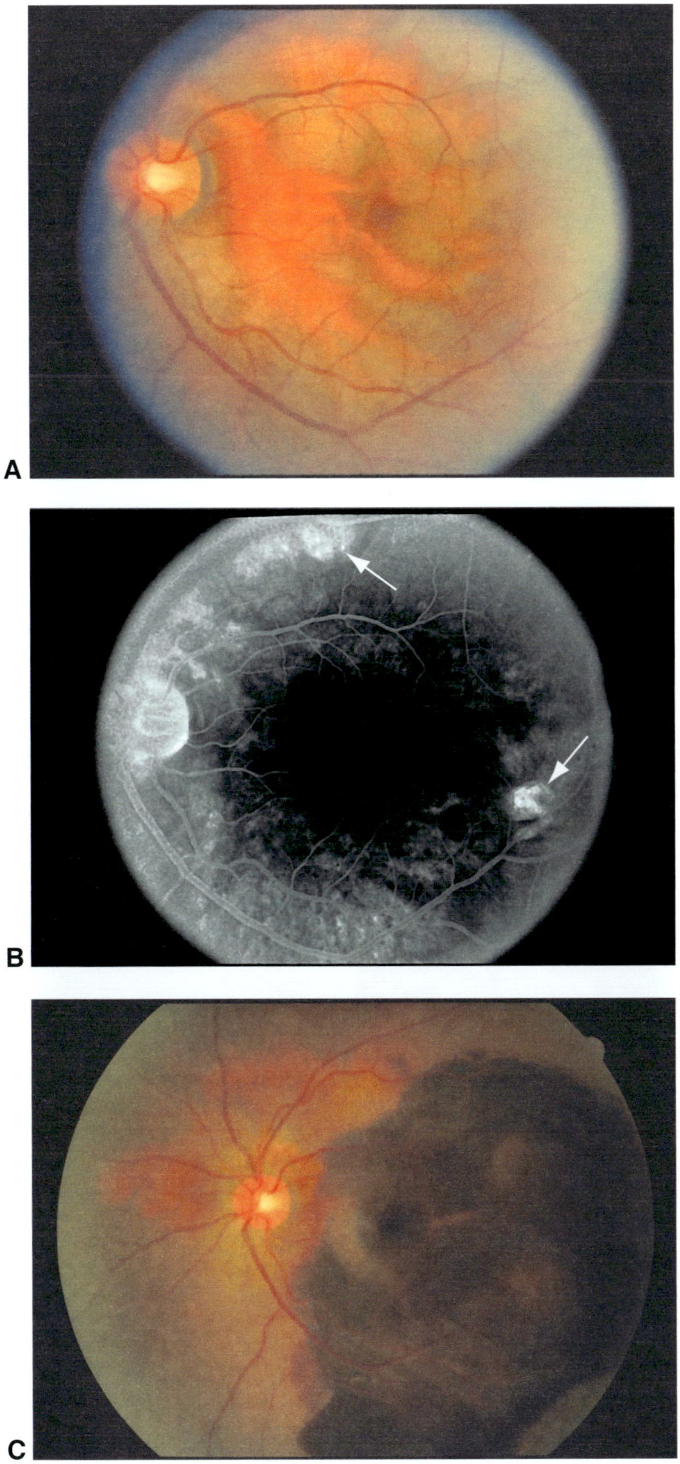

Figure 11-34 Polypoidal choroidal vasculopathy (PCV). **A,** Elevated, red-orange nodular and tubular lesions in the peripapillary and macular regions. **B,** Late fluorescein angiogram (860 seconds) shows hyperfluorescent polypoidal lesions *(arrows)* without apparent leakage. **C,** Dense subretinal hemorrhage in same patient as in **A** and **B.** Note the persistent red-orange lesions nasal and superior to the optic disc. *(Courtesy of Robert H. Rosa, Jr, MD.)*

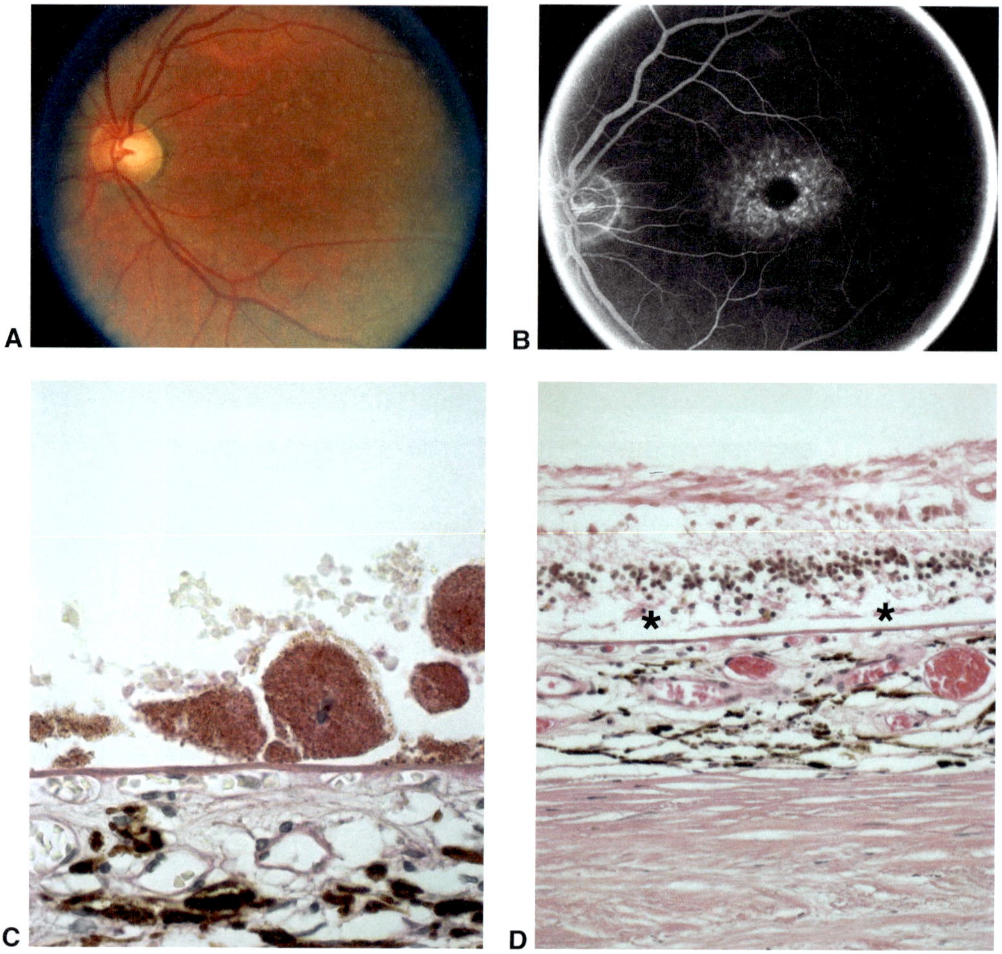

Figure 11-35 Stargardt disease. **A,** Fundus photograph shows characteristic retinal flecks and pigment mottling in the macular region. **B,** Fluorescein angiogram (midphase) shows late hyperfluorescence in a "bull's-eye" pattern in the central macula. Note the dark choroid (eg, absence of normal background choroidal blush), which is characteristic of Stargardt disease. **C,** Histology with periodic acid–Schiff (PAS) stain discloses hypertrophic RPE cells with numerous PAS-positive cytoplasmic granules containing lipofuscin. This histopathologic finding corresponds to the retinal flecks seen clinically. **D,** In advanced stages of Stargardt disease, geographic RPE atrophy with loss of the photoreceptor cell layer *(asterisks)* may be observed. *(Courtesy of Sander Dubovy, MD.)*

Best disease

Best disease, or Best vitelliform macular dystrophy, is a dominantly inherited, early-onset macular degenerative disease that exhibits some histopathologic similarities to AMD. The diagnosis of Best disease is based on the presence of a vitelliform (resembling the yolk of an egg) lesion (see Fig 12-10 in BCSC Section 12, *Retina and Vitreous*) or pigmentary changes in the central macula and a reduced ratio of the light peak to dark trough in the electro-oculogram. Mutations in the *VMD2* gene on chromosome 11 (11q13) encoding the bestrophin protein have been identified in Best disease. The gene product, bestrophin, localizes to the basolateral plasma membrane of the RPE and represents a family of chloride ion channels. Investigators have reported that bestrophins are volume-sensitive and may play a role in cell volume regulation in the RPE cells.

Fischmeister R, Hartzell HC. Volume sensitivity of the bestrophin family of chloride channels. *J Physiol.* 2005;562(Pt 2):477–491.

Marmorstein AD, Marmorstein LY, Rayborn M, Wang X, Hollyfield JG, Petrukhin K. Bestrophin, the product of the Best vitelliform macular dystrophy gene (VMD2), localizes to the basolateral plasma membrane of the retinal pigment epithelium. *Proc Natl Acad Sci USA.* 2000;97(23):12758–12763.

Pattern dystrophies

The term *pattern dystrophies* refers to a heterogeneous group of inherited macular disorders characterized by varying patterns of pigment deposition in the macula at the level of the RPE. Recognized pattern dystrophies include butterfly-shaped pattern dystrophy (BPD), adult-onset foveomacular vitelliform dystrophy (AFMVD), reticular dystrophy, and fundus pulverulentus. BPD is characterized by a butterfly-shaped, irregular, depigmented lesion at the level of the RPE. AFMVD is characterized by the presence of slightly elevated, symmetric, round to oval, yellow lesions at the level of the RPE, which are typically smaller than the vitelliform lesion characteristic of Best disease (Fig 11-36). Optical coherence tomography (OCT) has demonstrated elevation of the photoreceptor layer, with localization of the dystrophic material between the photoreceptors and RPE. The most common genetic mutation associated with the pattern dystrophies is in the *RDS/peripherin* gene. Histologic studies reveal central loss of the RPE and photoreceptor cell layer, with a moderate number of pigment-containing macrophages in the subretinal space and outer neurosensory retina (see Fig 11-36). To either side, the RPE is distended with lipofuscin. Basal laminar and linear deposits are present throughout the macular region. The pathologic finding of pigment-containing cells with lipofuscin in the subretinal space correlates clinically with the vitelliform appearance. See BCSC Section 12, *Retina and Vitreous,* for further discussion.

Dubovy SR, Hairston RJ, Schatz H, et al. Adult-onset foveomacular pigment epithelial dystrophy: clinicopathologic correlation of three cases. *Retina.* 2000;20(6):638–649.

Diffuse Photoreceptor Dystrophies

Inherited dystrophies affecting the rods and cones are discussed in greater detail elsewhere in the BCSC (see BCSC Section 12, *Retina and Vitreous*). Only the most common diffuse photoreceptor dystrophy, retinitis pigmentosa, is discussed here.

Retinitis pigmentosa (RP) is a group of inherited retinal diseases characterized by photoreceptor and RPE dysfunction resulting in progressive visual field loss. The genetics of RP are complex. It can be sporadic, autosomal dominant, autosomal recessive, or X-linked. Mutations in the rhodopsin gene *(RHO)* are the most common cause of autosomal dominant RP. Ophthalmoscopic findings include pigment arranged in a bone spicule–like configuration around the retinal arterioles, arteriolar narrowing, and optic

A

B

C

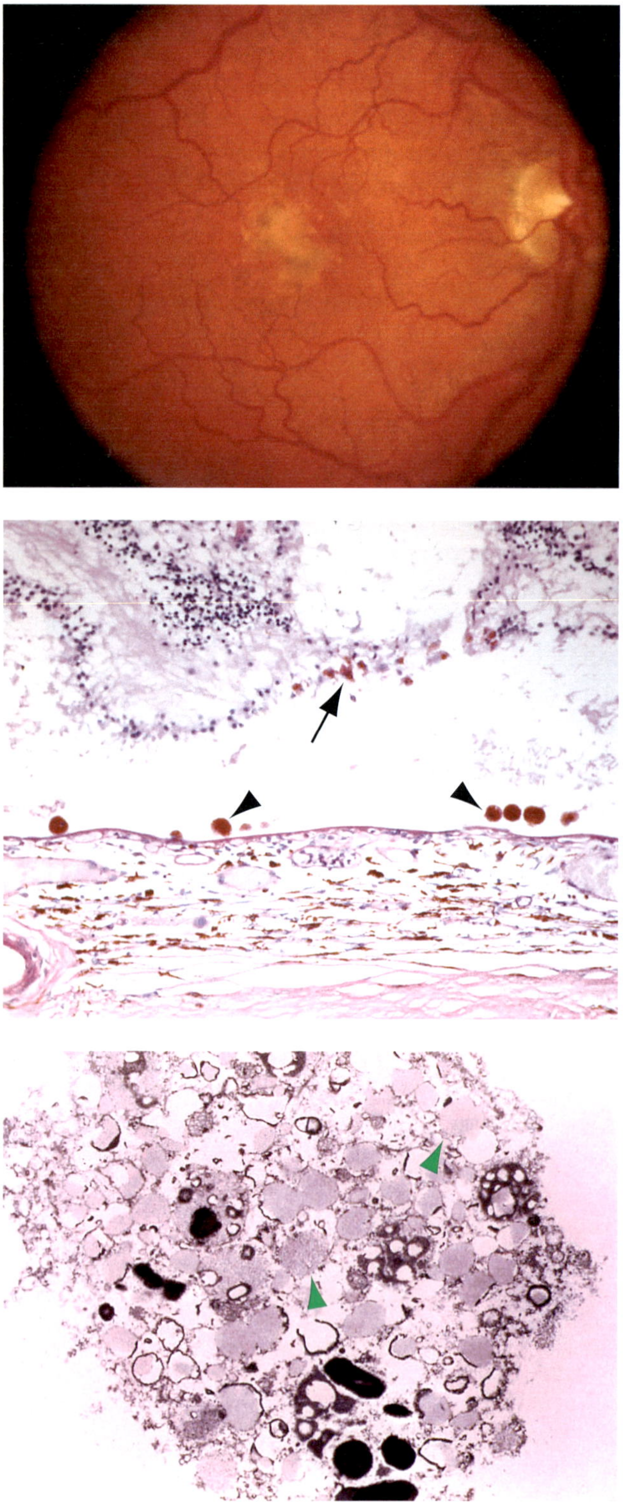

Figure 11-36 Adult-onset foveomacular vitelliform dystrophy. **A,** Yellowish, egg yolk–like lesion in the central macula. **B,** Histologic findings include pigment-containing cells in the subretinal space *(arrowheads)* and outer neurosensory retina *(arrow)*. **C,** Electron microscopy shows pigment-containing cells filled with lipofuscin *(arrowheads)*. *(Courtesy of Sander Dubovy, MD.)*

disc atrophy (Fig 11-37A). The disease is characterized primarily by the loss of rod photoreceptor cells by apoptosis. Cones are seldom directly affected by the identified mutations; however, they degenerate secondarily to rods. The term *retinitis pigmentosa* is a misnomer, because clear evidence of inflammation is lacking. Microscopically, photoreceptor cell loss occurs, as well as RPE hyperplasia with migration into the retina around retinal vessels (Fig 11-37B). The arterioles, though narrowed clinically, show no histologic abnormality initially. Later, thickening and hyalinization of the vessel walls appear. The optic nerve may show diffuse or sectoral atrophy, with gliosis as a late change.

Ben-Arie-Weintrob Y, Berson EL, Dryja TP. Histopathologic-genotypic correlations in retinitis pigmentosa and allied diseases. *Ophthalmic Genet.* 2005;26(2):91–100.

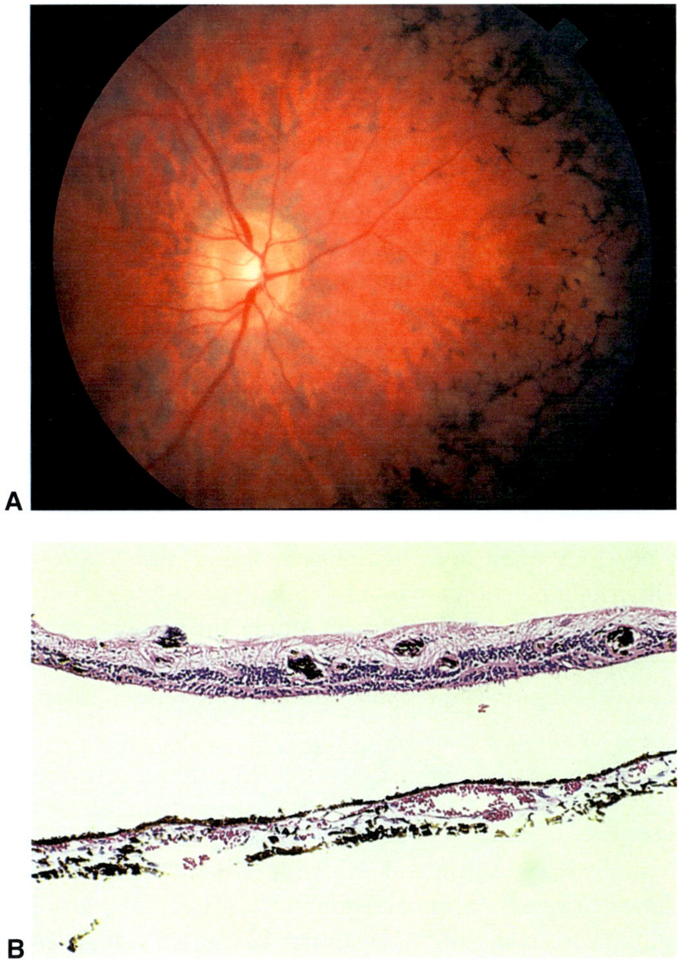

Figure 11-37 Retinitis pigmentosa. **A,** Fundus photograph shows mild optic disc atrophy, marked retinal arteriolar narrowing, and bone-spicule pigmentation in the fundus. **B,** Histologically, note the marked photoreceptor cell loss and RPE pigment migration into the retina in a perivascular distribution, corresponding to the bone spicule–like pattern seen clinically. The retina is artifactitiously detached. *(Part A courtesy of Robert H. Rosa, Jr, MD.)*

Neoplasia

Retinoblastoma

Retinoblastoma is the most common primary intraocular malignancy in childhood, occurring in 1 in 14,000–20,000 live births; the incidence varies slightly from country to country. Chapter 19 in this volume discusses retinoblastoma at length, from a more clinical point of view. Several other volumes of the BCSC cover various aspects of this topic as well; consult the *Master Index*. For American Joint Committee on Cancer (AJCC) definitions and staging of retinoblastoma, see the appendix at the back of this text.

Pathogenesis

Although retinoblastoma was once considered to be of glial origin (lesions clinically simulating retinoblastoma were formerly called *pseudogliomas*), the neuroblastic origin of this tumor from the nucleated layers of the retina has been well established. Immunohistochemical studies have demonstrated that tumor cells stain positive for neuron-specific enolase, rod–outer segment photoreceptor–specific S antigen, and rhodopsin. Tumor cells also secrete an extracellular substance known as *interphotoreceptor retinoid-binding protein,* a product of normal photoreceptors. Retinoblastoma tumor cells grown in culture have been shown to express a red and a green photopigment gene, as well as cone cell alpha subunits of transducin. These findings further support the concept that retinoblastoma may be a neoplasm of cone cell lineage. However, immunohistochemical and molecular studies cast some doubt on the hypothesis that a single cell type is the progenitor of retinoblastoma. The presence of small amounts of glial tissue within retinoblastoma suggests that tumor cells may possess the ability to differentiate into astroglia or that the resident glial cells proliferate in response to primary neoplastic cells.

The so-called *retinoblastoma gene,* localized to the long arm of chromosome 13, is deceptively named, as it does not actively cause retinoblastoma. The normal gene *suppresses* the development of retinoblastoma (and possibly other tumors, such as osteosarcoma). Retinoblastoma develops when both homologous loci of the suppressor gene become nonfunctional either by a deletion error or by mutation. Although 1 normal gene is sufficient to suppress the development of retinoblastoma, the presence of 1 normal gene and 1 abnormal gene is apparently an unstable situation that may lead to mutation in the normal gene and the loss of tumor suppression, thus allowing retinoblastoma to develop.

Dryja TP, Cavenee W, White R, et al. Homozygosity of chromosome 13 in retinoblastoma. *N Engl J Med.* 1984;310(9):550–553.

Histologic features

Histologically, retinoblastoma consists of cells with round, oval, or spindle-shaped nuclei that are approximately twice the size of a lymphocyte (Fig 11-38). Nuclei are hyperchromatic and surrounded by an almost imperceptible amount of cytoplasm. Mitotic activity is usually high, although pyknotic nuclei may make this difficult to assess. As tumors expand into the vitreous or subretinal space, they frequently outgrow their blood supply, creating a characteristic pattern of necrosis with the formation of pseudorosettes (viable

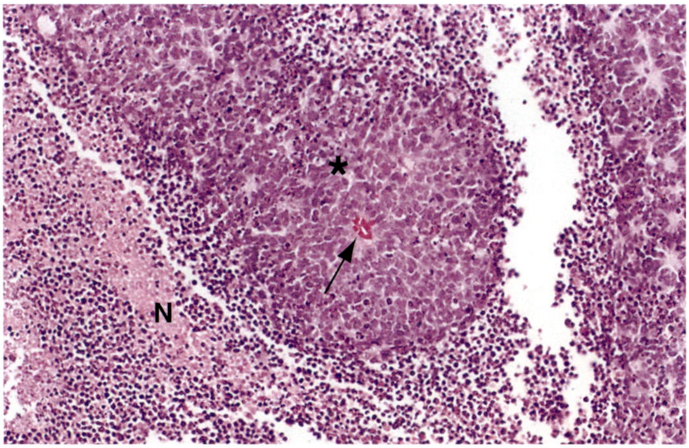

Figure 11-38 Retinoblastoma. Note the viable tumor cells *(asterisk)* surrounding a blood vessel *(arrow)* and the alternating zones of necrosis *(N)*. This histologic arrangement is referred to as a *pseudorosette*.

tumor cells surrounding a blood vessel); calcification is a common finding in areas of necrosis (Fig 11-39). Cuffs of viable cells course along blood vessels with regions of ischemic necrosis beginning 90–120 μm from nutrient vessels. DNA released from necrotic cells may be detected within tumor vessels and within blood vessels in tissues remote from the tumor, such as the iris. Neovascularization of the iris can complicate retinoblastoma (Fig 11-40).

Cells shed from retinoblastoma tumors remain viable in the vitreous and subretinal space, and they may eventually give rise to implants throughout the eye. It may be difficult

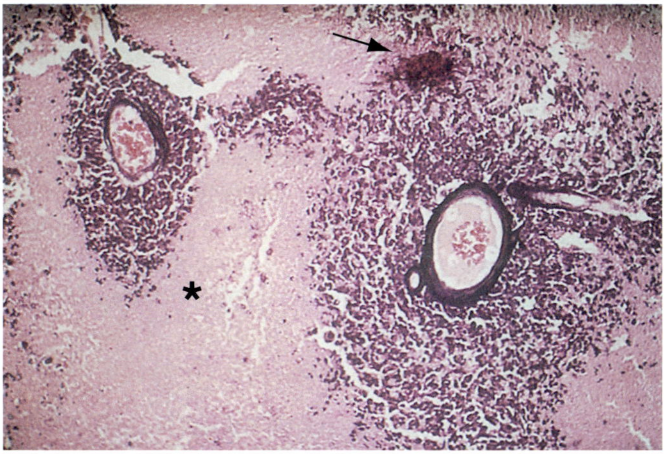

Figure 11-39 Retinoblastoma. Zones of viable tumor (usually surrounding blood vessels) alternate with zones of tumor necrosis *(asterisk)*. Calcium *(arrow)* is present in the necrotic area. The basophilic material surrounding the blood vessels is DNA, presumably liberated from the necrotic tumor.

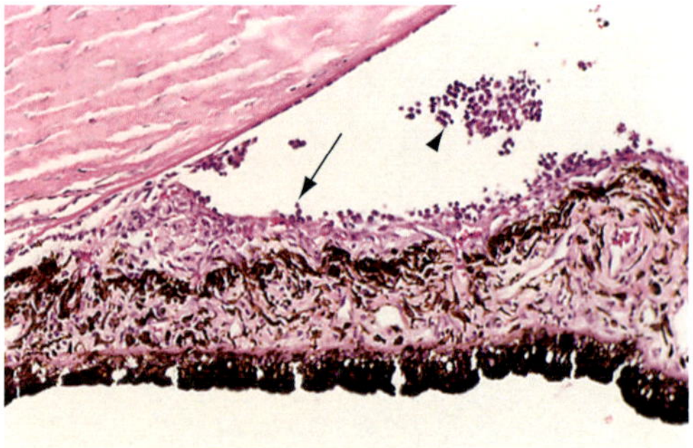

Figure 11-40 Retinoblastoma. Note the thick iris neovascular membrane *(arrow)* and the free-floating tumor cells *(arrowhead)* in the anterior chamber.

to determine histologically whether multiple intraocular foci of the tumor represent multiple primary tumors, implying a systemic distribution of the abnormal gene, or tumor seeds (see Chapter 19, Fig 19-7).

The formation of highly organized *Flexner-Wintersteiner rosettes* is a characteristic feature of retinoblastoma that does not occur in other neuroblastic tumors, with the rare exception of some pinealoblastomas and ectopic intracranial retinoblastomas. Flexner-Wintersteiner rosettes are expressions of retinal differentiation. The cells of these rosettes surround a central lumen lined by a refractile structure. The refractile lining corresponds to the external limiting membrane of the retina that represents sites of attachments between photoreceptors and Müller cells. The rosette is characterized by a single row of columnar cells with eosinophilic cytoplasm and peripherally situated nuclei (Fig 11-41A). The chromatin of cell nuclei in rosettes is usually looser than that of nuclei from undifferentiated cells in adjacent tumor.

A less commonly encountered rosette, without features of retinal differentiation, known as the *Homer Wright rosette,* can be found in other neuroblastic tumors, such as neuroblastoma and medulloblastoma of the cerebellum, as well as in retinoblastoma. The lumen of a Homer Wright rosette is filled with a tangle of eosinophilic cytoplasmic processes (Fig 11-41B).

Evidence of photoreceptor differentiation has also been documented for another flowerlike structure known as a *fleurette.* Fleurettes are curvilinear clusters of cells composed of rod and cone inner segments that are often attached to abortive outer segments (Fig 11-41C). The fleurette expresses a greater degree of retinal differentiation than does the Flexner-Wintersteiner rosette. In a typical retinoblastoma, the undifferentiated tumor cells greatly outnumber the fleurettes and Flexner-Wintersteiner rosettes, and differentiation is not an important prognostic indicator.

Progression

The most common route for retinoblastoma tumor to escape from the eye is by way of the optic nerve. Direct infiltration of the optic nerve can lead to extension into the brain. Cells that spread into the leptomeninges can gain access to the subarachnoid space, with the potential for seeding throughout the central nervous system (Fig 11-42). Invasion of the optic nerve is a poor prognostic sign (Fig 11-43). See Chapter 19 for a discussion of prognosis.

Massive uveal invasion, in contrast, theoretically increases the risk of hematogenous dissemination. Spread to regional lymph nodes may be seen when a tumor involving the

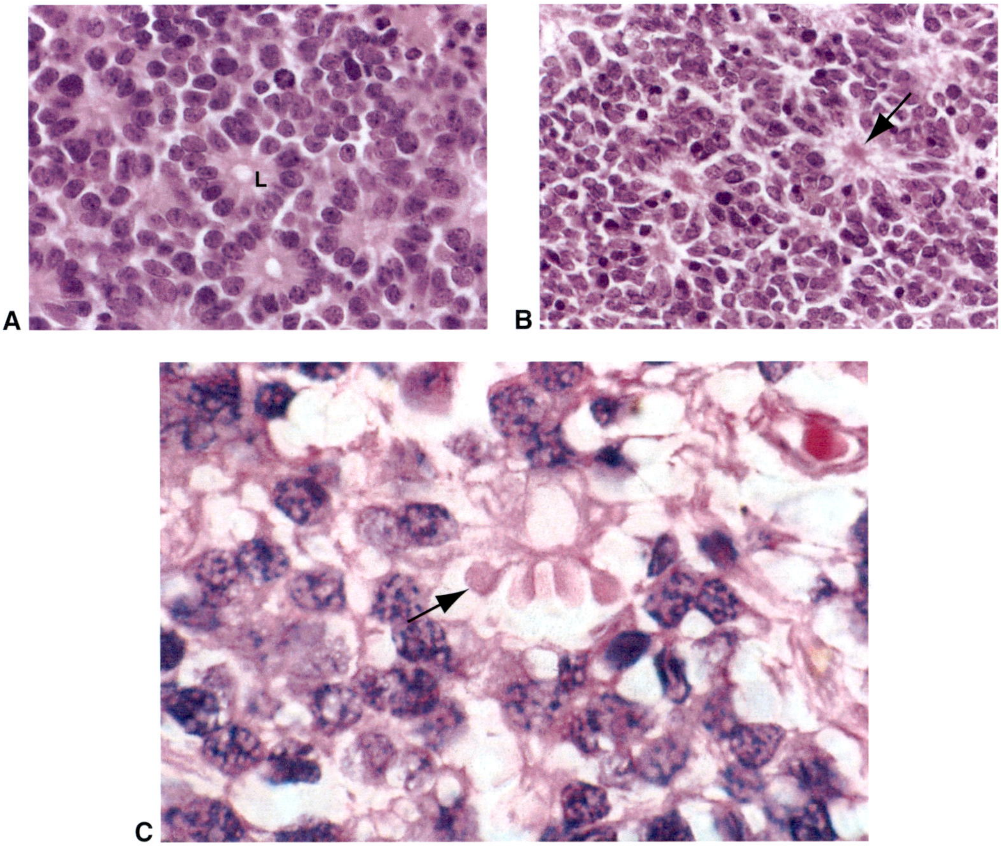

Figure 11-41 Retinoblastoma rosettes. **A,** Flexner-Wintersteiner rosettes: note the central lumen *(L)*. **B,** Homer Wright rosettes: note the neurofibrillary tangle *(arrow)* in the center of these structures. **C,** The fleurette *(arrow)* demonstrates bulbous cellular extension of retinoblastoma cells that represent differentiation along the lines of photoreceptor inner segments.

anterior segment grows into the conjunctival substantia propria, especially when the trabecular meshwork is involved.

Retinocytoma

Retinocytoma is characterized histologically by numerous fleurettes admixed with individual cells that demonstrate varying degrees of photoreceptor differentiation (Fig 11-44). Retinocytoma should be distinguished from the spontaneous regression of retinoblastoma that is the end result of coagulative necrosis. See the discussion in Chapter 19.

Also referred to as *retinoma,* retinocytoma differs from retinoblastoma in the following ways:

- Retinocytoma cells have more cytoplasm and more evenly dispersed nuclear chromatin than do retinoblastoma cells. Mitoses are not observed in retinocytoma.
- Although calcification may be identified in retinocytoma, necrosis is usually absent.

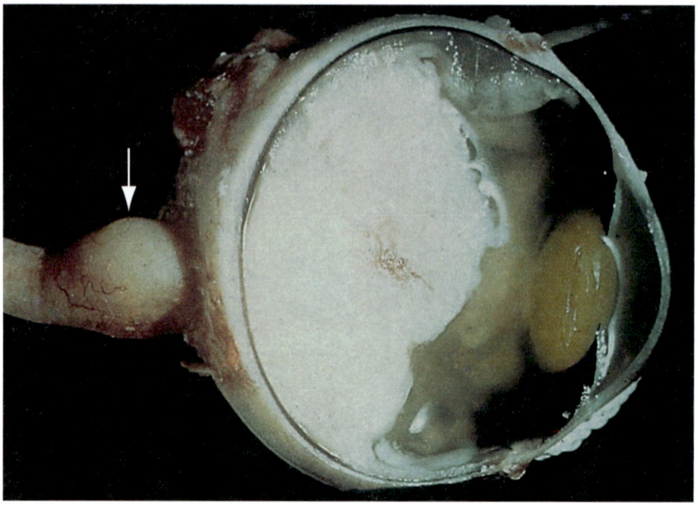

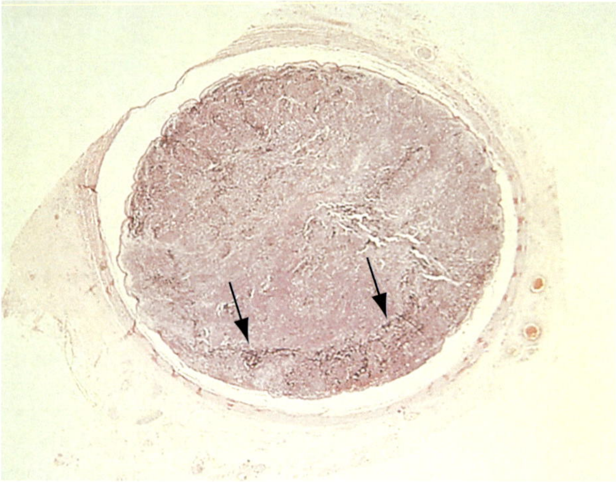

Figure 11-42 Retinoblastoma. **A,** Massive invasion of the globe posteriorly by retinoblastoma with bulbous enlargement of the optic nerve *(arrow)* caused by direct extension. **B,** A cross section of the optic nerve taken at the surgical margin of transection. Tumor *(arrows)* is present in the nerve at this point, and the prognosis is poor.

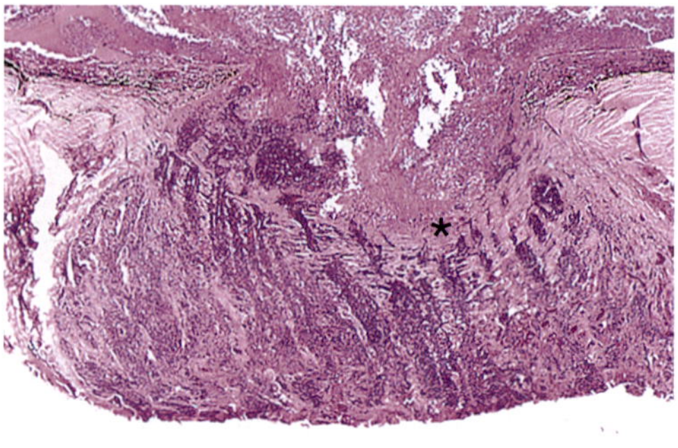

Figure 11-43 Retinoblastoma has invaded the optic nerve and extended to the margin of resection posterior to the lamina cribrosa *(asterisk).* This is an extremely poor prognostic sign.

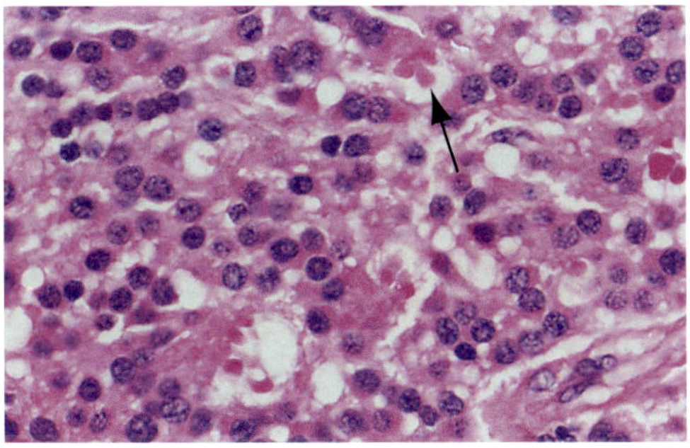

Figure 11-44 Retinocytoma. Note the exquisite degree of photoreceptor differentiation with apparent stubby inner segments *(arrow).*

Medulloepithelioma

Also known as *diktyoma,* medulloepithelioma is a congenital neuroepithelial tumor arising from primitive medullary epithelium. This tumor usually occurs in the ciliary body but has also been documented in the retina and optic nerve. Clinically, medulloepithelioma may appear as a lightly pigmented or amelanotic, cystic mass in the ciliary body, with erosion into the anterior chamber and iris root (see Part II, Intraocular Tumors, Chapter 19, Fig 19-12). Although the tumor develops before the medullary epithelium shows substantial signs of differentiation, cells are organized into ribbonlike structures that have a distinct cellular polarity (Fig 11-45). These ribbonlike structures are composed of undifferentiated round to oval cells possessing little cytoplasm. Cell nuclei are stratified in 3 to 5 layers, and the entire structure is lined on one side by a thin basement membrane. One surface secretes a mucinous substance, rich in hyaluronic acid, that resembles primitive vitreous. Stratified sheets of cells are capable of forming mucinous cysts that are clinically characteristic. Homer Wright and Flexner-Wintersteiner rosettes can also be seen.

Medulloepitheliomas that contain solid masses of neuroblastic cells indistinguishable from retinoblastoma are more difficult to classify. Medulloepitheliomas that have substantial numbers of undifferentiated cells with high mitotic rates and that demonstrate tissue invasion are considered malignant, although patients treated with enucleation have high

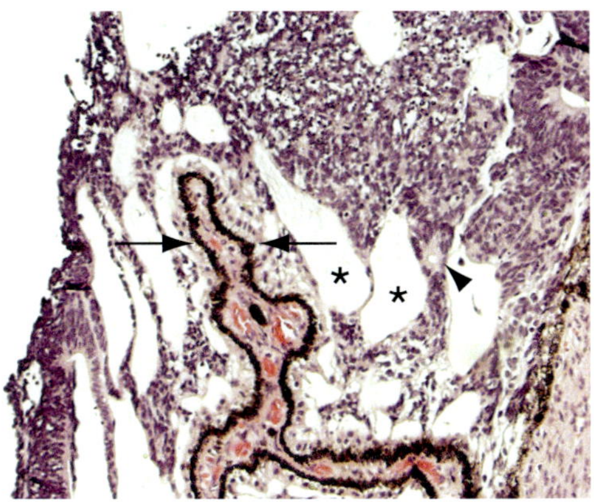

Figure 11-45 Medulloepithelioma. Histology shows a ciliary process *(between arrows)* surrounded by ribbons, cords, and small sheets of blue tumor cells with pockets of vitreous *(asterisks)* and occasional Flexner-Wintersteiner rosettes *(arrowhead).* *(Courtesy of George J. Harocopos, MD.)*

survival rates, and "malignant" medulloepithelioma typically follows a relatively benign course if the tumor remains confined to the eye.

Heteroplastic tissue, such as cartilage or smooth muscle, may be found in medulloepitheliomas. Tumors composed of cells from 2 different embryonic germ layers are referred to as *teratoid medulloepitheliomas.* Malignant teratoid medulloepitheliomas demonstrate either solid areas of undifferentiated neuroblastic cells or sarcomatous transformation of heteroplastic elements.

Fuchs Adenoma

Fuchs adenoma, an acquired tumor of the nonpigmented epithelium of the ciliary body, may be associated with sectoral cataract and may simulate other iris or ciliary body neoplasms. Fuchs adenomas consist of hyperplastic, nonpigmented ciliary epithelium arranged in sheets and tubules with alternating areas of PAS-positive basement membrane material.

Combined Hamartoma of the Retina and RPE

A combined hamartoma of the retina and RPE is characterized clinically by the presence of a slightly elevated, variably pigmented mass involving the RPE, peripapillary retina, optic nerve, and overlying vitreous (see Chapter 17, Fig 17-15). Frequently, a preretinal membrane is present that distorts the tumor's inner retinal surface. The lesion is often diagnosed in childhood, supporting a probable hamartomatous origin, but it is possible that the vascular changes are primary, with secondary changes in the adjacent RPE.

The tumor is characterized by thickening of the optic nerve head and peripapillary retina, with an increased number of vessels. The RPE is hyperplastic and frequently migrates into a perivascular location. Vitreous condensation and fibroglial proliferation may be present on the surface of the tumor.

Adenomas and Adenocarcinomas of the RPE

Neoplasia of the RPE is uncommon and is distinguished from hyperplasia of the RPE principally by the absence of a history of, or pathologic features suggesting, prior trauma or eye disease. *Adenomas* of the RPE typically retain characteristics of RPE cells, including basement membranes, cell junctions, and microvilli. *Adenocarcinomas* are distinguished from adenomas by greater anaplasia, mitotic activity, and invasion of the choroid or retina. No metastases have ever been documented to occur in patients with RPE adenocarcinomas.

Spencer WH, ed. *Ophthalmic Pathology: An Atlas and Textbook.* 4th ed. Philadelphia: Saunders; 1997:1291–1313.

CHAPTER 12

Uveal Tract

Topography

The *iris, ciliary body,* and *choroid* constitute the uveal tract (Fig 12-1). The uveal tract is embryologically derived from mesoderm and neural crest. Firm attachments between the uveal tract and the sclera exist at only 3 sites:

- scleral spur
- exit points of the vortex veins
- optic nerve

Iris

The iris is located in front of the crystalline lens. It separates the anterior segment of the eye into 2 compartments, the anterior chamber and the posterior chamber, and forms a circular aperture (pupil) that controls the amount of light transmitted into the eye. The iris is composed of 5 layers:

- anterior border layer
- stroma
- muscular layer
- anterior pigment epithelium
- posterior pigment epithelium

The anterior border layer represents a condensation of iris stroma and melanocytes and is coarsely ribbed with numerous crypts (Fig 12-2). The stroma contains blood vessels, nerves, melanocytes, fibrocytes, and clump cells. The clump cells are both macrophages

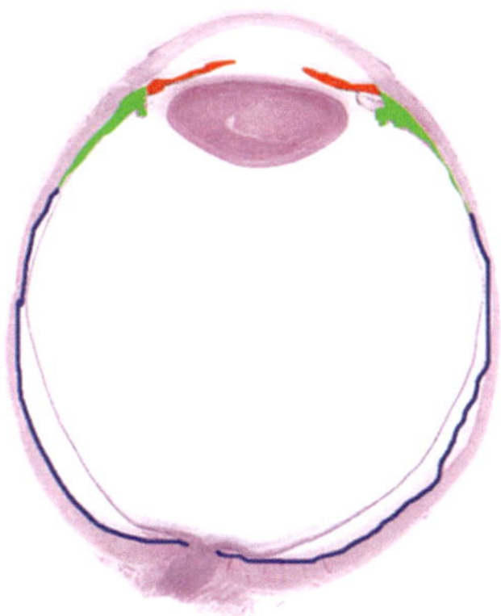

Figure 12-1 Uveal topography. The uveal tract consists of the iris *(red),* the ciliary body *(green),* and the choroid *(blue*). *(Courtesy of Nasreen A. Syed, MD.)*

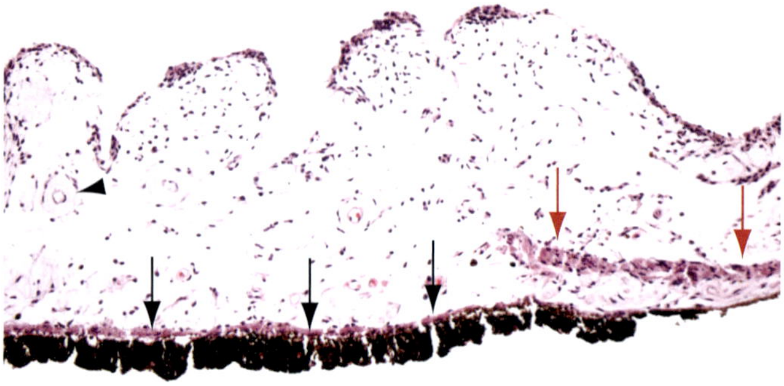

Figure 12-2 Histologic appearance of the iris: the anterior border layer is thrown into numerous crypts and folds. The sphincter muscle *(red arrows)* is present at the pupillary border, whereas the dilator muscle *(black arrows)* lies just anterior to the posterior pigment epithelium. Normal iris vessels demonstrate a thick collagen cuff *(arrowhead)*. *(Courtesy of Nasreen A. Syed, MD.)*

containing phagocytosed pigment (type I, or clump cells of Koganei) and variants of smooth-muscle cells (type II clump cells). The vessels within the stroma have a thick collar of collagen. The muscular layer is made up of the dilator muscle and the sphincter muscle. Both are smooth muscle under autonomic control; however, the dilator muscle is unique in that it is derived from the anterior layer of pigment epithelium. The posterior iris is lined by a double layer of cuboidal epithelium arranged in an apex-to-apex configuration. The cytoplasm of these cells is packed with melanin granules. Iris color is determined by the number and size of the melanin pigment granules in the anterior stromal melanocytes.

Ciliary Body

The ciliary body, which is approximately 6.0–6.5 mm wide, extends from the base of the iris and becomes continuous with the choroid at the ora serrata. The ciliary body is composed of 2 areas:

- the *pars plicata,* which contains the ciliary processes
- the *pars plana*

The inner portion of the ciliary body is lined by a double layer of epithelial cells, the inner nonpigmented layer and the outer pigmented layer (Fig 12-3). The zonular fibers of the lens attach to the ciliary processes. The ciliary smooth muscle has 3 types of fibers: *longitudinal (Brücke muscle), radial,* and *the innermost circular (Müller muscle).* These muscle groups function as a unit during accommodation.

Choroid

The choroid is the pigmented vascular tissue that forms the middle coat of the posterior part of the eye. It extends from the ora serrata anteriorly to the optic nerve posteriorly and consists of 3 principal layers:

- lamina fusca (suprachoroid layer)

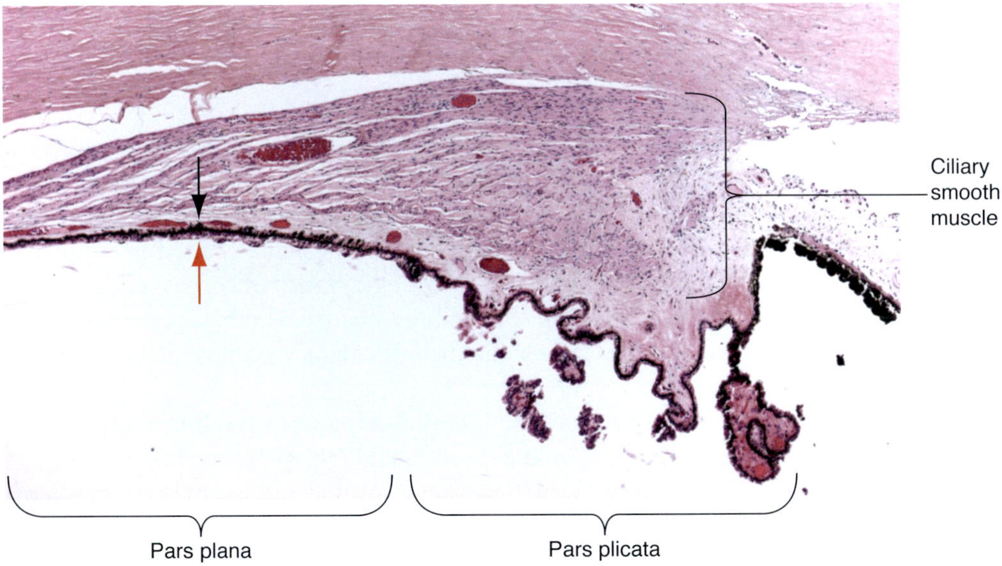

Figure 12-3 Normal ciliary body. The inner face of the ciliary body is lined with a double layer of epithelium. The inner layer is nonpigmented *(red arrow)* and the outer layer is pigmented *(black arrow)*. *(Courtesy of Nasreen A. Syed, MD.)*

- stroma
- choriocapillaris

The choriocapillaris is the blood supply for the retinal pigment epithelium (RPE) and the outer retinal layers (Fig 12-4).

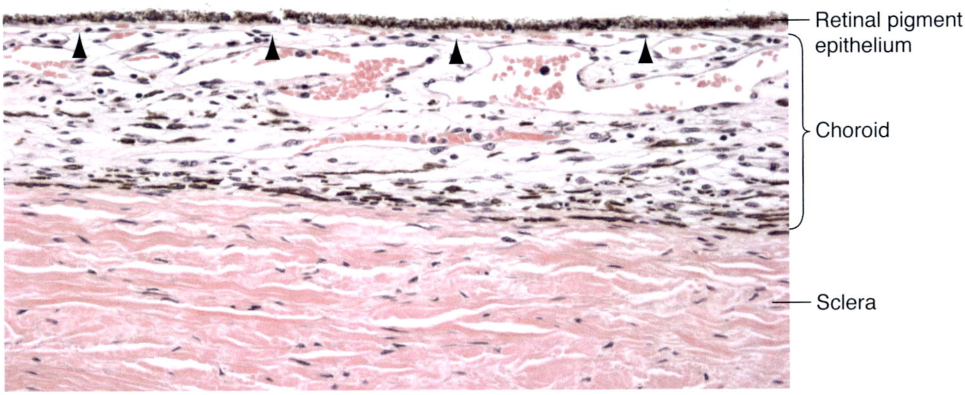

Figure 12-4 The choroid is a vascular, pigmented structure present between the retinal pigment epithelium and the sclera. The layer closest to the pigment epithelium is composed of capillaries and is known as the *choriocapillaris (arrowheads)*. *(Courtesy of Nasreen A. Syed, MD.)*

Congenital Anomalies

Aniridia

True aniridia, or complete absence of the iris, is rare. Most cases of aniridia are incomplete, with a narrow rim of rudimentary iris tissue present. Aniridia is usually bilateral, though sometimes asymmetric. Histologically, the rudimentary iris consists of underdeveloped ectodermal–mesodermal neural crest elements. The angle is often incompletely developed, and peripheral anterior synechiae with an overgrowth of corneal endothelium are often present, most likely accounting for the high incidence of glaucoma associated with aniridia. Other ocular findings in aniridia include cataract, corneal pannus, and foveal hypoplasia.

Both autosomal dominant and sporadic inheritance patterns for aniridia have been described. An association between sporadic aniridia and Wilms tumor has been linked to 11p13 deletions and to mutations in the *PAX6* gene, located in the same region. Microcephaly, mental retardation, and genitourinary abnormalities have also been described in association with aniridia.

See also BCSC Section 2, *Fundamentals and Principles of Ophthalmology,* and Section 6, *Pediatric Ophthalmology and Strabismus.*

Hingorani M, Hanson I, van Heyningen V. Aniridia. *Eur J Hum Genet.* 2012;20(10): 1011–1017.

Coloboma

A coloboma—the absence of part or all of an ocular tissue—may affect the iris, ciliary body, choroid, or all 3 structures. Histologically, colobomas appear as an area nearly or entirely devoid of tissue. See BCSC Section 2, *Fundamentals and Principles of Ophthalmology,* and Section 6, *Pediatric Ophthalmology and Strabismus,* for further discussion of uveal colobomas.

Inflammations

BCSC Section 9, *Intraocular Inflammation and Uveitis,* discusses the conditions described in the following sections and also explains in depth the immunologic processes involved.

Infectious

The uveal tract may be involved in infectious processes that appear restricted to a single intraocular structure or that may be part of a generalized inflammation affecting several or all coats of the eye. If the eye is the primary source of the infection, as with posttraumatic bacterial infection, the infection is termed *exogenous.* If, however, the infection originates elsewhere in the body, such as with a ruptured diverticulum, and subsequently spreads hematogenously to involve the uveal tract, the infection is referred to as *endogenous.* A wide variety of organisms can cause infections of the uveal tract, including bacteria, fungi, viruses, and protozoa.

Histopathology often shows a mixed acute and chronic inflammatory infiltrate within the choroid, ciliary body, or iris stroma. In cases of viral, fungal, or protozoal (eg, toxoplasmosis) agents, the presence of epithelioid histiocytes is typical (granulomatous inflammation). Special stains (see Table 3-2) for microorganisms (tissue Gram, Gomori methenamine silver, PAS [periodic acid–Schiff], Ziehl-Neelsen) may be helpful if infection is suspected.

Noninfectious

Sympathetic ophthalmia

Sympathetic ophthalmia is a rare bilateral granulomatous panuveitis that occurs after accidental or surgical injury to 1 eye (the *exciting,* or *inciting, eye*) followed by a latent period and development of uveitis in the uninjured globe (the *sympathizing eye*). The inflammation in the sympathizing eye may occur as early as 9 days or as late as 50 years following the suspected triggering incident. Enucleation of the inciting eye, if blind, is thought to help control inflammation or reduce the risk of inflammation in the other eye.

Histologically, a diffuse granulomatous inflammatory reaction is present within the uveal tract and is composed of lymphocytes and epithelioid histiocytes containing phagocytosed melanin pigment (Figs 12-5, 12-6). Plasma cells are usually scant, suggesting a cell-mediated response. Typically, the choriocapillaris is spared. Varying degrees of inflammation may be present in the anterior chamber, such as collections of histiocytes deposited on the corneal endothelium *(mutton-fat keratic precipitates). Dalen-Fuchs nodules,* which are collections of epithelioid histiocytes and lymphocytes between the RPE and the Bruch membrane, may be seen in some cases (Fig 12-7). However, Dalen-Fuchs nodules may be present in other diseases, such as Vogt-Koyanagi-Harada syndrome, and thus are not pathognomonic of sympathetic ophthalmia.

Vogt-Koyanagi-Harada syndrome

Vogt-Koyanagi-Harada (VKH) syndrome is a rare cause of posterior or diffuse uveitis and may have both ocular and systemic manifestations. The syndrome occurs more

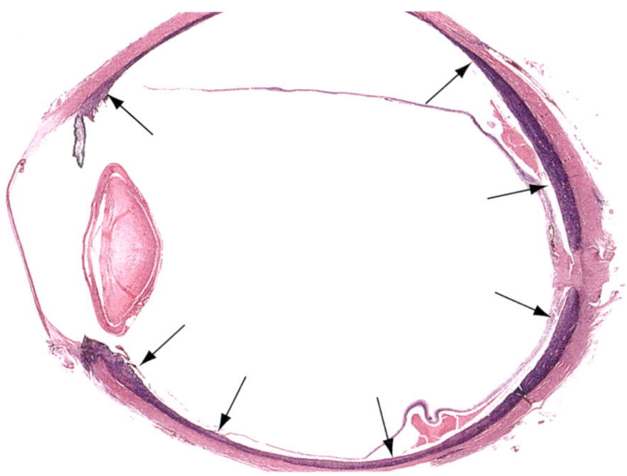

Figure 12-5 Sympathetic ophthalmia. Diffuse infiltration of the uveal tract by chronic inflammatory cells *(arrows)*. *(Courtesy of Hans E. Grossniklaus, MD.)*

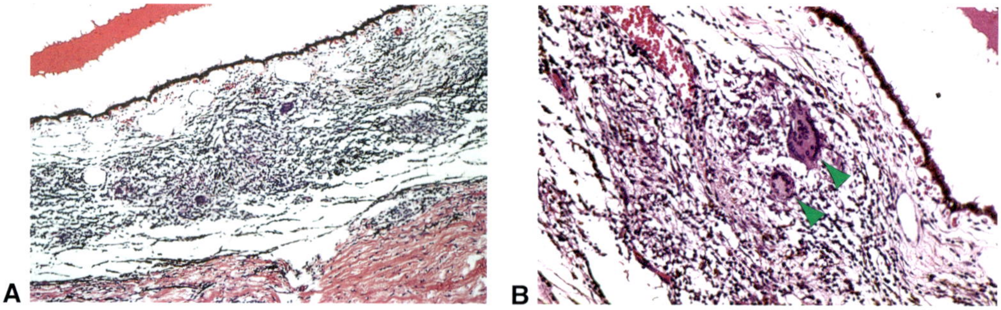

Figure 12-6 Sympathetic ophthalmia. **A,** Diffuse granulomatous inflammation within the choroid. **B,** Higher magnification shows the presence of multinucleated giant cells *(arrowheads).* *(Courtesy of Hans E. Grossniklaus, MD.)*

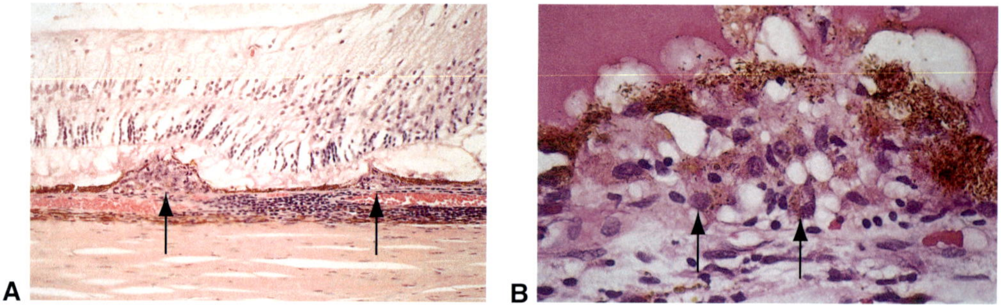

Figure 12-7 Dalen-Fuchs nodules in sympathetic ophthalmia. **A,** Focal collections of inflammatory cells are located between the RPE and Bruch membrane *(arrows).* **B,** Higher magnification demonstrates the presence of epithelioid histiocytes containing cytoplasmic pigment *(arrows)* within the nodules. *(Courtesy of Hans E. Grossniklaus, MD.)*

commonly in patients with Asian or Native American ancestry and usually affects individuals between 30 and 50 years of age.

A chronic, diffuse granulomatous uveitis resembles that seen in sympathetic ophthalmia. However, in VKH, the entire choroid, including the choriocapillaris, tends to be involved by the inflammatory reaction. The granulomatous inflammation may extend to involve the retina. Because the disease is one of exacerbation and remission, chorioretinal scarring and RPE hyperplasia and/or atrophy may also be observed.

Sarcoidosis

Sarcoidosis is a multisystem granulomatous disease characterized by inflammatory nodules, which can occur in various organs and tissues. The uveal tract is the most common site of ocular involvement by sarcoidosis. Anteriorly, inflammatory nodules of the iris may be seen, either at the pupillary margin *(Koeppe nodules)* or elsewhere on the iris *(Busacca nodules).* In the posterior segment, chorioretinitis, periphlebitis, and chorioretinal nodules may be seen. Periphlebitis may appear clinically as inflammatory lesions described as *candlewax drippings.* The optic nerve may be edematous because of inflammatory infiltration.

Histologically, the classic sarcoid nodule is composed of noncaseating granulomas. These are collections of epithelioid histiocytes, sometimes accompanied by multinucleated giant cells, that have a surrounding cuff of lymphocytes (Fig 12-8). *Noncaseating* refers to the lack of necrosis in the center of the nodule. In the uvea, the inflammatory infiltrate may show a more diffuse distribution of lymphocytes and epithelioid histiocytes (granulomatous inflammation). The multinucleated giant cells may demonstrate *asteroid bodies* (star-shaped, acidophilic bodies) and *Schaumann bodies* (spherical, basophilic, calcified bodies). Neither asteroid nor Schaumann bodies are pathognomonic for sarcoidosis.

Juvenile xanthogranuloma

Juvenile xanthogranuloma is an uncommon inflammatory condition that occurs in children. The skin and uvea are commonly affected areas and, in the uveal tract, lesions may present as a solid mass, mimicking a tumor. Histologically, the lesions have a characteristic appearance with the presence of lipid-laden histiocytes, Touton giant cells, lymphocytes, and occasional eosinophils (Fig 12-9). The lesions are often vascularized, and these blood vessels tend to be fragile. This results in intralesional hemorrhage and, in the iris, may result in spontaneous hyphema.

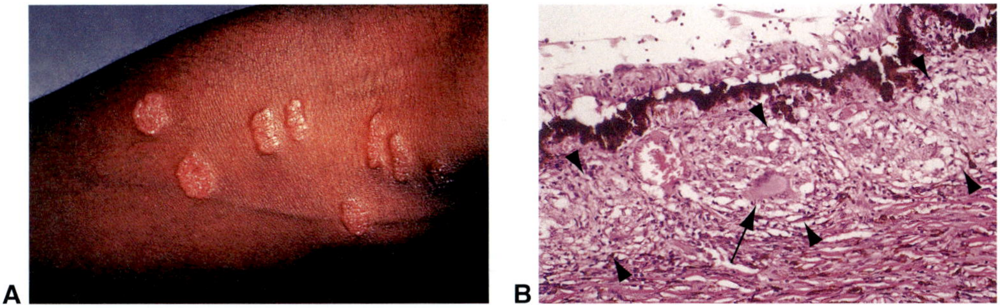

Figure 12-8 Sarcoidosis. **A,** Gross appearance of multiple discrete nodules on the skin of the upper extremity. **B,** Histology of sarcoid nodule showing epithelioid histiocytes *(between arrowheads)* and multinucleated giant cells *(arrow)*. *(Part A courtesy of Curtis E. Margo, MD; part B courtesy of Hans E. Grossniklaus, MD.)*

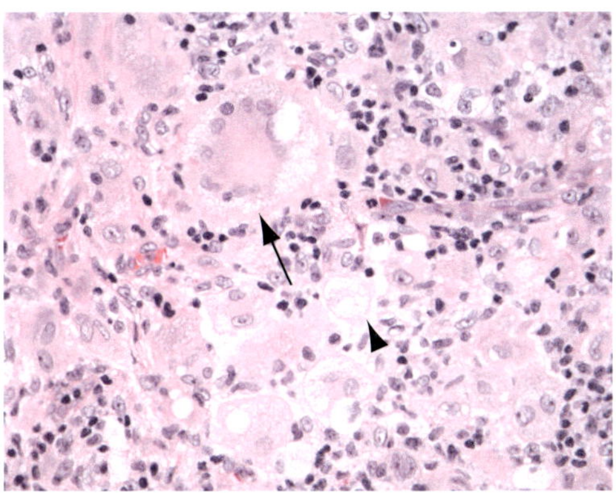

Figure 12-9 Juvenile xanthogranuloma. Touton giant cells *(arrow)*, foamy histiocytes *(arrowhead)*, and lymphocytes are admixed. *(Courtesy of Nasreen A. Syed, MD.)*

Degenerations

Rubeosis Iridis

Rubeosis iridis, or neovascularization of the iris, is a common finding in surgically enucleated blind eyes. It may be associated with a wide variety of conditions (Table 12-1). Histologically, the new vessels tend to lack supporting tissue and do not possess the encircling thick fibrous cuff seen in normal iris vessels. The vessels grow on the anterior surface of the iris and may extend to involve the angle. The neovascular membrane has a fibrous component consisting of myofibroblasts, which contract and eventually lead to angle closure due to formation of peripheral anterior synechiae. Neovascularization of the angle often results in *neovascular glaucoma,* a secondary type of glaucoma. Contraction of the membranes may also lead to *ectropion uveae,* an anterior displacement or dragging of the posterior iris pigment epithelium at the pupillary border. The anterior surface of the iris often becomes flattened. In advanced cases, atrophy of the dilator muscle, attenuation of the pigment epithelium, and stromal fibrosis occur (Fig 12-10).

Hyalinization of the Ciliary Body

Over time, the ciliary body processes become hyalinized and fibrosed, with loss of stromal cellularity. The thin, delicate processes become blunted and attenuated, and the stroma becomes more eosinophilic. This process is a normal aging change of the ciliary body and is not considered pathologic, although it does contribute functionally to the development of presbyopia.

Table 12-1 Conditions Associated With Rubeosis Iridis

Vascular disorders
- Central retinal vein occlusion
- Central retinal artery occlusion
- Branch retinal vein occlusion
- Carotid occlusive disease

Ocular diseases
- Intraocular inflammation
  - Infectious (eg, severe corneal ulcer)
  - Noninfectious (eg, uveitis)
- Retinal detachment
- Coats disease
- Secondary glaucoma

Surgery and radiation therapy
- Retinal detachment surgery
- Radiation

Systemic diseases
- Diabetes mellitus
- Sickle cell disease

Neoplastic diseases
- Retinoblastoma
- Melanoma of the choroid/iris
- Metastatic carcinoma

Trauma

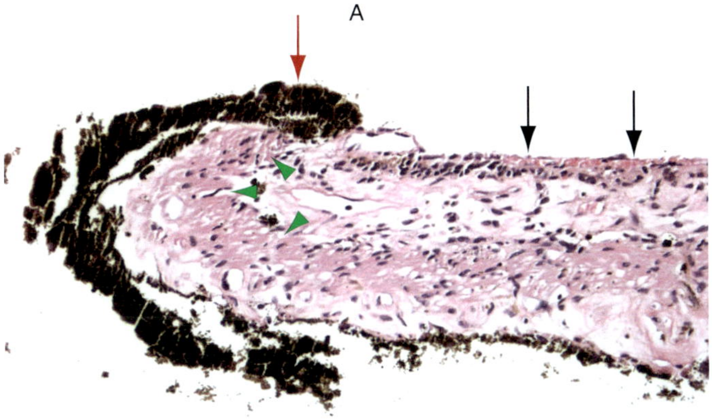

Figure 12-10 Iris neovascularization (rubeosis). Small blood vessels sprout from existing iris vasculature, typically on the surface of the iris *(black arrows).* Note the flat anterior surface of the iris (*A* = anterior, *P* = posterior). The contractile component of the neovascular membrane may result in dragging of the iris pigment epithelium *(red arrow)* and sphincter muscle *(arrowheads)* anteriorly at the pupillary margin, in turn resulting in *ectropion uveae.* *(Courtesy of Nasreen A. Syed, MD.)*

Choroidal Neovascularization

Choroidal neovascularization is discussed at length in Chapter 11 and in BCSC Section 12, *Retina and Vitreous.*

Neoplasia

Uveal neoplasms are also discussed in detail in Chapters 17, 18, and 20. The discussion of uveal neoplasms in this chapter focuses primarily on histopathology.

Iris

Nevus

An *iris nevus* represents a localized proliferation of melanocytic cells that generally appears as a darkly pigmented lesion of the iris stroma with minimal distortion of the iris architecture (see Chapter 17, Fig 17-1). An iris nevus appears histologically as a collection of branching dendritic cells or spindle cells, usually with melanin granules in the cytoplasm. The nuclei of these cells are typically oblong or ovoid with a bland appearance and indistinct nucleoli. Less commonly, epithelioid nevus cells may be present. A variety of growth patterns and cytologic appearances is possible, but cellular atypia and significant mitotic activity are not present. The nevus cells are present as an aggregate within the stroma and occasionally are also present in a plaquelike distribution on the surface of the iris. Occasionally, the cells may extend into the adjacent angle structures.

Melanoma

Melanomas arising in the iris tend to follow a nonaggressive clinical course compared to posterior (ciliochoroidal) melanomas. The majority of iris melanomas occur in the inferior sectors of the iris (see Chapter 17, Fig 17-3). The lesions can be quite vascularized and may occasionally cause spontaneous hyphema.

Iris melanomas are composed of spindle melanoma cells, epithelioid melanoma cells, or a combination of these. Histologically, spindle cells possess plump, spindle-shaped nuclei that have a coarse, granular appearance and prominent nucleoli. These cells are the equivalent of spindle-B cells in posterior melanoma (see the "Melanoma" section under Choroid and Ciliary Body). Epithelioid cells are polyhedral in shape, with large, round nuclei that have a clumped chromatin pattern and prominent eosinophilic nucleoli. Both types of cells tend to have a high nuclear-to-cytoplasmic ratio. The cytoplasm of melanoma cells can range from lightly to heavily pigmented. Typically, they grow as a solid mass in the stroma, sometimes with a surface plaque. Occasionally, iris melanomas may demonstrate satellite lesions or a diffuse growth pattern that replaces normal stroma (Fig 12-11). The modified Callender classification for posterior melanomas (see the discussion later in the chapter) is not applicable to iris melanomas in terms of prognostic significance.

Although iris melanomas may grow in a locally aggressive fashion, they rarely metastasize. One exception occurs when melanomas grow to diffusely involve the entire iris stroma. In such cases, the melanoma may extend posteriorly into the chamber angle and involve the ciliary body.

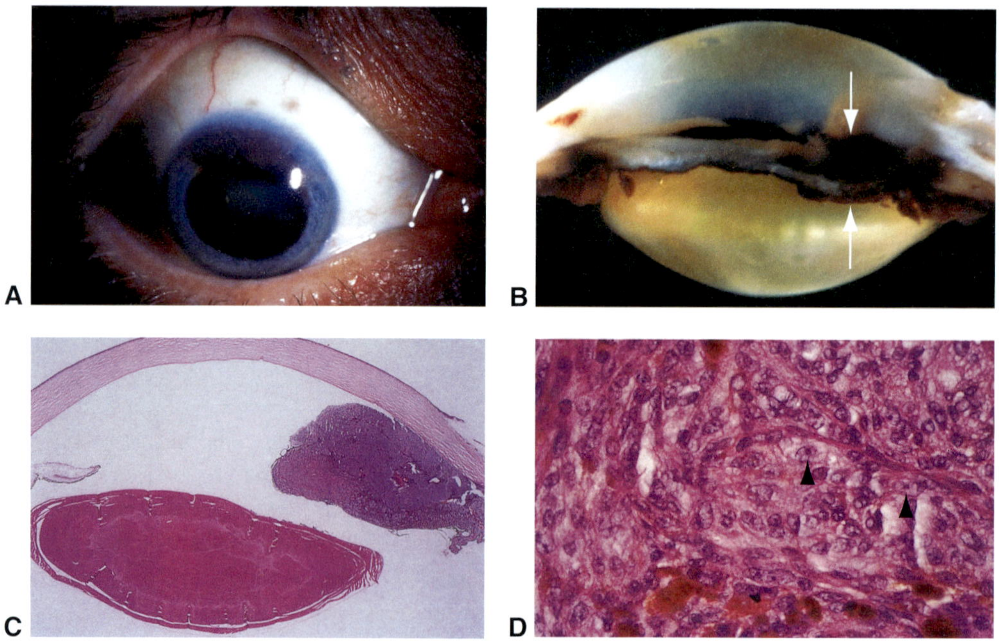

Figure 12-11 **A,** Clinical appearance of iris melanoma. The pigmented tumor is seen between 10:30 and 1:00. **B,** Gross appearance of pigmented iris mass *(between arrows)*. **C,** Low magnification shows the iris melanoma completely replacing the normal iris stroma, extending into the anterior chamber, touching the posterior cornea, and occluding the angle. **D,** Histology of iris melanoma shows numerous plump epithelioid melanoma cells containing prominent nucleoli *(arrowheads)*. *(Courtesy of Hans E. Grossniklaus, MD.)*

Choroid and Ciliary Body

Nevus

Most nevi of the uveal tract occur in the choroid (see Chapter 17, Fig 17-2). One review of 100 nevi showed that fewer than 6% involved the ciliary body; the remainder were present in the choroid. Four types of nevus cells have been described. They are

- *plump polyhedral:* abundant cytoplasm filled with pigment and a small, round to oval nucleus with bland appearance
- *slender spindle* (Fig 12-12): cytoplasm contains scant pigment and a small, dark, elongated nucleus
- *plump fusiform dendritic:* morphology is intermediate between plump polyhedral and slender spindle
- *balloon cells:* abundant, foamy cytoplasm that lacks pigment and has a bland nucleus

Depending on the size and location of the nevus, it may exert nonspecific effects on adjacent ocular tissues. The associated choriocapillaris may become compressed or obliterated, and drusen may be seen overlying the nevus. Less commonly, localized serous detachments of the overlying RPE or neurosensory retina develop.

Most choroidal nevi remain stationary over long periods of observation. However, the presence of nevus cells associated with some melanomas supplies evidence that melanomas may arise from choroidal nevi.

Melanocytoma

The melanocytoma is a specific type of uveal tract nevus (magnocellular nevus) that warrants separate consideration. These jet-black lesions may occur anywhere in the uveal tract, but they most commonly appear in the peripapillary region (see Chapter 17, Fig 17-12).

Histologically, a melanocytoma is composed of plump polyhedral cells with small nuclei and abundant cytoplasm. Because the nevus cells are so heavily pigmented, it is usually necessary to obtain bleached sections to accurately study the cytologic features. Areas of cystic degeneration or necrosis may be observed.

Melanoma

Melanoma arising from the ciliary body and choroid is the most common primary intraocular malignancy in adults. When this tumor achieves significant size, it may extend

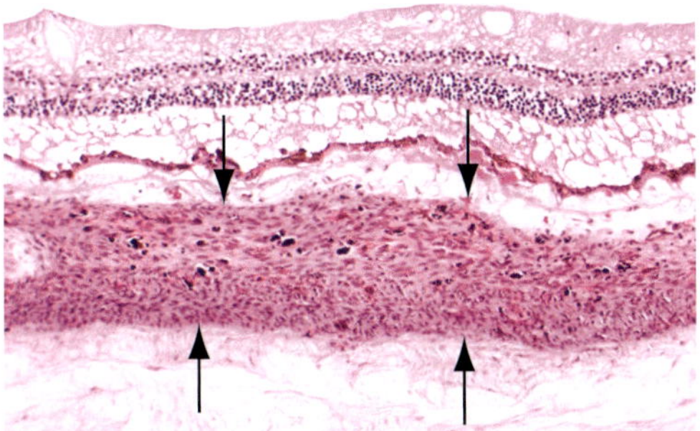

Figure 12-12 Spindle cell choroidal nevus *(between arrows)* is composed of slender, spindle-shaped cells with thin, homogeneous nuclei. *(Courtesy of Nasreen A. Syed, MD.)*

beyond its site of origin (ie, from the choroid to the ciliary body and vice versa). Unlike iris melanomas, ciliary body and choroidal melanomas exhibit similar features and are usually considered to be the same type of tumor, with similar histologic features and prognostic implications.

Histologically, ciliary body and choroidal melanomas are composed of spindle cells and/or epithelioid cells (Figs 12-13, 12-14, 12-15). Less commonly, balloon cells similar to those seen in nevi may be present. Spindle cell melanomas consist primarily of spindle-B melanoma cells. They may also contain spindle-A cells; however, a tumor consisting entirely of spindle-A cells is considered a nevus. Melanoma cells can vary considerably with regard to cytoplasmic melanin content. The mitotic rate in melanomas tends to be low, and

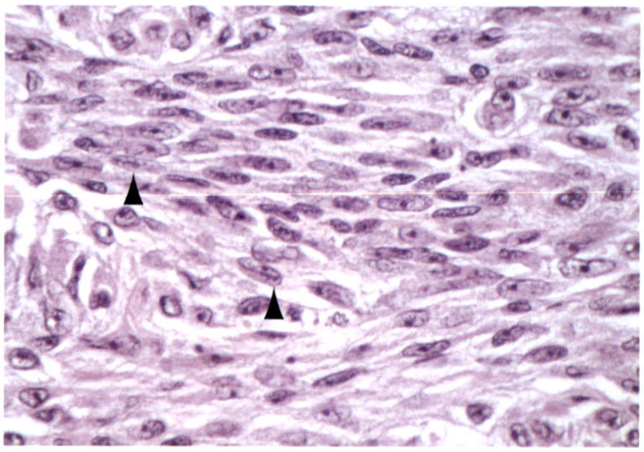

Figure 12-13 Spindle-A cells have slender, elongated nuclei with small nucleoli. A central stripe may be present down the long axis of the nucleus *(arrowheads)*. Tumors composed exclusively of spindle-A cells are considered to be nevi. *(Courtesy of Nasreen A. Syed, MD.)*

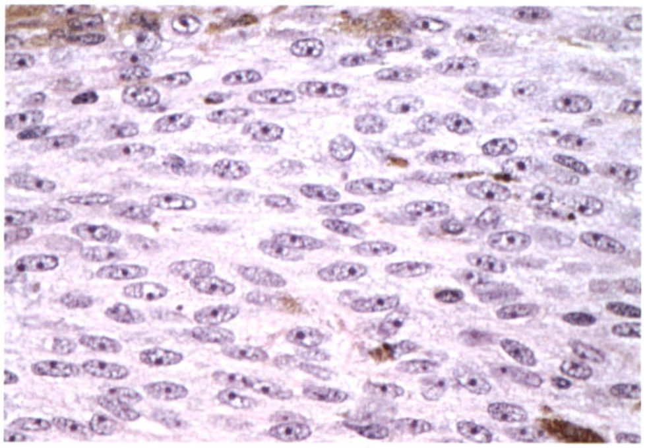

Figure 12-14 Compared with spindle-A cells, spindle-B cells demonstrate a higher nuclear-to-cytoplasmic ratio; more coarsely granular chromatin; and plumper, large nuclei. Nucleoli are prominent and mitoses are present, though not in large numbers. Tumors composed of a mix of spindle-A and spindle-B cells are designated *spindle cell melanomas*. *(Courtesy of Nasreen A. Syed, MD.)*

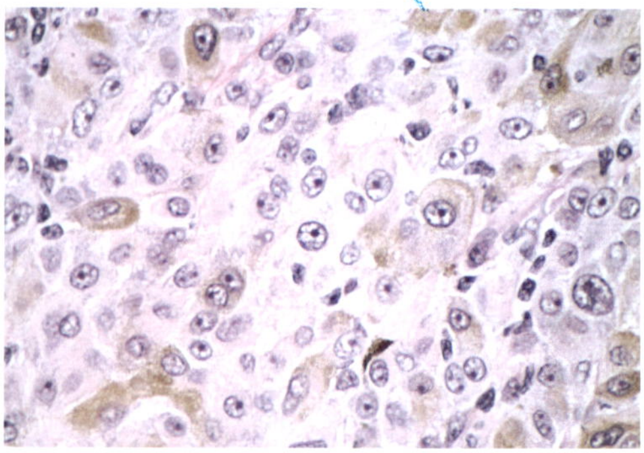

Figure 12-15 Epithelioid melanoma cells. Cells resemble epithelium because of abundant eosinophilic cytoplasm and enlarged oval to polygonal nuclei. Epithelioid melanoma cells often lack cohesiveness and demonstrate marked pleomorphism, including the formation of multinucleated tumor giant cells. Nuclei have a conspicuous nuclear membrane, very coarse chromatin, and large nucleoli. *(Courtesy of Nasreen A. Syed, MD.)*

these tumors may exhibit various amounts of necrosis. Pigment-laden macrophages or a lymphocytic inflammatory infiltrate (tumor-infiltrating lymphocytes) may be present.

Melanomas typically start as dome-shaped lesions and, as they grow and break through the Bruch membrane, they acquire a mushroom or collar-button shape (Fig 12-16). Less commonly, choroidal lesions may grow in a diffuse pattern, replacing normal choroid without achieving significant height. In the ciliary body, the equivalent of the diffuse pattern is the *ring melanoma,* in which the tumor extends for the entire circumference of the ciliary body (Figs 12-17, 12-18).

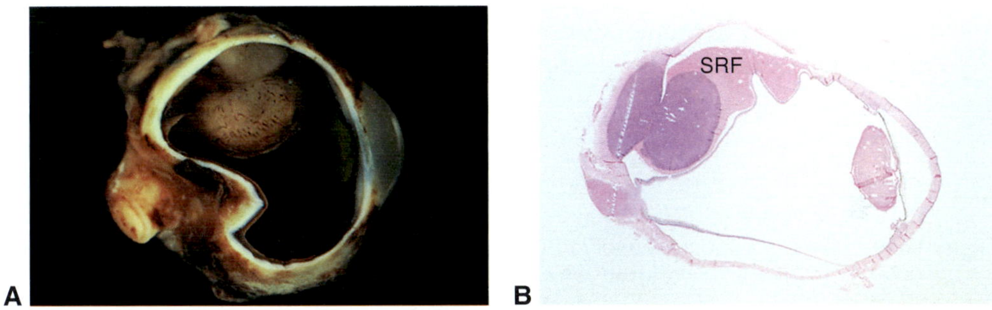

Figure 12-16 Choroidal melanoma with rupture through the Bruch membrane. **A,** Gross appearance. **B,** Microscopic appearance. Note the subretinal fluid *(SRF)* adjacent to the tumor.

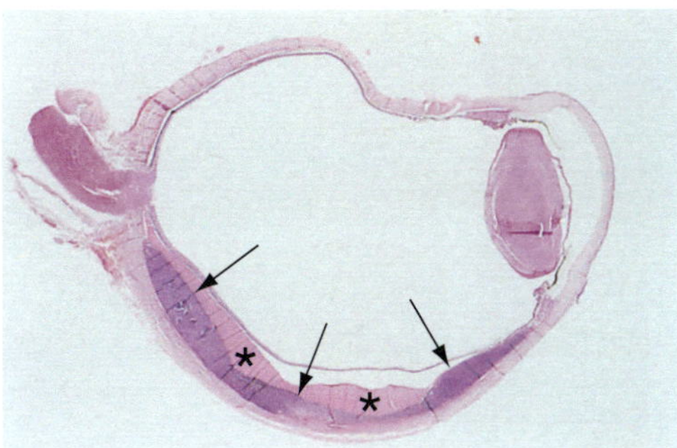

Figure 12-17 Some melanomas grow in a diffuse placoid fashion, replacing normal choroid, without achieving significant height *(arrows).* Note the eosinophilic proteinaceous material *(asterisks)* interposed between the retina and the tumor, corresponding to exudative retinal detachment overlying the tumor.

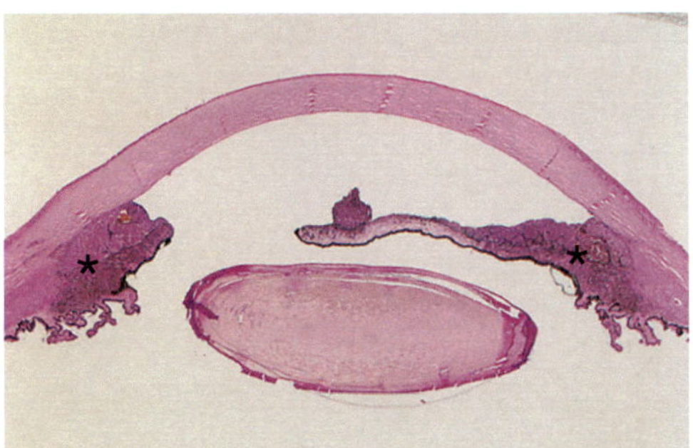

Figure 12-18 By definition, a ring melanoma *(asterisks)* follows the major arterial circle of the iris circumferentially around the eye.

Choroidal melanomas may also cause serous detachments of the overlying and adjacent retina, with subsequent degenerative changes in the outer segments of the photoreceptors (Fig 12-19). Melanomas may extend through scleral emissary channels to gain access to the episcleral surface and the orbit (Fig 12-20). Less commonly, aggressive melanomas may directly invade the underlying sclera or overlying retina (see Fig 12-19). Direct invasion of the anterior chamber may lead to secondary glaucoma. In addition, tumor necrosis may lead to the liberation of melanin pigment, which can then gain access to the anterior chamber and angle, causing a type of secondary glaucoma called *melanomalytic glaucoma.*

Several factors that can be identified on pathologic examination have been significantly correlated with survival in patients with choroidal and ciliary body melanomas. The 2 most important variables associated with survival are

- the size of the largest tumor dimension in contact with the sclera
- the cell type making up the tumor

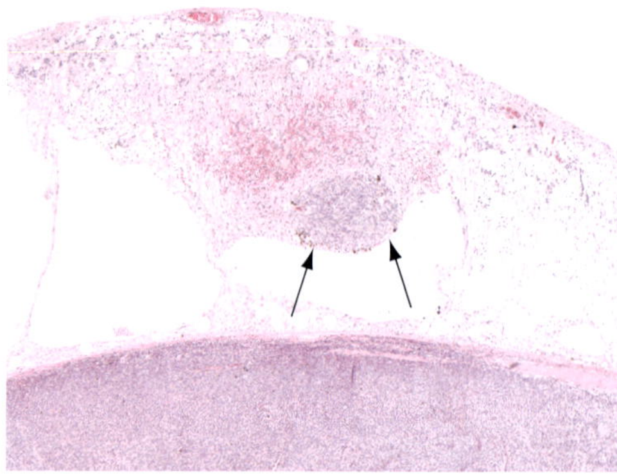

Figure 12-19 Invasion of neurosensory retina by melanoma *(arrows).* Note the atrophy of overlying outer retina, cystoid edema, and intraretinal hemorrhage. *(Courtesy of Nasreen A. Syed, MD.)*

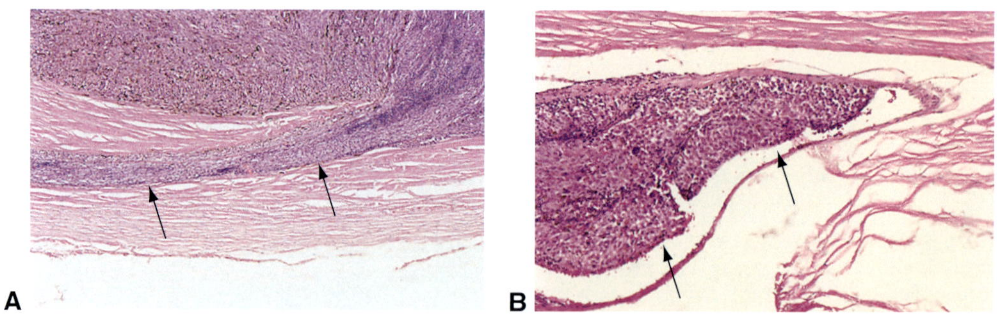

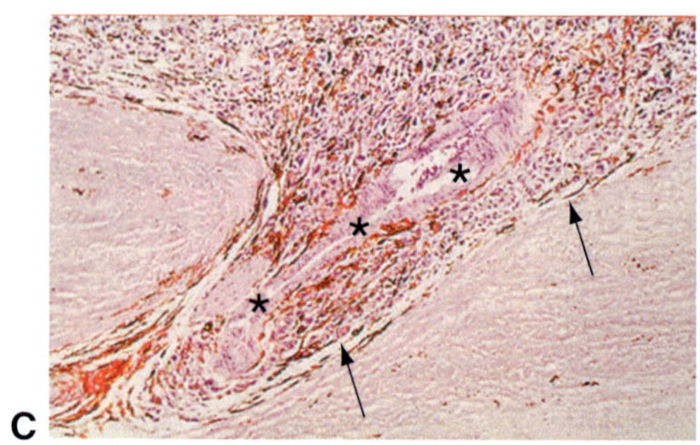

Figure 12-20 **A,** Note the melanoma cells tracking along scleral emissary canals *(arrows).* **B,** Melanoma is found within the vortex vein *(arrows).* **C,** Some melanomas *(arrows)* track along the outer sheaths of posterior ciliary vessels *(asterisks)* and nerves.

The modified Callender classification is used for the cytologic classification of uveal melanomas:

- spindle cell melanoma
- epithelioid melanoma
- mixed-cell type (mixture of spindle and epithelioid cells)

Occasionally, a melanoma undergoes extensive necrosis, which precludes classification.

Spindle cell melanoma has the best prognosis, and epithelioid melanoma the worst. Melanomas of mixed-cell type have an intermediate prognosis. Some authors have suggested that survival following enucleation decreases with increasing proportions of epithelioid cells in mixed-cell melanomas. Totally necrotic melanomas assume the same prognosis as mixed-cell melanomas.

The modified Callender classification has some disadvantages. First, there is continuing controversy about the minimum number of epithelioid cells needed for a melanoma to be classified as mixed-cell type. Second, the scheme is difficult to reproduce, even among experienced ophthalmic pathologists. This difficulty arises because the cytologic features of the melanoma cells reflect a continuous spectrum.

Cytomorphometric measurements of melanoma cells have been studied. One such measurement is the *mean of the 10 largest melanoma cell nucleoli (MLN).* This parameter has been shown to correlate well with mortality after enucleation. The correlation with morphometry is enhanced further when combined with the largest dimension of scleral contact by tumor.

Intrinsic tumor extravascular matrix patterns have also been studied and shown to have prognostic significance. Tumors containing more complex extravascular matrix patterns such as closed loops or networks (3 loops located back-to-back) are associated with an increased incidence of subsequent metastases (Fig 12-21).

Cytogenetic studies of uveal melanoma have shown that approximately half of uveal melanomas demonstrate monosomy of chromosome 3. A smaller proportion demonstrates

A
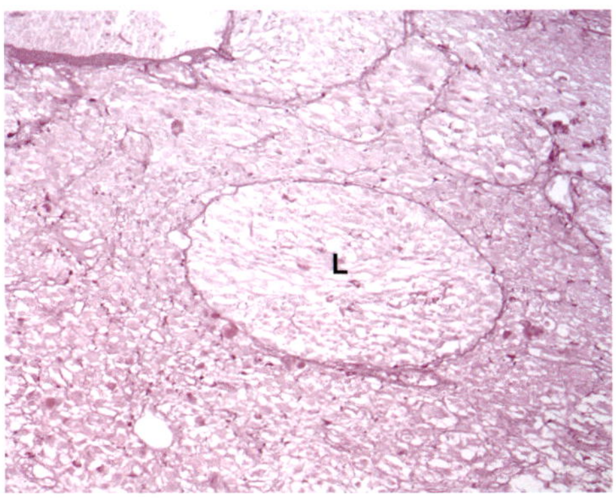

B
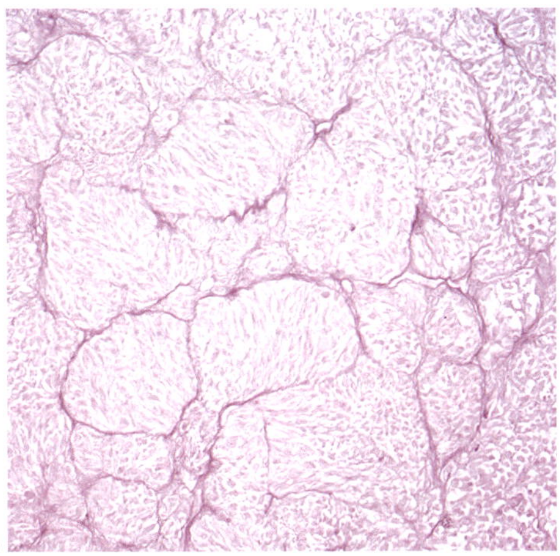

Figure 12-21 Extravascular matrix patterns in uveal melanoma. **A,** Closed loop *(L).* **B,** Network: 3 or more back-to-back loops. *(Courtesy of Nasreen A. Syed, MD.)*

changes in chromosome 8, with either gain or loss of a chromosome. Monosomy 3 and trisomy 8 are associated with increased mortality from the tumor. A commercially available test using gene expression profiling allows prognostic classification of uveal melanoma tumors. The test requires a small amount of fresh or paraffin-embedded tissue and classifies these tumors as either Class 1 (low metastatic potential) or Class 2 (high metastatic potential).

Other factors associated with an increased mortality rate include extrascleral extension, anterior or juxtapapillary location of the tumor, and the presence of tumor-infiltrating lymphocytes. Invasion through the Bruch membrane does not affect survival.

Lymphatic spread of ciliary body and choroidal melanomas is rare. Metastases almost invariably result from the hematogenous spread of melanoma to the liver. The reason for the propensity of melanomas to spread to the liver is unknown, although more than 95% of tumor-related deaths have liver involvement. In as many as one-third of tumor-related deaths, the liver is the sole site of metastasis.

Some types of uveal melanomas show biologic behavior that cannot be predicted according to the criteria just discussed. Survival rates of patients with diffuse ciliary body melanomas (ring melanoma) are particularly poor. These relatively flat tumors are almost always of mixed-cell type, and they may grow circumferentially without becoming significantly elevated. Diffuse choroidal melanomas similarly have a poor prognosis.

See Chapter 17. Also see the appendix for the American Joint Committee on Cancer (AJCC) staging form for uveal melanoma.

Metastatic Tumors

Metastatic lesions are the most common intraocular tumors in adults. These lesions most often involve the choroid, but any ocular structure can be affected. Unlike primary uveal melanoma, metastatic lesions are often multiple and may be bilateral. Although these lesions typically assume a flattened growth pattern, rare cases of collar-button or mushroom-shaped lesions have been reported. The most common primary tumors metastasizing to the eye are breast carcinoma in women and lung carcinoma in men (Fig 12-22), although tumors from many different primary sites have been reported. Histologically, metastatic tumors may recapitulate the appearance of the primary lesion, or they may appear less differentiated. Special histochemical and immunohistochemical stains can be helpful in diagnosing the metastatic lesion and determining its origin. The importance of a careful clinical history cannot be overemphasized. See Chapter 20 for further discussion.

Other Uveal Tumors

Hemangioma

Hemangiomas of the choroid occur in 2 specific forms. The *localized* choroidal hemangioma typically occurs in patients without systemic disorders. The *diffuse* choroidal hemangioma is generally seen in patients with Sturge-Weber syndrome (encephalofacial angiomatosis).

Histologically, both the diffuse and localized hemangiomas show collections of variably sized vessels within the choroid (Fig 12-23). The lesions may appear as predominantly

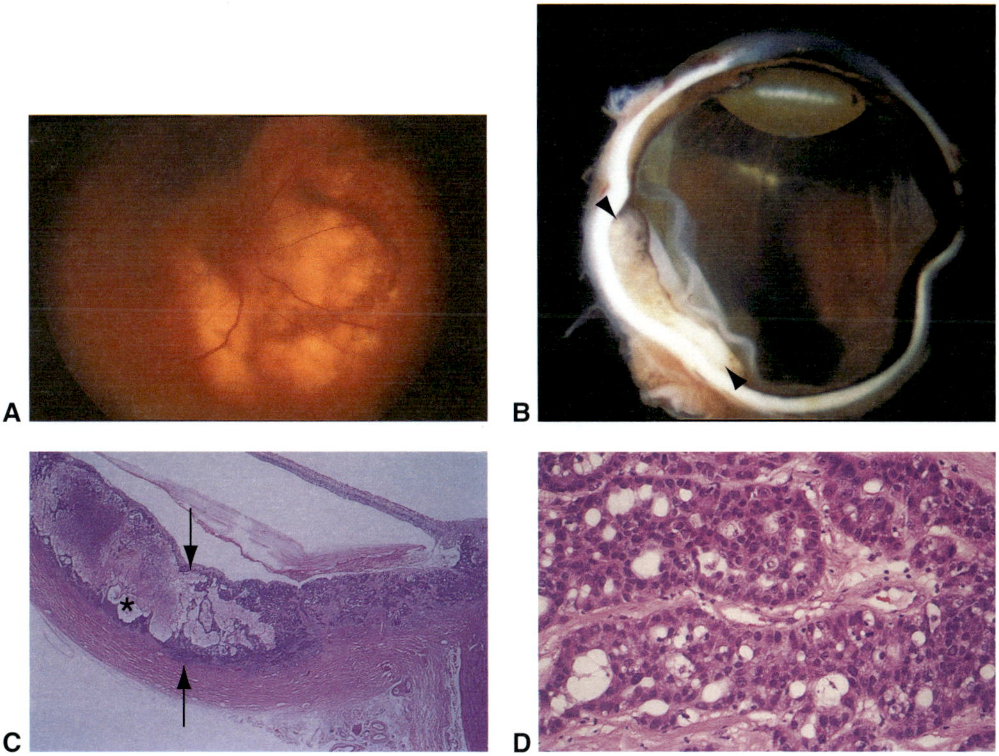

Figure 12-22 **A,** Clinical appearance of a metastatic lesion from a primary lung tumor. **B,** Gross appearance of lesion *(between arrowheads).* **C,** Choroidal metastasis from lung adenocarcinoma; histology shows adenocarcinoma *(between arrows)* with mucin production *(asterisk).* Note overlying retinal detachment. **D,** Higher magnification depicts a well-differentiated adenocarcinoma with distinct glandular appearance. *(Courtesy of Hans E. Grossniklaus, MD.)*

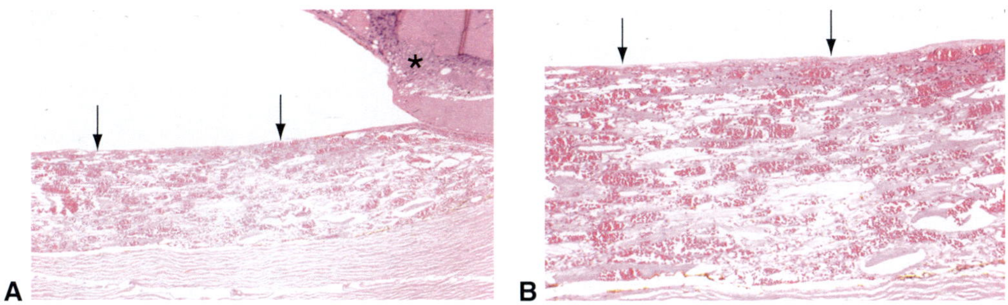

Figure 12-23 Choroidal hemangioma with a large number of thin-walled, variably sized vessels within the choroid. **A,** Low-magnification view illustrating exudative retinal detachment overlying the lesion *(asterisk). Arrows* designate the Bruch membrane. **B,** Higher magnification; *arrows* designate Bruch membrane. *(Courtesy of Nasreen A. Syed, MD.)*

capillary hemangiomas or cavernous hemangiomas or a mixed pattern. The adjacent and overlying choroid may show compressed melanocytes, hyperplastic RPE, and fibrous tissue proliferation. See also Chapter 18 and Figures 18-1 and 18-2 in this volume and BCSC Section 12, *Retina and Vitreous.*

Choroidal osteoma

Choroidal osteomas are benign bony tumors that typically arise from the juxtapapillary choroid and are seen in adolescent to young adult patients, more commonly in females. The characteristic lesion appears yellow to orange and has well-defined margins (see Chapter 17, Fig 17-13). Histologically, the tumor is composed of compact bone located in the peripapillary choroid. The intratrabecular spaces are filled with a loose connective tissue containing large and small blood vessels, vacuolated mesenchymal cells, and scattered mast cells. The bony trabeculae contain osteocytes, cement lines, and occasional osteoclasts. See Chapter 17 for further discussion.

Lymphoid proliferation

The choroid may be the site of lymphoid proliferation, either as a primary ocular process or in association with systemic lymphoproliferative disease.

Uveal lymphoid infiltration (formerly *reactive lymphoid hyperplasia*) of the uveal tract is similar to the spectrum of low-grade lymphoid lesions that occur in the orbit (see Chapter 14) and conjunctiva. There may be diffuse involvement of the uveal tract by a mixture of lymphocytes and plasma cells, and lymphoid follicles may be present. In addition, there may be a similar infiltrate located along the posterior episclera. Lymphocyte typing reveals a polymorphic population without clonal restriction; this finding distinguishes inflammatory pseudotumor from lymphoma.

Lymphoma of the uveal tract occurs almost exclusively in association with systemic lymphoma (Fig 12-24) as an extranodal site. The classification of lymphomas is discussed in Chapter 14.

Grossniklaus HE, Martin DF, Avery R, et al. Uveal lymphoid infiltration: report of four cases and clinicopathologic review. *Ophthalmology.* 1998;105(7):1265–1273.

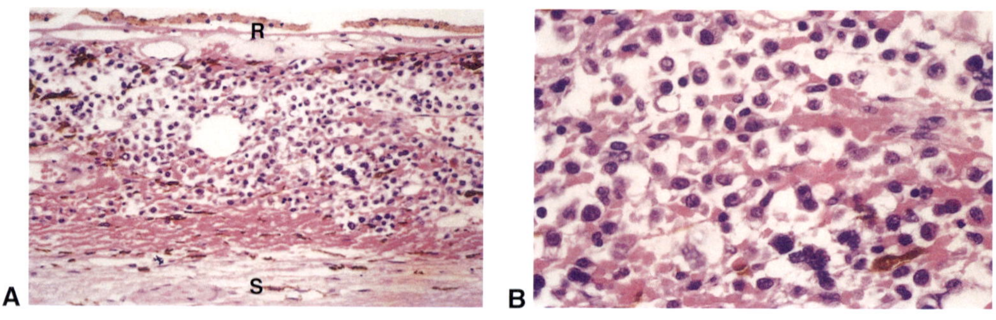

Figure 12-24 **A,** Diffuse expansion of choroid by lymphoma. *R* = RPE, *S* = sclera. **B,** Higher magnification depicts atypical lymphocytes. *(Courtesy of Hans E. Grossniklaus, MD.)*

Neural sheath tumors

Neurilemomas (schwannomas) and neurofibromas are rare tumors of the uveal tract. Multiple neurofibromas may occur in the ciliary body, iris, and choroid in patients with neurofibromatosis. The histopathologic features of these tumors are discussed in Chapter 14.

Leiomyoma

Neoplasms arising from the smooth muscle of the ciliary body have been reported only rarely. When they occur, they may be confused with amelanotic melanoma or neurofibroma clinically. Histologically, they consist of a proliferation of tightly packed slender spindle cells lacking pigment. Immunohistochemical stains may be useful in making the diagnosis, as leiomyomas express smooth muscle–related antigens. By light and transmission electron microscopy, these tumors sometimes exhibit both myogenic and neurogenic features. In such cases, the term *mesectodermal leiomyoma* is employed.

Trauma

The uveal tract is frequently involved in cases of ocular trauma. *Prolapse* of uveal tissue through a perforating ocular injury is a common association. *Rupture* of the choroid may occur as the result of a blunt or penetrating injury. The pattern of the rupture most frequently appears as semicircular lines circumscribing the optic nerve head in the peripapillary region. If the macula is involved, the prognosis for vision recovery is guarded. Subretinal neovascularization can occur as a late complication. More severe injury may cause rupture of both the choroid and the retina, a condition termed *chorioretinitis sclopetaria.*

Choroidal detachment, either localized or diffuse, may occur after traumatic globe rupture or surgery. Serous or hemorrhagic fluid accumulates in the suprachoroidal space between the choroid and the sclera. Depending on the etiology, the fluid may spontaneously resorb, allowing for reattachment of the choroid. In other cases, surgical drainage of the fluid may be required.

CHAPTER 13

Eyelids

Topography

The eyelids extend from the eyebrow superiorly to the cheek inferiorly and can be subdivided into orbital and tarsal components. At the level of the tarsus, the eyelid consists of 4 main histologic layers, from anterior to posterior:

- skin
- orbicularis oculi muscle
- tarsus
- palpebral conjunctiva

A surgical plane of dissection through an incision along the gray line of the eyelid margin is possible between the orbicularis and the tarsus, functionally dividing the eyelid into anterior and posterior lamellae (Fig 13-1). See also BCSC Section 7, *Orbit, Eyelids, and Lacrimal System.*

The skin of the eyelids is thinner than that of most other body sites. It consists of an epidermis of keratinizing stratified squamous epithelium, which also contains melanocytes and antigen-presenting Langerhans cells; and a dermis of loose collagenous connective tissue, which contains the following:

- cilia and associated sebaceous glands (of Zeis)
- apocrine sweat glands (of Moll)
- eccrine sweat glands
- pilosebaceous units

Eyelid elevation is effected by the *levator palpebrae superioris,* of which only the aponeurotic portion is present in the eyelid, and *Müller muscle* (smooth muscle connecting the upper border of the tarsus with the levator). Eyelid closure is accomplished by the *orbicularis oculi* (striated skeletal muscle). The *tarsal plate,* a thick plaque of dense, fibrous connective tissue, contains the sebaceous meibomian glands. Also present near the upper border of the superior tarsal plate (and less so along the lower border of the inferior tarsal plate) are the accessory lacrimal glands of Wolfring; the accessory lacrimal glands of Krause are located in the conjunctival fornices. The *palpebral conjunctiva* is tightly adherent to the posterior surface of the tarsus.

Eyelid glands secrete their products in various ways. Apocrine sweat glands secrete sweat by decapitation of the apical portion of the cell. Eccrine sweat glands and lacrimal glands secrete without losing any part of the cell. Sebaceous glands are holocrine glands,

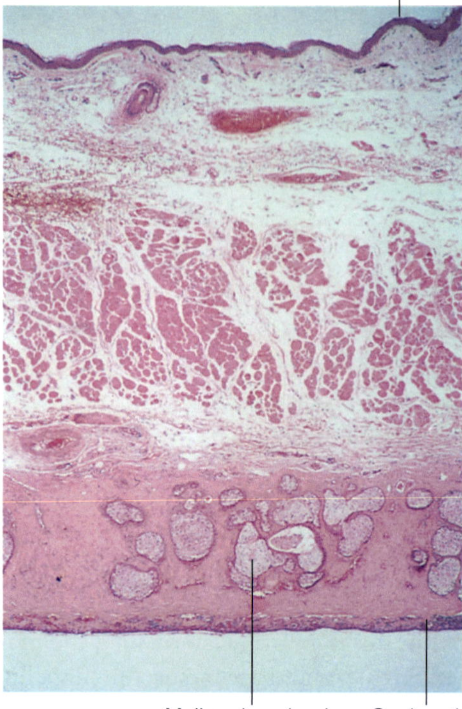

Figure 13-1 Cross section of a normal eyelid. Proceeding from top (anterior) to bottom (posterior), note the epidermis; the dermis, resting on the orbicularis; the tarsus, surrounding the meibomian glands; and the palpebral (tarsal) conjunctiva.

meaning that they shed the entire cell as they secrete. Table 13-1 lists the normal functions of the eyelid glands and some of the pathologic conditions related to them.

Following are several terms used commonly in dermatopathology:

- *acanthosis:* increased thickness (hyperplasia) of the stratum malpighii (consisting of the strata basale, spinosum, and granulosum) of the epidermis
- *hyperkeratosis:* increased thickness of the stratum corneum of the epidermis
- *parakeratosis:* retention of nuclei within the stratum corneum with corresponding absence of the stratum granulosum
- *papillomatosis:* formation of fingerlike upward projections of epidermis lining fibrovascular cores
- *dyskeratosis:* premature individual cell keratinization within the stratum malpighii
- *acantholysis:* loss of cohesion (dissolution of intercellular bridges) between adjacent epithelial cells
- *spongiosis:* widening of intercellular spaces between cells in the stratum malpighii due to edema

Table 13-1 Secretory Elements of the Eyelid: Function and Pathology

Secretory Element	Normal Function	Pathology
Conjunctival goblet cells	Mucin secretion to enhance corneal wetting	Numbers diminished in some dry-eye states Mucoepidermoid carcinoma
Accessory lacrimal glands of Krause and Wolfring	Basal tear secretion of the aqueous layer	Sjögren syndrome Graft-vs-host disease Rare tumors (benign mixed tumor)
Meibomian (sebaceous) glands	Secretion of lipid layer of tears to retard evaporation	Chalazion Sebaceous carcinoma
Sebaceous glands of Zeis	Lubrication of the cilia	External hordeolum Sebaceous carcinoma
Apocrine glands of Moll	Lubrication of the cilia	Ductal cyst (sudoriferous cyst, apocrine hidrocystoma) Apocrine carcinoma
Eccrine glands	Secretions for temperature control, electrolyte balance	Ductal cyst (sudoriferous cyst, eccrine hidrocystoma) Syringoma Sweat gland carcinoma

Congenital Anomalies

See also BCSC Section 7, *Orbit, Eyelids, and Lacrimal System.*

Distichiasis

Distichiasis is the aberrant formation within the tarsus of cilia that exit the eyelid margin through the orifices of the meibomian glands. The pathogenesis of distichiasis is thought to be an anomalous formation within the tarsus of a complete pilosebaceous unit rather than the normal sebaceous (meibomian) gland. Histologically, hair follicles can be seen within the tarsal plate. The tarsus may be rudimentary, and the glands of Moll are often hypertrophic. See BCSC Section 6, *Pediatric Ophthalmology and Strabismus,* and Section 8, *External Disease and Cornea,* for additional discussion.

Phakomatous Choristoma

A rare congenital tumor, phakomatous choristoma (Zimmerman tumor) is formed from the aberrant location of lens epithelium within the inferonasal portion of the lower eyelid. These cells may undergo cytoplasmic enlargement, identical to the "bladder" cell in a cataractous lens. PAS-positive basement membrane material is produced, recapitulating the lens capsule (Fig 13-2). The nodule formed is usually present at birth and enlarges slowly. Complete excision is the usual treatment.

Dermoid Cyst

Dermoid cysts may occur in the eyelid, but they are more common in the orbit and are discussed in Chapter 14.

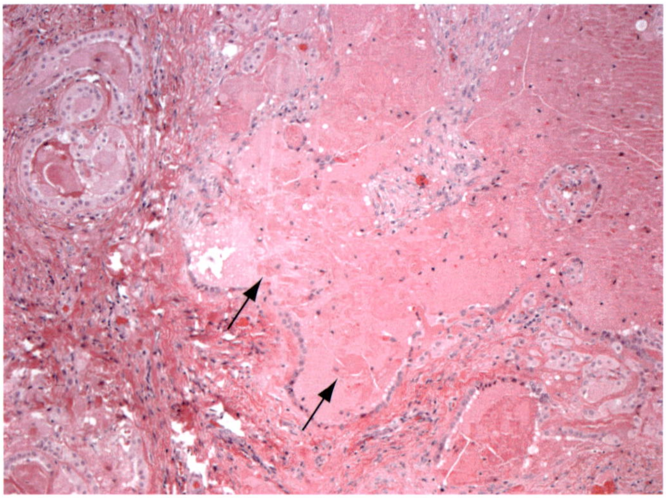

Figure 13-2 Phakomatous choristoma of the eyelid. The dermis displays a disorganized proliferation of lens epithelium and occasional "bladder" cells *(arrows)*. Note the large amount of eosinophilic material that represents lens nuclear/cortical proteins. *(Courtesy of Nasreen A. Syed, MD.)*

Inflammations

Infectious

Depending on the causative agent, infections of the eyelids may produce disease that is localized (eg, hordeolum), multicentric (eg, papillomas), or diffuse (cellulitis). Routes of infection may be primary inoculation through a bite or wound, direct spread from a contiguous site such as a paranasal sinus infection, or hematogenous dissemination from a remote site. Infectious agents may be

- bacterial, such as *Staphylococcus aureus* in hordeolum and infectious blepharitis
- viral, such as molluscum contagiosum due to a poxvirus
- fungal, such as blastomycosis, coccidioidomycosis, or aspergillosis

Hordeolum

Also known as a *stye,* hordeolum is a primary, acute, self-limited inflammatory process typically involving the glands of Zeis and, less often, the meibomian glands of the eyelids. A small abscess, or focal collection of neutrophils and necrotic debris (pus), forms at the site of infection. Lesions may drain spontaneously or require surgical drainage.

Cellulitis

The diffuse spread of acute inflammatory cells through tissue planes is known as *cellulitis. Preseptal cellulitis* involves the tissues of the eyelid anterior to the orbital septum, the fibrous membrane connecting the borders of the tarsal plates to the bony orbital rim. The condition can be due to infected skin lesions or bacterial infection of the paranasal sinuses. Histologically, there is neutrophilic infiltration of the soft tissues, accompanied by interstitial edema and, occasionally, necrosis (Fig 13-3).

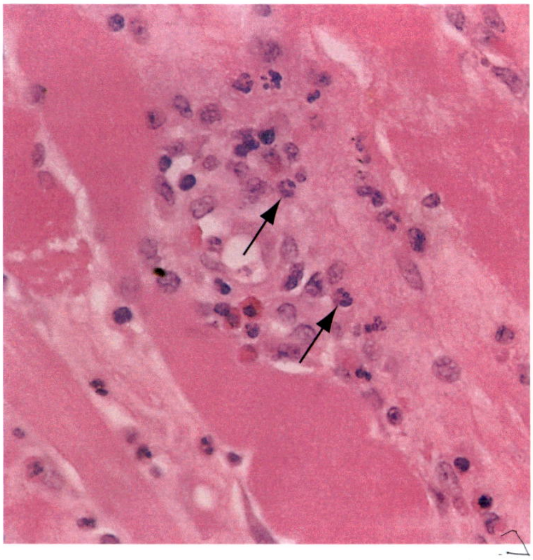

Figure 13-3 Neutrophils *(arrows)* dissect between the skeletal muscle fibers of the orbicularis in this biopsy of a preseptal cellulitis of the eyelid.

Viral infections

Human papillomavirus may infect the skin of the eyelids and typically manifests as *verruca vulgaris,* commonly known as a *wart.* Clinically, it is usually an elevated papillary lesion. Histologically, the lesions demonstrate hyperkeratosis and acanthosis and exhibit a papillary growth pattern. Infected cells may demonstrate cytoplasmic clearing (koilocytosis). A mixed inflammatory infiltrate is typically present in the superficial dermis (Fig 13-4).

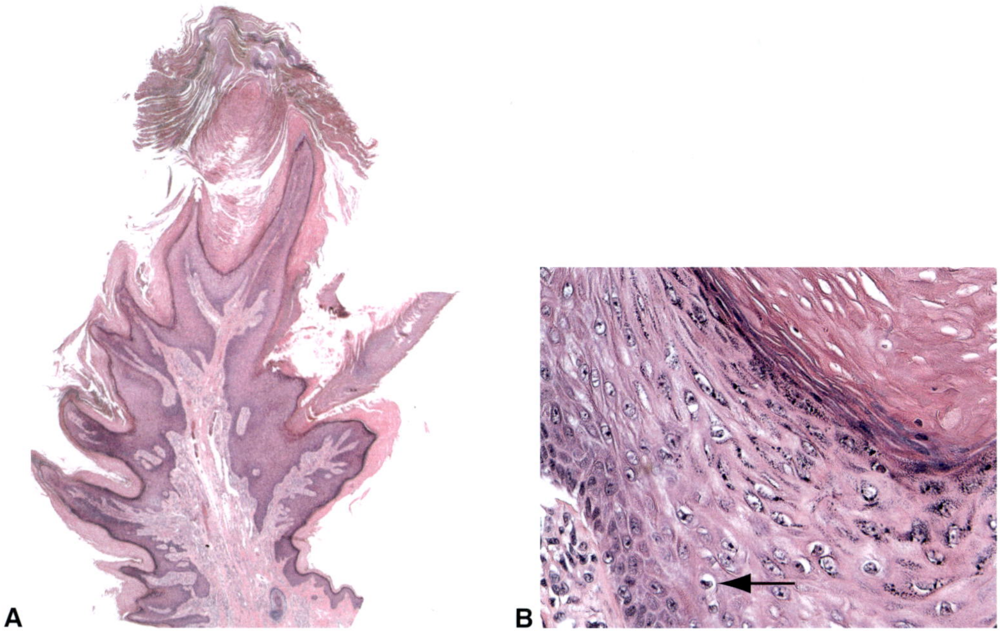

Figure 13-4 **A,** Verruca vulgaris is a form of infection of the eyelid with human papillomavirus (HPV). The lesion has a papillary growth pattern with fingerlike projections. **B,** Occasional koilocytes with nuclear contraction and cytoplasmic clearing are present *(arrow). (Courtesy of Nasreen A. Syed, MD.)*

Molluscum contagiosum is caused by a member of the poxvirus family. Dome-shaped, waxy epidermal nodules with central umbilication form and, if present on the eyelid margin, may cause a secondary follicular conjunctivitis (Fig 13-5). Histologically, the lesions are distinctive, with a nodular proliferation of infected epithelium producing a central focus of necrotic cells that are extruded to the skin surface. As the replicating virus fills the cytoplasm, the nucleus is displaced peripherally by large viral inclusions (molluscum bodies) and finally disappears as the cells are shed (Fig 13-6).

Noninfectious

Chalazion

A chalazion is a chronic, often painless nodule of the eyelid that occurs when the lipid secretions of the meibomian glands or, less often, the glands of Zeis are discharged into the

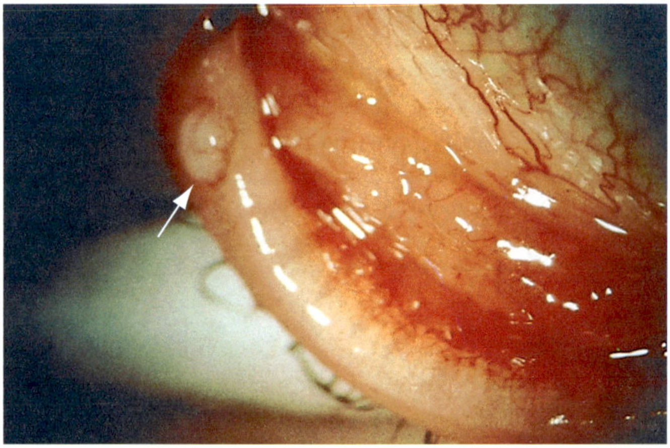

Figure 13-5 Molluscum contagiosum involving the eyelid margin *(arrow)*. Note the associated follicular conjunctivitis.

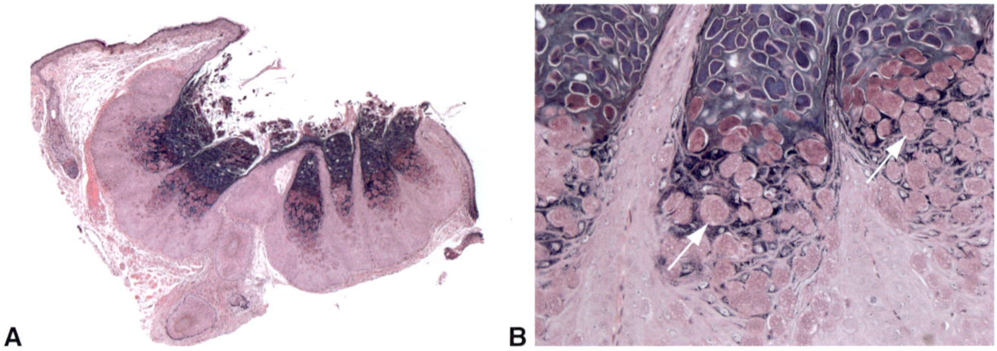

Figure 13-6 Molluscum contagiosum. **A,** Note the cup-shaped, thickened epidermis with a central crater. **B,** Note the eosinophilic inclusion bodies *(arrows)* becoming basophilic as they migrate to the surface. *(Courtesy of Nasreen A. Syed, MD.)*

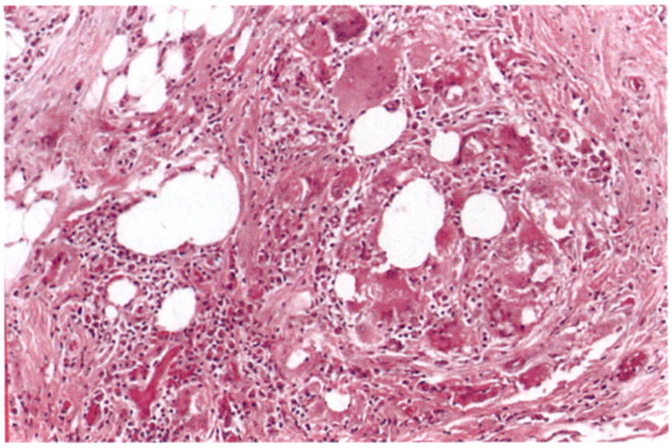

Figure 13-7 Chalazion. Granulomatous inflammation (epithelioid histiocytes and multinucleated giant cells) surrounds clear spaces formerly occupied by lipid (lipogranuloma).

surrounding tissues, inciting a lipogranulomatous reaction (Fig 13-7). Because the lipid is dissolved by solvents during routine tissue processing, histologic sections show histiocytes and multinucleated giant cells enveloping optically clear ("lipid dropout") spaces. Lymphocytes, plasma cells, and neutrophils are also often present.

Degenerations

Xanthelasma

Xanthelasmas are single or multiple soft yellow plaques occurring in the medial canthal region of the eyelids. Associated hyperlipoproteinemic states, particularly hyperlipoproteinemia types II and III, are present in 30%–40% of patients with xanthelasma. These eyelid xanthomas consist of collections of histiocytes with foamy lipid-laden cytoplasm distributed diffusely, often around blood vessels, within the dermis (Fig 13-8). Associated inflammation is minimal to nonexistent.

Amyloid

The term *amyloid* refers to a heterogeneous group of extracellular proteins that exhibit birefringence and dichroism under polarized light when stained with Congo red (see

A 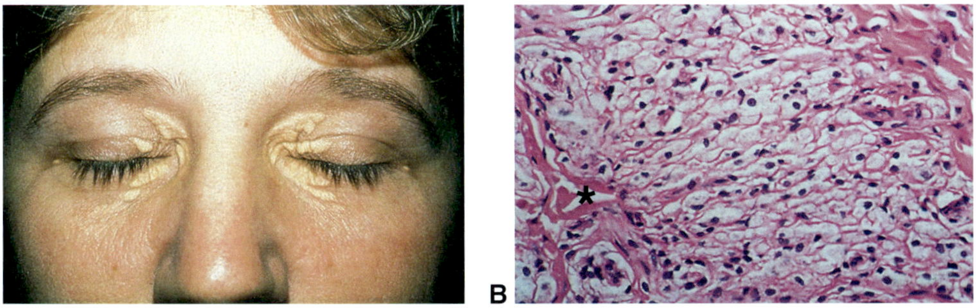 B

Figure 13-8 **A,** Patient with prominent xanthelasma. Note the yellow papules on the medial aspect of the upper and lower eyelids. **B,** Note the foam cells (filled with lipid) surrounding a venule *(asterisk)*. *(Part A from* External Disease and Cornea: A Multimedia Collection. *San Francisco: American Academy of Ophthalmology; 1994:slide 10.)*

Chapter 5 and Fig 5-13). These features result from the 3-dimensional configuration of the proteins into a β-pleated sheet. Examples of proteins that may form amyloid deposits include

- immunoglobulin light chain fragments (AL amyloid) in plasma cell dyscrasias
- transthyretin mutations in familial amyloid polyneuropathy (FAP) types I and II (see Chapter 10)
- gelsolin mutations in FAP type IV (Meretoja syndrome [lattice corneal dystrophy type II])

Amyloid within the skin of the eyelid is highly indicative of a systemic disease process, either primary or secondary, whereas deposits elsewhere in the ocular adnexa but not in the eyelid are more likely a localized disease process.

Amyloid deposits in the skin are usually multiple, bilateral, symmetric, waxy yellow-white nodules. The deposition of amyloid within blood vessel walls in the skin causes increased vascular fragility and often results in intradermal hemorrhages, accounting for the purpura seen clinically (Fig 13-9). On routine histologic sections, amyloid appears as an amorphous, eosinophilic extracellular deposit, usually within vessel walls but also in soft tissue and around peripheral nerves and sweat glands. Stains useful in demonstrating amyloid deposits include Congo red, crystal violet, and thioflavin T. Electron microscopy reveals the deposits to be composed of randomly oriented extracellular fibrils measuring 7–10 nm in diameter (see Fig 10-11).

Other systemic diseases with eyelid manifestations are listed in Table 13-2.

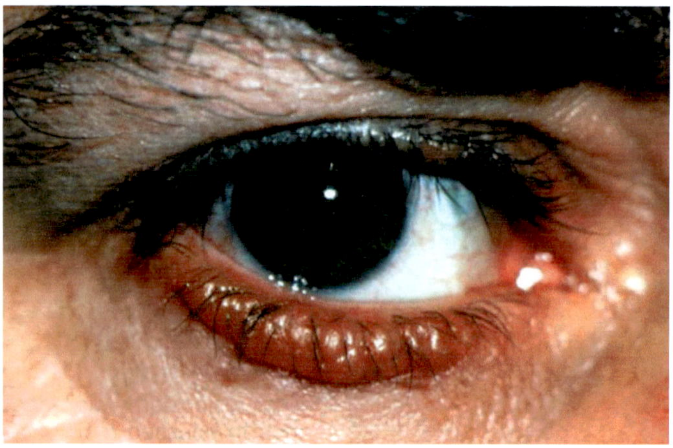

Figure 13-9 Cutaneous amyloid in a patient with multiple myeloma. Note the waxy elevation and the associated purpura of the lower eyelid. *(Courtesy of John B. Holds, MD.)*

Table 13-2 Eyelid Manifestations of Systemic Diseases

Systemic Condition	Eyelid Manifestation
Erdheim-Chester disease	Xanthelasma, xanthogranuloma
Hyperlipoproteinemia	Xanthelasma
Amyloidosis	Waxy papules, ptosis, purpura
Sarcoidosis	Papules
Wegener granulomatosis	Edema, ptosis, lower eyelid retraction
Scleroderma	Reduced mobility, taut skin
Polyarteritis nodosa	Focal infarct
Systemic lupus erythematosus	Telangiectasias, edema
Dermatomyositis	Edema, erythema
Relapsing polychondritis	Papules
Carney complex	Myxoma
Fraser syndrome	Cryptophthalmos
Treacher Collins syndrome	Lower eyelid coloboma

Modified from Wiggs JL, Jakobiec FA. Eyelid manifestations of systemic disease. In: Albert DM, Jakobiec FA, eds. *Principles and Practice of Ophthalmology.* Philadelphia: Saunders; 1994:1859.

Cysts

Epidermoid and Dermoid Cysts

Epidermoid cysts, also known as *epidermal inclusion cysts,* are common in the eyelids. They may arise spontaneously or as a result of the entrapment of epidermis beneath the skin surface following traumatic laceration or surgical incision. Epidermoid cysts are lined with stratified squamous keratinizing epithelium and contain keratin (Fig 13-10). Dermoid cysts (discussed earlier in this chapter) are similar to epidermoid cysts histologically, but they have skin adnexal structures such as hair follicles and sebaceous glands in the wall. The lumen contains hair and sebum in addition to keratin.

Ductal Cysts

Within the eyelid are the ducts of numerous structures, including the apocrine and eccrine sweat glands and the lacrimal gland. Any of these ducts may give rise to 1 or more

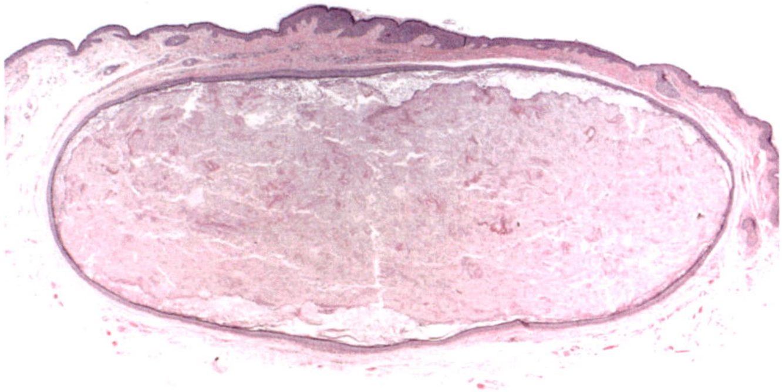

Figure 13-10 An epidermoid, or epidermal inclusion cyst, is present in the dermis. The cyst lining resembles epidermis, and the lumen contains keratin. *(Courtesy of Nasreen A. Syed, MD.)*

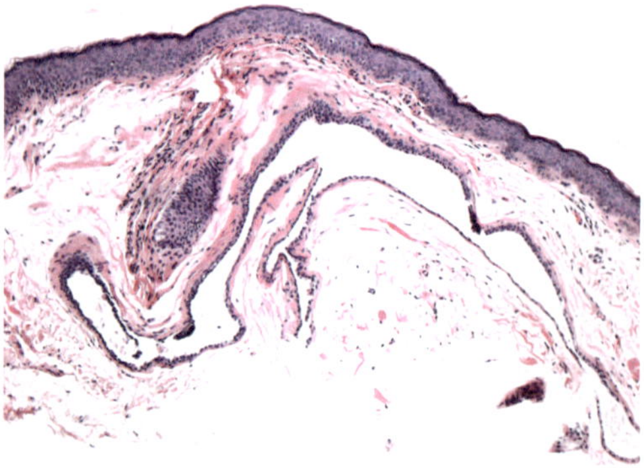

Figure 13-11 An apocrine hidrocystoma is typically lined with a double layer of cuboidal epithelium. Epithelial cells may demonstrate decapitation secretion. *(Courtesy of Nasreen A. Syed, MD.)*

cysts. Ducts are typically lined with a double layer of cuboidal epithelium, as are ductal cysts. The lumen of the cyst typically appears empty histologically. Cysts arising from sweat ducts are referred to as either *apocrine* or *eccrine hidrocystomas* (Fig 13-11). A cyst arising from the duct of the lacrimal gland is called a *dacryops.*

Neoplasia

Epidermal Neoplasms

Seborrheic keratosis

Seborrheic keratosis, a common benign epithelial proliferation, occurs in middle age. Clinically, it is a well-circumscribed, oval, dome-shaped to verrucoid "stuck-on" papule, varying from pink to brown in color. Histologically, several architectural patterns are possible, although all demonstrate hyperkeratosis, acanthosis, and some degree of papillomatosis. The acanthosis is a result of the proliferation of either polygonal or basaloid squamous cells without dysplasia.

A characteristic finding in most types of seborrheic keratoses is the formation of pseudohorn cysts, which are concentrically laminated collections of surface keratin within the acanthotic epithelium (Fig 13-12). Irritated seborrheic keratosis, also termed

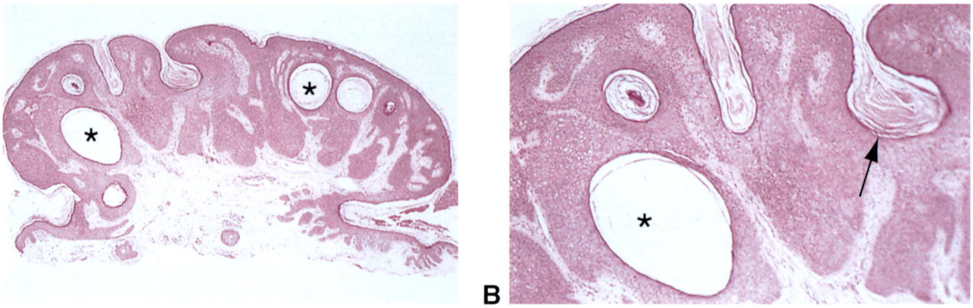

A

B

Figure 13-12 Seborrheic keratosis. **A,** The epidermis is acanthotic with a papillary configuration. Note the keratin-filled cysts *(asterisks).* **B,** When serial histologic sections are studied, pseudohorn cysts *(asterisk)* within the epidermis are seen to represent crevices or infoldings of epidermis *(arrow).* *(Courtesy of Hans E. Grossniklaus, MD.)*

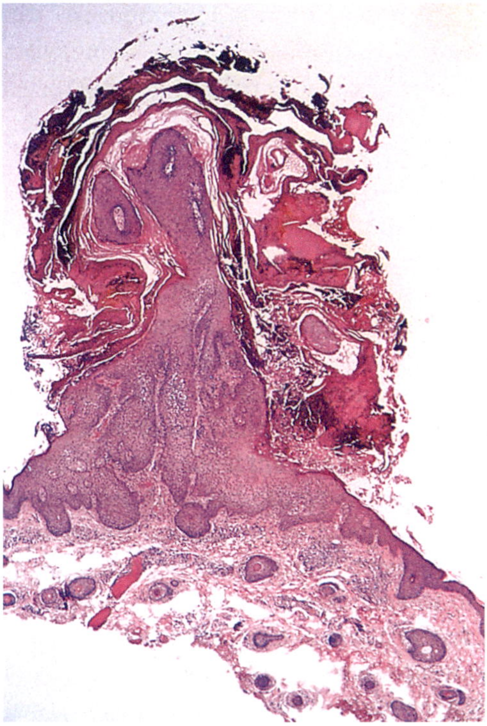

Figure 13-13 Irritated seborrheic keratosis, also known as *inverted follicular keratosis.* Clinically, this lesion appeared as a cutaneous horn.

inverted follicular keratosis, shows nonkeratinizing squamous epithelial whorling, or squamous "eddies," instead of pseudohorn cysts (Fig 13-13). Heavy melanin phagocytosis by keratinocytes may impart a dark brown color to an otherwise typical seborrheic keratosis, which may then be confused clinically with melanoma.

Sudden onset of multiple seborrheic keratoses is known as the *Leser-Trélat sign* and is associated with a malignancy, usually a gastrointestinal adenocarcinoma; these keratoses may in fact represent evolving acanthosis nigricans. Table 13-3 lists other systemic malignancies with cutaneous manifestations.

Table 13-3 Eyelid Neoplasms in Association With Systemic Malignancies

Syndrome	Eyelid Manifestation
Muir-Torre syndrome (visceral carcinoma, usually colon)	Keratoacanthoma, sebaceous neoplasm (adenoma, carcinoma)
Cowden disease (breast carcinoma; fibrous hamartomas of breast, thyroid, GI tract)	Multiple trichilemmomas
Basal cell nevus syndrome (medulloblastoma, fibrosarcoma)	Multiple basal cell carcinomas

Modified from Wiggs JL, Jakobiec FA. Eyelid manifestations of systemic disease. In: Albert DM, Jakobiec FA, eds. *Principles and Practice of Ophthalmology.* Philadelphia: Saunders; 1994:1859.

Keratoacanthoma

Keratoacanthoma is a rapidly growing epithelial proliferation with a potential for spontaneous involution. There is strong evidence supporting the idea that keratoacanthomas are a variant of a well-differentiated squamous cell carcinoma. These studies are based on expression of proliferation markers (cyclins and cyclin-dependent kinases) and oncoproteins (mutated p53) that are expressed similarly by both entities. Dome-shaped nodules with a keratin-filled central crater may attain a considerable size, up to 2.5 cm in diameter, within a matter of weeks to months (Fig 13-14). The natural history is typically spontaneous involution over several months, resulting in a slightly depressed scar.

Histologically, keratoacanthomas show a cup-shaped invagination of well-differentiated squamous cells forming irregularly configured nests and strands and inciting a chronic inflammatory host response. The proliferating epithelial cells undermine the adjacent normal epidermis. At the deep aspect of the proliferating nodules, mitotic activity and nuclear atypia may occur, making the distinction between keratoacanthoma and invasive squamous cell carcinoma problematic. If unequivocal invasion is present, the lesion should be considered a well-differentiated squamous cell carcinoma. Many dermatopathologists and ophthalmic pathologists have ceased to use the term *keratoacanthoma* altogether and prefer to call this lesion *well-differentiated keratinizing squamous cell carcinoma* because of the possibility of perineural invasion and metastasis. When the clinical differential diagnosis is keratoacanthoma versus squamous cell carcinoma, the lesion should be completely excised to permit optimal histologic examination of the lateral and deep margins of the tumor–host interface.

Actinic keratosis

Actinic keratoses are precancerous squamous lesions that appear, clinically, as erythematous, scaly macules or papules in middle age on sun-exposed skin, particularly on the face

A B

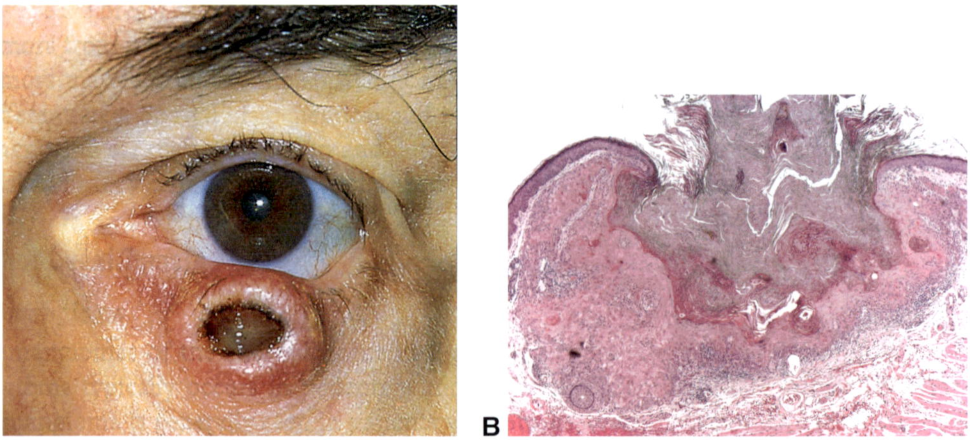

Figure 13-14 **A,** Patient with keratoacanthoma. Note the cuplike configuration. In this case, the central crater was originally filled with keratin. **B,** Low-power histologic section illustrating the central keratin crater and the downward (invasive) growth pattern. *(Part B courtesy of Nasreen A. Syed, MD.)*

and the dorsal surfaces of the hands. Actinic keratoses range from a few millimeters up to 1 cm in greatest dimension. Hyperkeratotic types may form a cutaneous horn, and hyperpigmented types may clinically simulate lentigo maligna. Squamous cell carcinoma may develop from preexisting actinic keratosis; thus, biopsy of suspicious lesions and long-term follow-up are necessary in patients with this condition. However, when squamous cell carcinoma arises in actinic keratosis, the risk of subsequent metastatic dissemination is very low (0.5%–3.0%).

Histologically, there are 5 subtypes, ranging from hypertrophic to atrophic; all types demonstrate changes in the epidermis with hyperkeratosis and parakeratosis. Cellular atypia such as nuclear hyperchromasia and enlargement, nuclear membrane irregularities, and increased nuclear-to-cytoplasmic ratio is present and ranges from mild (involving only the basal epithelial layers) to frank carcinoma in situ, or full-thickness involvement of the epidermis. Dyskeratosis (premature individual cell keratinization) and mitotic figures above the basal epithelial layer are often present (Fig 13-15). The underlying dermis shows solar elastosis (elastotic degeneration of collagen) (Fig 13-16), which manifests as fragmentation, clumping, and loss of eosinophilia of dermal collagen. A chronic inflammatory cell infiltrate is usually present in the superficial dermis. The base of the lesion must be examined histologically to determine whether invasive squamous cell carcinoma is present; for this reason, shave biopsy not including the base of the lesion is contraindicated.

Carcinoma

Basal cell carcinoma (BCC) is the most common malignant neoplasm of the eyelids, accounting for more than 90% of all eyelid malignancies. Exposure to sunlight is the main risk factor, although genetic factors can play a role in familial syndromes. The lower eyelid is more commonly involved than the upper eyelid, with the medial canthus being the second most common site of involvement. Tumors in the medial canthal area are more

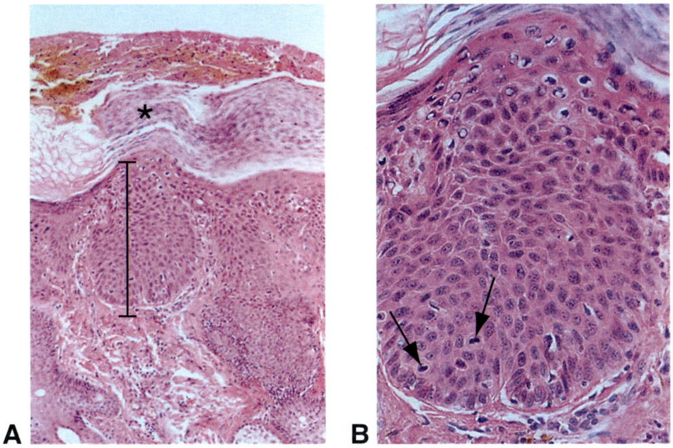

Figure 13-15 Actinic keratosis. **A,** Note the epidermal thickening (acanthosis *[I]*), disorganization within the epidermis (dysplasia), parakeratosis *(asterisk),* and inflammation within the dermis. **B,** Note the epidermal disorganization and mitotic figures *(arrows).*

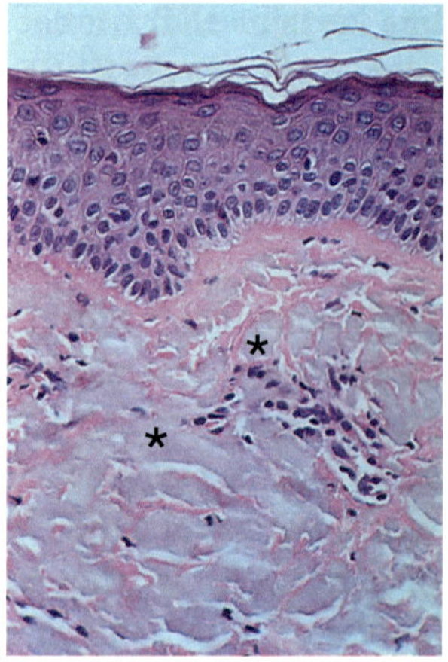

Figure 13-16 Solar elastosis. The collagen of the dermis appears bluish *(asterisks)* in this H&E stain, instead of pink. This is a histopathologic sign of ultraviolet light–induced damage.

likely to be deeply invasive and to involve the orbit. The most common type, nodular BCC (Fig 13-17A) is a slowly enlarging, slightly elevated lesion with ulceration and pearly, raised, rolled edges. The morpheaform, or sclerosing, variant of BCC is a flat or slightly depressed pale yellow indurated plaque; this type is often infiltrative, and its extent is difficult to determine clinically. A small percentage of BCCs are pigmented.

As the name implies, BCCs originate from the stratum basale, or stratum germinativum, of the epidermis and the outer root sheath of the hair follicle and occur only in hair-bearing tissue. Tumor cells are characterized by relatively bland, monomorphous nuclei and a high nuclear-to-cytoplasmic ratio. BCC forms cohesive islands with nuclear palisading of the peripheral cell layer. Frequently, a clear space surrounds the islands of tumor cells, presumably an artifact of tissue processing (Fig 13-17B). BCCs may exhibit a variety of histologic patterns, including keratotic (hair follicle), squamous (metatypical),

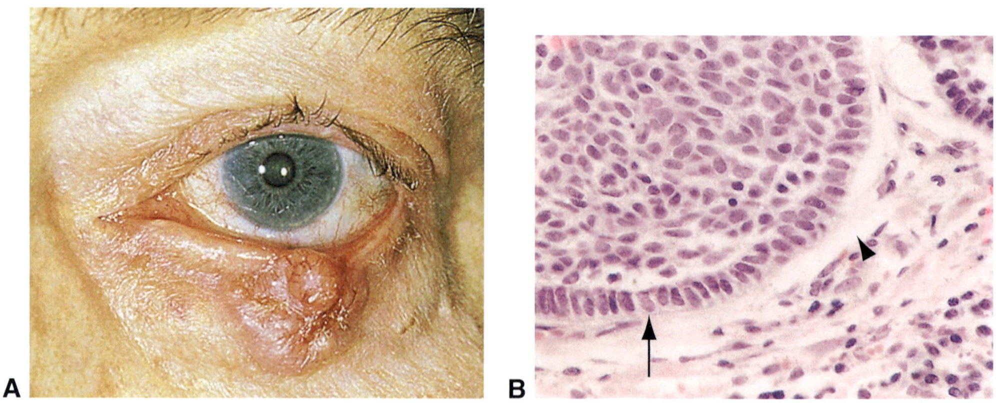

Figure 13-17 Basal cell carcinoma. **A,** Clinical appearance of the nodular type. **B,** Histologic appearance. Note the characteristic palisading of the cells around the outer edge of the tumor *(arrow)* and the artifactitious separation between the nest of tumor cells and the dermis (retraction artifact, *arrowhead*).

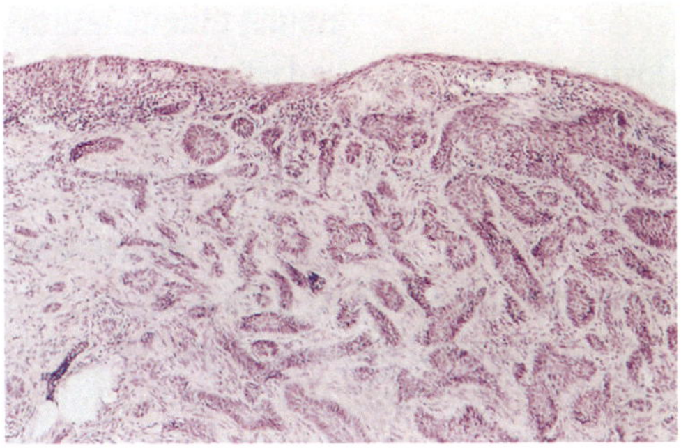

Figure 13-18 Basal cell carcinoma, morphea-form (sclerosing) type. Thin strands and cords of tumor cells are seen in a fibrotic (desmoplastic) dermis.

sebaceous, adenoid, and eccrine (syringoid) differentiation. The morphea (sclerosing) variant shows thin cords and strands of tumor cells set in a fibrotic stroma (Fig 13-18).

Complete excision is the treatment of choice, and surgical margin control is required. Typically, margin control is achieved with frozen sections or Mohs micrographic excision. Morbidity in BCCs is almost always the result of local spread; metastasis is extremely unusual.

Although *squamous cell carcinoma (SCC)* may occur in the eyelids, it is at least 10 and perhaps up to 40 times less common than BCC. Because most SCCs arise in solar-damaged skin, the lower eyelid is more frequently involved than the upper. However, the proportion of SCCs occurring in the upper eyelid is larger than the proportion of BCCs occurring in the upper eyelid. The clinical appearance of SCC is diverse, ranging from ulcers to plaques to fungating or nodular growths. Accordingly, the clinical differential diagnosis is a long list, and pathologic examination of excised tissue is necessary for accurate diagnosis.

Histologic examination shows atypical squamous cells forming nests and strands, extending beyond the epidermal basement membrane, infiltrating the dermis, and inciting a fibrotic tissue reaction (Fig 13-19). Tumor cells may be well differentiated (forming keratin and easily recognizable as squamous), moderately differentiated, or poorly differentiated (requiring ancillary studies to confirm the nature of the neoplasm). The presence of intercellular bridges between tumor cells should be sought when the diagnosis is in question. Perineural and lymphatic invasion may be present and should be reported when identified microscopically. The use of frozen section (conventional or Mohs microsurgery) or permanent section margin control is indicated to treat this tumor adequately. Regional lymph node metastasis is reported to occur in up to 20% of patients with SCC of the eyelid.

Chévez-Barrios P. Frozen section diagnosis and indications in ophthalmic pathology. *Arch Pathol Lab Med.* 2005;129(12):1626–1634.

Dermal Neoplasms

Capillary hemangiomas are common in the eyelids of children. They usually appear at or shortly after birth as a bright red lesion, grow over weeks to months, and involute by school age. Intervention is reserved for those lesions that affect vision because of ptosis or astigmatism, promoting amblyopia.

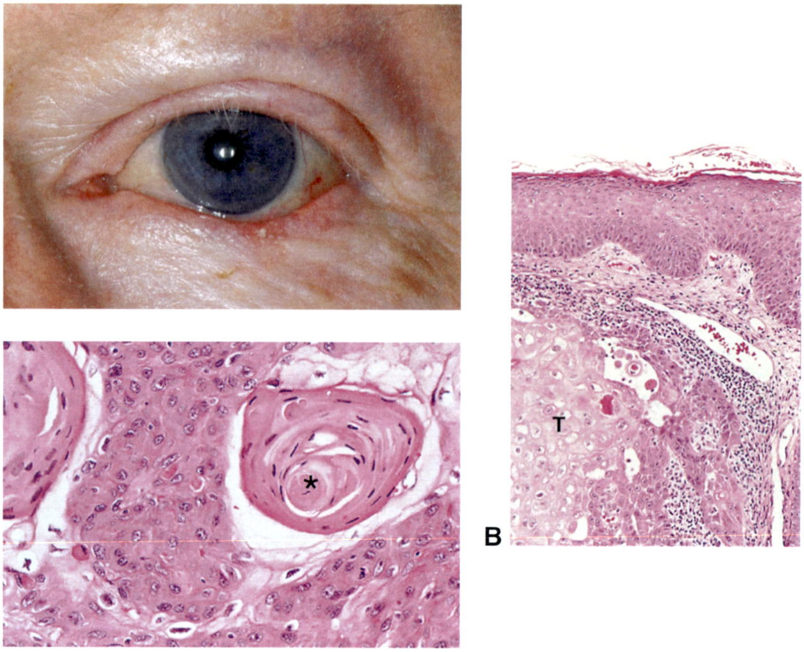

Figure 13-19 Squamous cell carcinoma. **A,** Clinical appearance. Note the focal loss of lashes and scaly appearance of the lower eyelid. **B,** Note the tumor cells *(T)* invading the dermis. **C,** Keratin *(asterisk)* is produced in this well-differentiated squamous cell carcinoma. *(Part A courtesy of Keith D. Carter, MD.)*

The histopathologic appearance depends on the stage of evolution of the hemangioma. Early lesions may be very cellular, with solid nests of plump endothelial cells and correspondingly little vascular luminal formation. Established lesions typically show well-developed, flattened, endothelium-lined capillary channels in a lobular configuration (Fig 13-20). Involuting lesions demonstrate increased fibrosis and hyalinization of capillary walls with luminal occlusion.

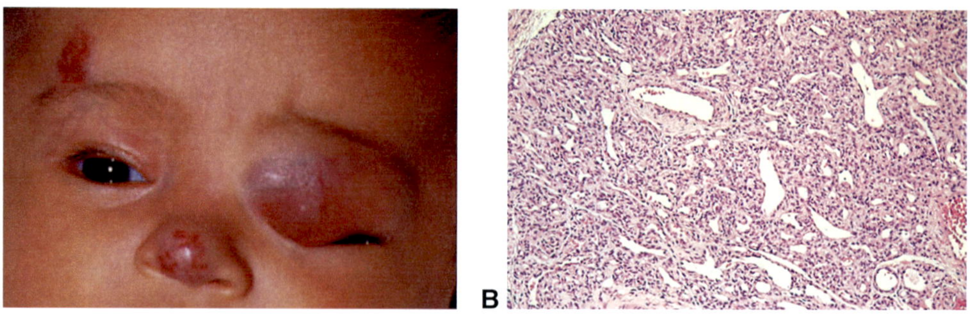

Figure 13-20 Capillary hemangioma. **A,** Infant with multiple capillary hemangiomas. **B,** Note the small capillary-sized vessels and the proliferation of benign endothelial cells. *(Part A courtesy of Sander Dubovy, MD.)*

Appendage Neoplasms

Syringoma

Syringoma is a common benign lesion of the lower eyelid and typically manifests as multiple tiny papules. Syringomas result from a malformation of the eccrine sweat gland ducts. Histologically, syringomas consist of multiple, comma-shaped or round ductules lined with a double layer of epithelium and containing a central lumen, often with secretory material (Fig 13-21).

Sebaceous hyperplasia

Sebaceous hyperplasia is an uncommon benign lesion of the eyelid and face. Clinically, it appears as a small, yellow papule. Histologically, it is typically a single enlarged sebaceous gland with numerous glandular lobules attached to a single central duct (Fig 13-22).

Sebaceous adenoma

Sebaceous adenoma is a rare benign lesion of the eyelid that typically manifests as a yellow, circumscribed nodule. Histologically, it is composed of multiple sebaceous lobules that are irregularly shaped and incompletely differentiated (Fig 13-23). Muir-Torre syndrome should be considered when sebaceous adenoma is diagnosed (see Table 13-3).

Sebaceous carcinoma

A sebaceous carcinoma most commonly involves the upper eyelid of elderly persons. It may originate in the meibomian glands of the tarsus, the glands of Zeis in the skin of

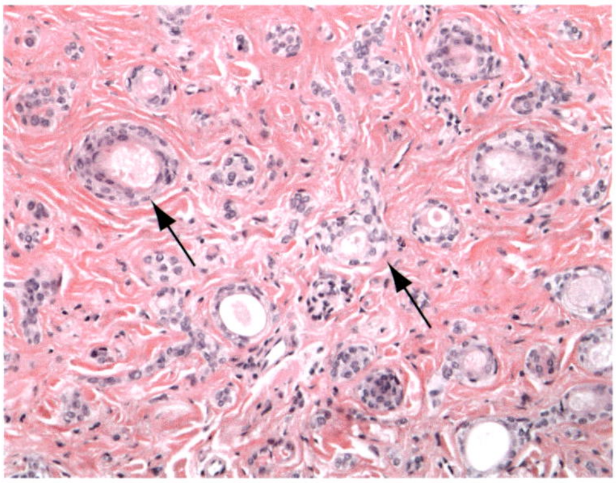

Figure 13-21 Histologically, syringoma is composed of small, epithelial-lined ductules that are round or comma-shaped *(arrows)*. *(Courtesy of Nasreen A. Syed, MD.)*

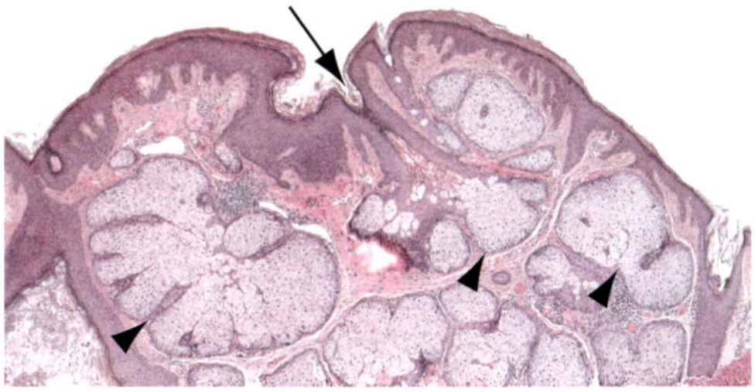

Figure 13-22 Sebaceous hyperplasia. Numerous sebaceous lobules *(arrowheads)* surround a hair follicle *(arrow)*. *(Courtesy of Nasreen A. Syed, MD.)*

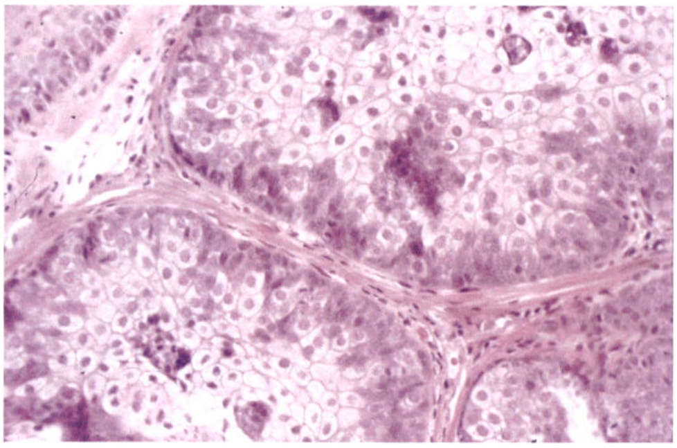

Figure 13-23 Sebaceous adenoma. Sebaceous lobules demonstrate focal proliferations of basophilic (blue) sebocytes. This lesion is most commonly associated with Muir-Torre syndrome. *(Courtesy of Nasreen A. Syed, MD.)*

the eyelid, or the sebaceous glands of the caruncle. Clinical diagnosis is often missed or delayed because of this lesion's propensity to mimic a chalazion or chronic blepharoconjunctivitis (Fig 13-24).

Histologically, well-differentiated sebaceous carcinomas are readily identified by the microvesicular foamy nature of the tumor cell cytoplasm (Fig 13-25A). Moderately differentiated tumors may exhibit some degree of sebaceous differentiation. Poorly differentiated tumors, however, may be difficult to distinguish from the other, more common epithelial malignancies. The demonstration of lipid within the cytoplasm of tumor cells by special stains, such as oil red O or Sudan black, is diagnostic, but it must be performed on tissue prior to processing and paraffin embedding.

When sebaceous carcinoma is suspected clinically, the pathologist should be alerted so that frozen section slides can be generated for lipid stains. Another feature, characteristic of but not pathognomonic for sebaceous cell carcinoma, is the dissemination of individual tumor cells and clusters of tumor cells within the epidermis or conjunctival epithelium, known as *pagetoid spread* (Fig 13-25B). Another pattern in the conjunctiva is that of complete replacement of conjunctival epithelium by tumor cells, or *sebaceous carcinoma in situ* (Fig 13-25C). A rare variant of sebaceous carcinoma involves only the epidermis and conjunctiva without demonstrable invasive tumor.

A 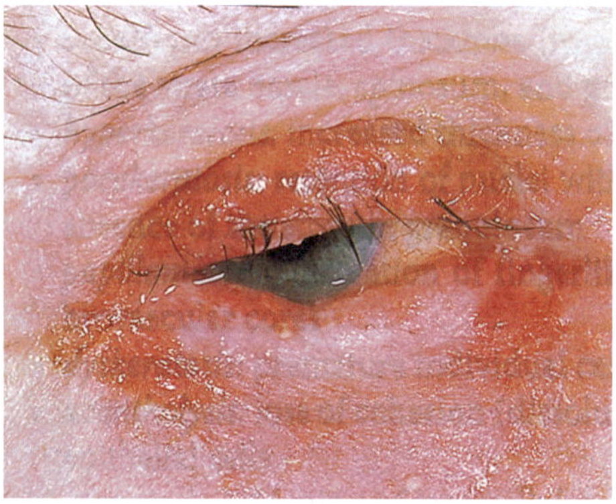 B 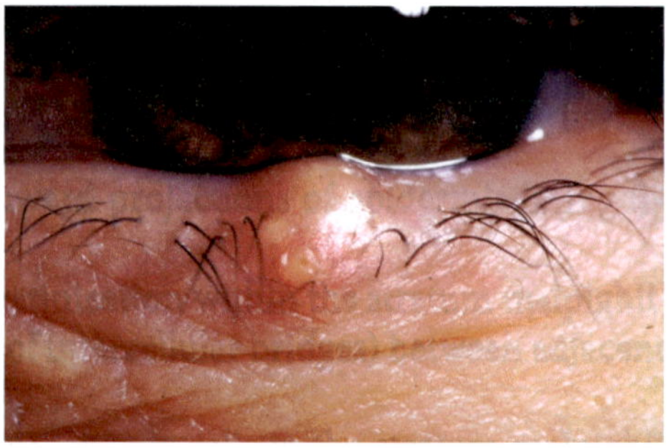

Figure 13-24 Sebaceous carcinoma. **A,** Note the eyelid erythema suggesting blepharitis. Note also the loss of eyelashes and the irregular eyelid thickening. **B,** This lesion mimics a chalazion of the lower eyelid. Focal lash loss is present. *(Part B courtesy of Roberta E. Gausas, MD.)*

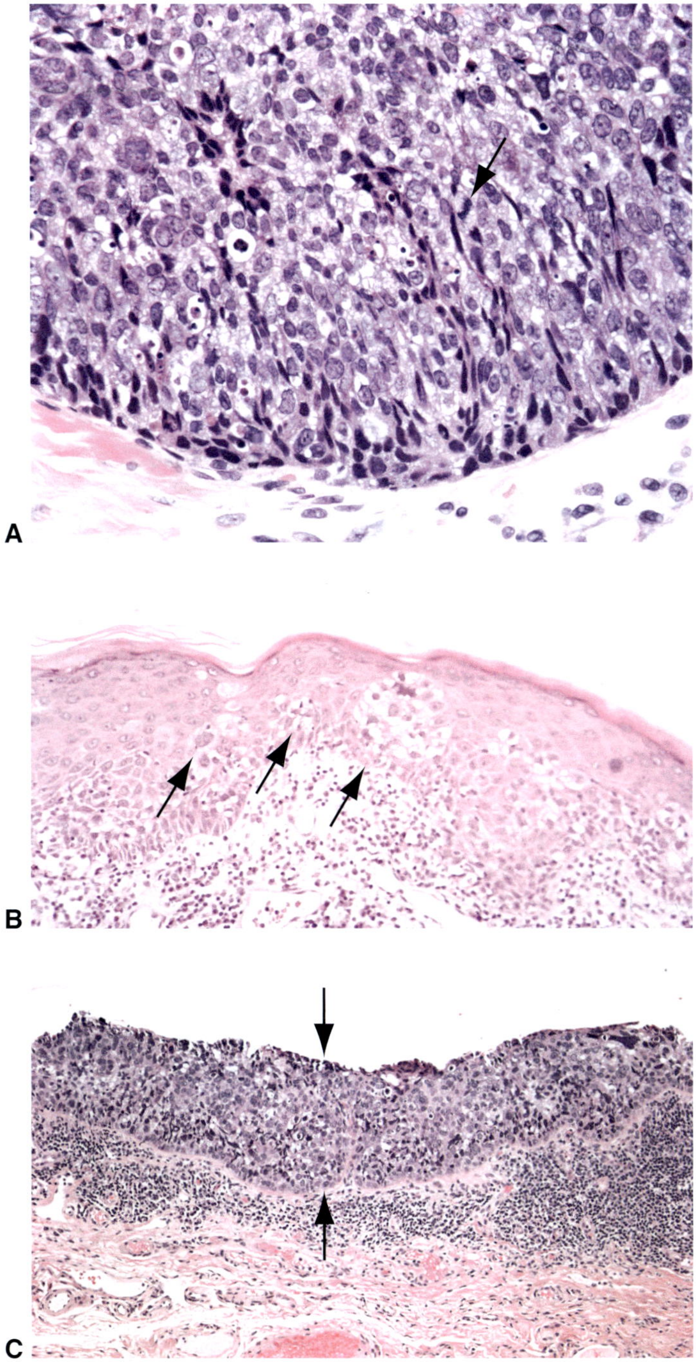

Figure 13-25 Sebaceous carcinoma, histology. **A,** Tumor cells often have hyperchromatic, atypical nuclei. The cytoplasm frequently has a foamy or vacuolated appearance. Note mitotic figure *(arrow)*. **B,** Pagetoid invasion of epidermis by individual tumor cells and small clusters of tumor cells *(arrows)*. **C,** Sebaceous carcinoma in situ with complete replacement of normal conjunctival epithelium by tumor cells *(between arrows)*. *(Courtesy of Nasreen A. Syed, MD.)*

Treatment recommendations include wide local excision of nodular lesions. Large or deeply invasive tumors may require exenteration. Frozen section control of surgical margins and Mohs micrographic surgery may provide suboptimal results because of difficulty in identifying intraepithelial spread. Permanent margins are often more reliable. Preoperative mapping by routine processing of multiple biopsies may afford a more accurate assessment of the extent of spread of the carcinoma. Survival rates for sebaceous carcinoma are worse than those for squamous cell carcinoma, but they have improved in recent years as a result of increased awareness, earlier detection, more accurate diagnosis, and appropriate treatment. Metastases first involve regional lymph nodes.

For American Joint Committee on Cancer definitions and staging of malignant neoplasms of the eyelid, see the appendix.

Melanocytic Neoplasms

The term *nevus* may refer to a variety of hamartomatous lesions of the skin or may refer to benign neoplastic proliferations of melanocytic cells. This discussion refers to the latter, *melanocytic nevi.* Melanocytic nevi commonly occur on the eyelids and may be visible at birth (congenital nevi) or become apparent in adolescence or adulthood. Congenital nevi tend to be larger than those appearing in later years, sometimes reaching substantial size. Nevi greater than 20 cm in diameter are referred to as *giant congenital melanocytic nevi.* The risk for development of melanoma in congenital nevi is proportional to the size of the nevus; close follow-up and/or excision of congenital nevi is warranted. Congenital nevi of the eyelid may develop in utero before the separation of the upper and lower eyelids and result in a "kissing" nevus (Fig 13-26). Nevi in adults often appear as dome-shaped lesions on the eyelid margin.

Histologically, most nevi are composed of nevus cells, specialized melanocytes that have a round rather than dendritic shape and tend to cluster together in nests. The cytoplasm of the nevus cell contains a variable amount of melanin pigment. Other characteristics of these cells include growth within and around adnexal structures, vessel walls, and the perineurium; and extension into the deep reticular dermis or subcutaneous tissue.

Nevi evolve with age and typically begin as macular (flat) lesions. Histologically, these lesions show nests of melanocytes along the epidermal–dermal junction and are consequently termed *junctional nevi* (Fig 13-27). Clinically, a junctional nevus is indistinguishable from an ephelis, or freckle; but in the latter, the basal layer of epidermal cells contains

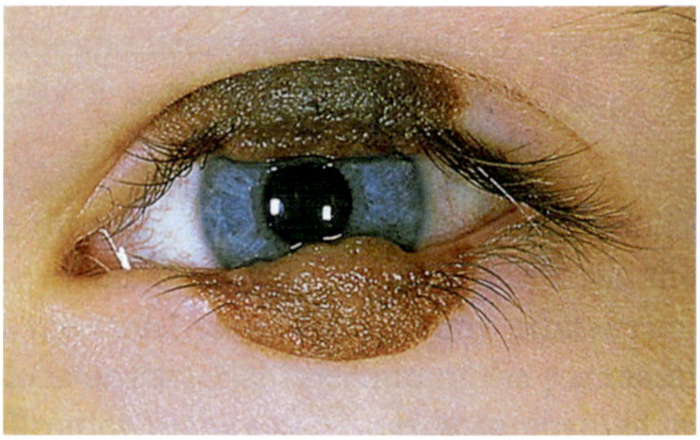

Figure 13-26 Congenital split, or "kissing," nevus of the eyelid.

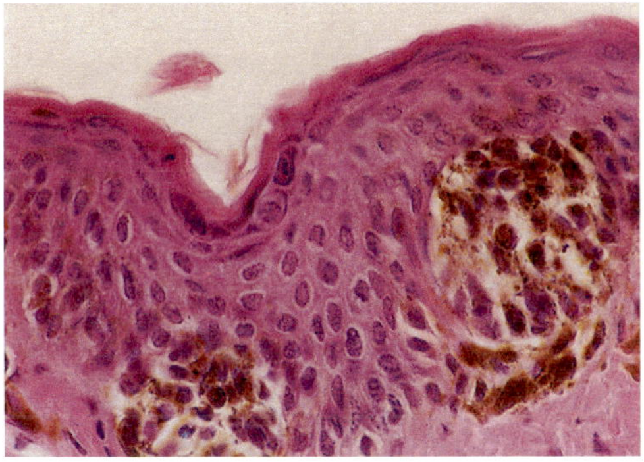

Figure 13-27 Junctional nevus. Nests of nevus cells are seen at the junction between epidermis and dermis.

the pigment. Typically in adolescence, the junctional nests of nevus cells begin to migrate into the superficial dermis, and the nevus becomes increasingly elevated clinically. At this stage, the nevus may increase in pigmentation as well. When both junctional and intradermal components are present, the histopathologic classification becomes *compound nevus* (Fig 13-28). Finally, sometime in adulthood, the junctional component disappears, leaving only nevus cells within the dermis, and the classification accordingly becomes *intradermal nevus* (Fig 13-29).

An evolution in the cytomorphology of the nevus cells also takes place: those in the superficial portion of the nevus are polygonal, or epithelioid, in shape (type A nevus cells). Within the midportion of the nevus, the cells become smaller, have less cytoplasm, and resemble lymphocytes (type B nevus cells). At the deepest levels, the nevus cells become spindled and appear similar to Schwann cells of peripheral nerves (type C nevus cells). Recognition of this "maturation" is useful in classifying melanocytic neoplasms as benign. Multinucleated giant melanocytes and interspersed adipose tissue are common in older nevi.

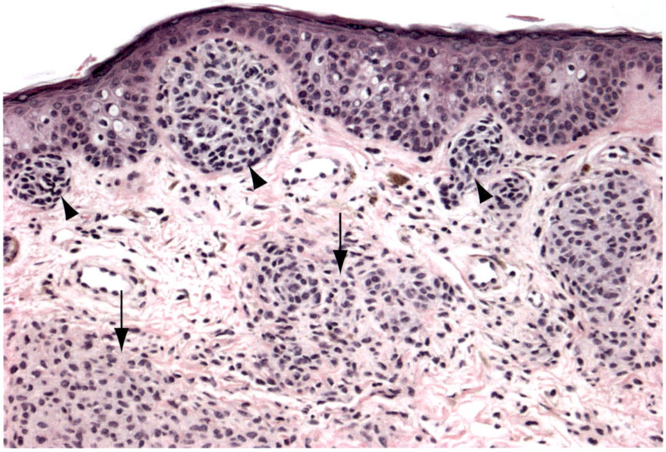

Figure 13-28 Compound nevus. Nests of nevus cells are present in the dermis *(arrows)* as well as at the junction of epidermis and dermis *(arrowheads)*. *(Courtesy of Nasreen A. Syed, MD.)*

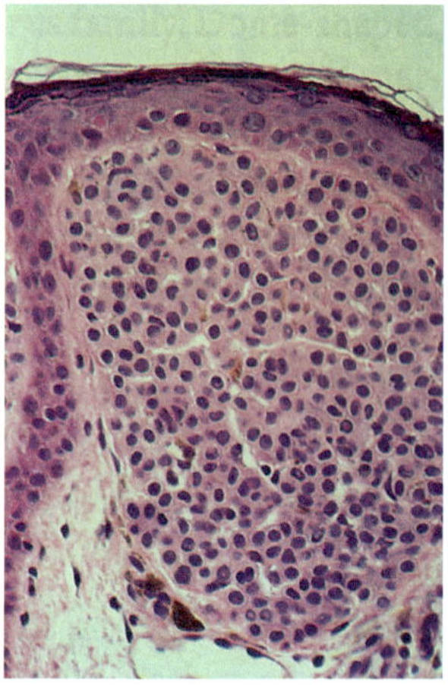

Figure 13-29 Intradermal nevus. The nests of nevus cells are confined to the dermis.

Nevi that show some clinical or pathologic atypicality include the Spitz nevus and the dysplastic nevus. *Spitz nevi* develop in late childhood or in adolescence and are uncommon after the second decade. In contrast to the clinical picture of the usual nevus, they may be larger (up to 1.0 cm) and have a tan-pink color. Histologically, they are usually compound and exhibit nuclear and cytoplasmic enlargement and pleomorphism, features suggesting malignancy. Other features suggesting malignancy, however, such as atypical mitotic figures, intraepidermal migration, and lack of maturation, are generally lacking.

Clinical features suggesting a *dysplastic nevus* may include size greater than 0.5 cm, irregular margins, and irregular pigmentation. Cytologic atypia is characterized by nuclear enlargement and hyperchromasia and prominent nucleoli. Clinically suspicious lesions should be completely excised. Persons with multiple dysplastic nevi are at increased risk for development of melanoma and may represent a genetic susceptibility, suggesting that family members should also be examined and observed closely.

Cutaneous melanoma is a rare occurrence on the eyelids. It may be associated with a preexisting nevus, or it may develop de novo. Clinical features suggesting malignancy are the same as those just mentioned for dysplastic nevi; in addition, invasive melanoma is heralded by a vertical (perpendicular to the skin surface) growth phase that results in an elevated or indurated mass. There are 4 main histologic subtypes of melanoma:

- superficial spreading
- lentigo maligna
- nodular
- acral-lentiginous

Superficial spreading is the most common type of cutaneous melanoma and demonstrates a radial (intraepidermal) growth pattern extending beyond the invasive component. Lentigo maligna melanoma occurs on the face of elderly individuals, with a long preinvasive phase, and is the most common type occurring on the eyelids. Acral-lentiginous melanoma, as the name implies, involves the extremities and is not seen on the eyelids (Fig 13-30).

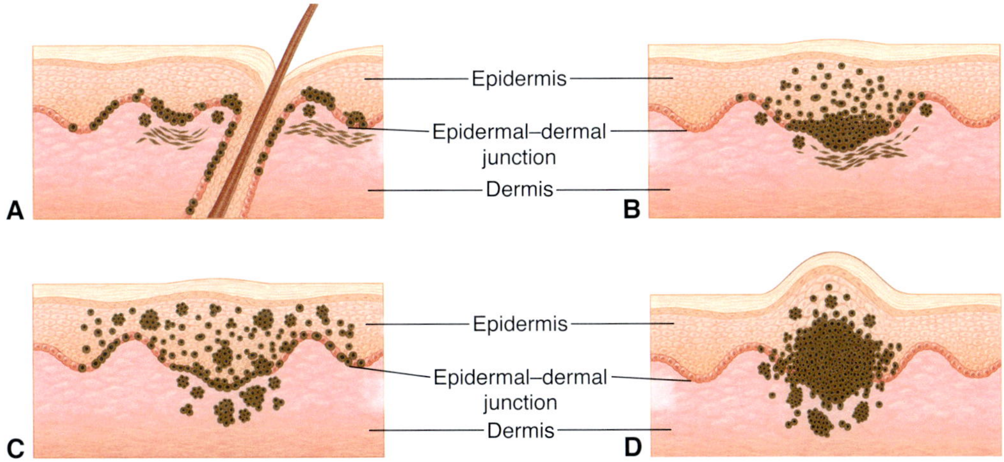

Figure 13-30 Schematic illustration of cutaneous melanoma types. **A,** Lentigo maligna melanoma. Atypical melanocytes (brown cells) proliferate predominantly in the basal layers of the epidermis in a linear or nested pattern, similar to primary acquired melanosis with atypia of the conjunctiva. Note the tendency of the melanocytes to involve the outer sheaths of the hair shafts. The invasive component is seen as brown cells (spindle and epithelioid) in the superficial dermis. **B,** Acral-lentiginous melanoma is similar to lentigo maligna melanoma, but atypical melanocytes are also present in the more superficial layers of the epidermis. **C,** In superficial spreading melanoma, tumor cell nests are present in all levels of the epidermis, often in a pagetoid fashion, with cells or clusters of cells scattered among epithelial cells. Lentigo maligna, acral-lentiginous, and superficial spreading melanomas spread horizontally (radial growth) through the skin, staying close to the epidermal–dermal junction. **D,** Nodular melanoma has a narrow intraepidermal component and more prominent vertical growth within the dermis; it is therefore more deeply invasive compared with the other types. *(Modified with permission from Spencer WH, ed.* Ophthalmic Pathology: An Atlas and Textbook. Vol 4. *Philadelphia: WB Saunders; 1996:2270. Illustration by Christine Gralapp.)*

Histologic features characteristic of melanoma include pagetoid intraepidermal spread of atypical melanocytic nests and single cells, nuclear abnormalities as listed earlier, lack of maturation in the deeper portions of the mass, and atypical mitotic figures. A bandlike lymphocytic host response along the base of the mass is more common in melanoma than in benign proliferations. Prognosis is correlated with depth of invasion (Breslow depth) in stage I (localized) disease. Metastases, when they occur, typically involve regional lymph nodes first.

CHAPTER 14

Orbit

Topography

Bony Orbit and Soft Tissues

Seven bones form the boundaries of the orbit (see Figures 1-1 through 1-3 in BCSC Section 7, *Orbit, Eyelids, and Lacrimal System*). These 7 bones are the frontal, zygomatic, palatine, lacrimal, sphenoid, ethmoid, and maxillary.

The orbital cavity is pear-shaped and has a volume of 30 cc. Structures and tissues occupying the cavity are the globe, lacrimal gland, muscles, tendons, fat, fascia, vessels, nerves, sympathetic ganglia, and cartilaginous trochlea. Inflammatory and neoplastic processes that increase the volume of the orbital contents lead to *proptosis* (protrusion) of the globe and/or *displacement* (dystopia) from the horizontal or vertical position. The degree and direction of ocular displacement help to localize the position of the mass.

The *lacrimal gland* is situated anteriorly in the superotemporal quadrant of the orbit. The gland is divided into orbital and palpebral lobes by the aponeurosis of the levator palpebrae superioris muscle. The acini of the glands are composed of low cuboidal epithelium. The ducts, which lie within the fibrovascular stroma, are lined by low cuboidal epithelium with a second outer layer of low, flat myoepithelial cells. See BCSC Section 2, *Fundamentals and Principles of Ophthalmology,* and Section 7, *Orbit, Eyelids, and Lacrimal System,* for additional discussion.

Congenital Anomalies

Dermoid and Other Epithelial Cysts

The major categories of orbital cysts of childhood include cysts of the surface epithelium, teratomatous cysts, neural cysts, secondary cysts (mucocele), inflammatory cysts (parasitic), and noncystic lesions with a cystic component. Congenital cysts of the surface epithelium are subdivided into *dermoid cysts* and *simple epithelial (epidermoid) cysts.* Dermoid cysts are the most common and are believed to arise as embryonic epithelial nests that became entrapped during embryogenesis. They may protrude through the frontozygomatic and frontomaxillary sutures to take a dumbbell shape. Most manifest in childhood as a mass in the superotemporal quadrant of the orbit. Rupture of cyst contents may produce a marked granulomatous reaction. Histologically, a dermoid cyst is encapsulated

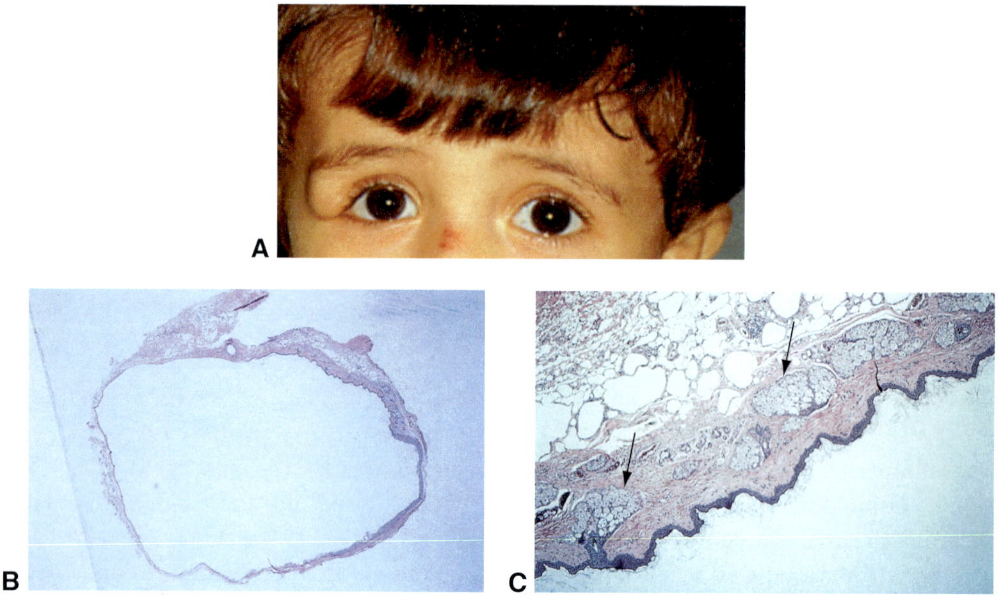

Figure 14-1 **A,** Clinical appearance of dermoid cyst of the right orbit. Note the typical superotemporal location. **B,** Low-power photomicrograph discloses a cyst lined by keratinized stratified squamous epithelium. **C,** The wall of the cyst contains sebaceous glands *(arrows)* and adnexal structures. *(Part A courtesy of Sander Dubovy, MD; parts B and C courtesy of Hans E. Grossniklaus, MD.)*

and lined by keratinized stratified squamous epithelium. The cyst contains keratin and hair, and its walls are lined with dermal appendages and adnexal structures, including sebaceous glands, hair follicles, and sweat glands (Fig 14-1). If the cyst wall does not have adnexal structures, the term *simple epithelial (epidermoid) cyst* is applied. Simple epithelial cysts may also be lined by respiratory, conjunctival, or apocrine epithelium.

Inflammations

The term *orbital inflammatory disease (OID)* broadly describes a variety of pathologic processes and clinical presentations related to inflammation of orbital tissue. OID may be idiopathic or secondary to a systemic inflammatory disease (such as Graves), retained foreign body, or infectious disease. OID includes the spectrum of bacterial or fungal infections, diffuse inflammation of multiple tissues (eg, sclerosing orbititis, diffuse anterior OID), and preferential involvement of specific orbital structures (eg, orbital myositis, optic perineuritis). Conditions masquerading as OID include congenital orbital mass lesions and orbital neoplastic disease such as lymphoma or rhabdomyosarcoma. These need to be ruled out before the diagnosis of OID is considered.

Noninfectious

Nonspecific orbital inflammation

Nonspecific orbital inflammation (NSOI, also referred to as *idiopathic orbital inflammation [IOI]* and *orbital inflammatory syndrome [sclerosing orbititis]*) refers to a space-occupying inflammatory disorder that simulates a neoplasm (thus, it is sometimes known as *orbital pseudotumor*) but has no recognizable cause. This disorder accounts for approximately 5% of orbital lesions. Clinically, patients have an abrupt course and usually complain of pain. The condition may affect children as well as adults. The inflammatory response may be diffuse or compartmentalized. When localized to an extraocular muscle, the condition is called *orbital myositis* (Fig 14-2); when localized to the lacrimal gland, it is frequently called *dacryoadenitis.*

In the early stages, inflammation predominates, with a polymorphous inflammatory response (eosinophils, neutrophils, plasma cells, lymphocytes, and macrophages) that is often perivascular and that frequently infiltrates muscle and fat, producing fat necrosis. In later stages, fibrosis is the predominant feature, often with interspersed lymphoid follicles bearing germinal centers. The fibrosis may inexorably replace orbital fat and encase extraocular muscles and the optic nerve (Fig 14-3). Immunophenotypic and molecular genetic analyses

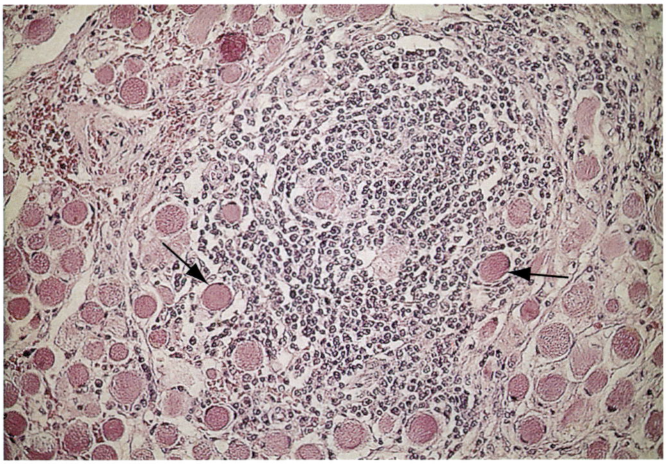

Figure 14-2 Nonspecific orbital inflammation (NSOI; orbital inflammatory syndrome). Note the skeletal muscle fibers *(arrows)* surrounded by a dense infiltrate of chronic inflammatory cells. Unlike thyroid eye disease, in which the tendons of the muscles typically are spared, this condition can affect any orbital structure, including the muscle tendons.

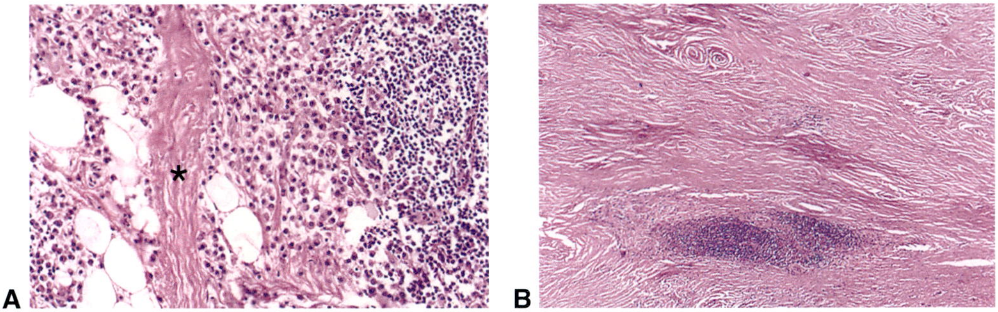

Figure 14-3 Nonspecific orbital inflammation. **A,** Note the mixture of inflammatory cells and the bundle of collagen *(asterisk)* running through the orbital fat. **B,** Diffuse fibrosis dominates the histologic picture of this fibrosing orbititis, considered by some authorities to represent a later stage of the condition illustrated in part **A.**

can differentiate NSOI from lymphoid tumors based on whether the proliferation of lymphocytes is polyclonal (NSOI) or monoclonal (lymphoma). CD20 and CD25 receptors have been demonstrated and may provide the basis for future treatments. Immunoglobulin G4 (IgG4)–positive plasmacytic infiltrates have recently become a marker for a sclerosing variant of fibroinflammatory diseases. The nature of the pathologic findings dictates the recommended treatment. See also BCSC Section 7, *Orbit, Eyelids, and Lacrimal System.*

Thyroid eye disease

Thyroid eye disease (TED), also known as *Graves disease, thyroid ophthalmopathy,* and *thyroid-associated orbitopathy,* is related to thyroid dysfunction and is the most common cause of unilateral or bilateral proptosis (exophthalmos) in adults. Signs and symptoms of TED are related to inflammation of the orbital connective tissue, inflammation and fibrosis of the extraocular muscles, and adipogenesis. The muscles appear firm and white, and the tendons are usually not involved. A cellular infiltrate of mononuclear cells, lymphocytes, plasma cells, mast cells, and fibroblasts involves the interstitial tissues of the extraocular muscles, most commonly the inferior and medial rectus muscles (Fig 14-4). In patients with and without TED, orbital fibroblasts are phenotypically distinct in that they express CD40 receptors generally found on B cells, and other surface receptors that typically play a role in modulating the inflammatory response. When the B-cell receptor is attached by T-cell–bound CD154, fibroblast inflammatory genes are up-regulated, including interleukin-6 (IL-6), IL8, and prostaglandin E_2 (PGE_2). In turn, synthesis of hyaluronan and glycosaminoglycans (GAG) is increased. This up-regulation of orbital fibroblasts is 100-fold greater than that seen in nonorbital fibroblasts in response to the same stimulus. As a result of the increased bulk, the optic nerve may be compromised at the orbital apex, and optic nerve head swelling may result. Late stages of TED are associated with progressive fibrosis that results in restriction of ocular movement and severe eyelid retraction with resultant exposure keratitis.

In addition, orbital fibroblasts expressing thyrotropin receptor (TSH-R) are found in TED. The number of TSH-R immunostained cells is high in early disease, decreases with disease duration, and is positively correlated with serum TSH-R antibody levels at the onset of TED. Stimulation of TSH-R results in up-regulation of TSH-R mRNA. Because orbital fibroblasts are derived from the neural crest and are pluripotent, the enhanced signaling promotes adipocyte differentiation and adipogenesis.

Finally, studies have identified circulating IgG in patients with TED. IgG recognizes and activates the insulin-like growth factor I (IGF-I) receptor expressed on the surface of numerous cell types, including fibroblasts. The stimulation of this factor by the circulating IgG may contribute to the development of TED by stimulating orbital fibroblasts to secrete glycosaminoglycans, cytokines, and chemoattractants.

See also BCSC Section 1, *Update on General Medicine,* and Section 7, *Orbit, Eyelids, and Lacrimal System.*

Bahn RS. Understanding the immunology of Graves' ophthalmopathy. Is it an autoimmune disease? *Endocrinol Metab Clin North Am.* 2000;29(2):287–296.

Gerding MN, van der Meer JWC, Broenink M, Bakker O, Wiersinga WM, Prummel MF. Association of thyrotropin receptor antibodies with the clinical features of Graves' ophthalmopathy. *Clin Endocrinol.* 2000;52(3):267–271.

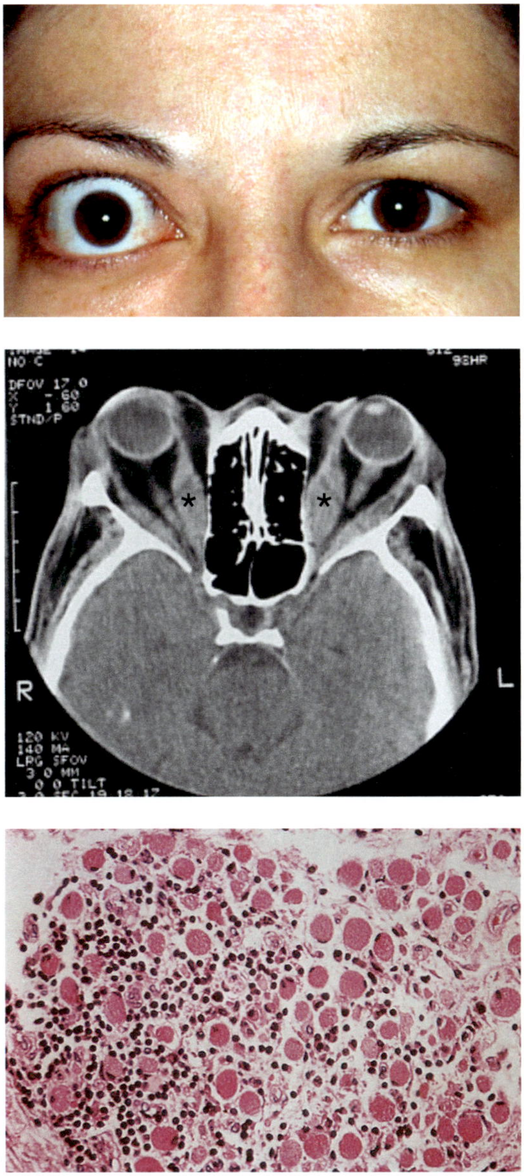

A B C

Figure 14-4 Thyroid eye disease. **A,** Clinical appearance demonstrating asymmetric proptosis and eyelid retraction, most prominent on the right side. **B,** CT scan (axial view) showing fusiform enlargement of the extraocular muscles *(asterisks).* **C,** The muscle bundles of the extraocular muscle are separated by fluid, accompanied by an infiltrate of mononuclear inflammatory cells. *(Parts A and B courtesy of Sander Dubovy, MD.)*

Kazim M, Goldberg RA, Smith TJ. Insights into the pathogenesis of thyroid-associated orbitopathy: evolving rationale for therapy. *Arch Ophthalmol.* 2002;120(3):380–386.

Wiersinga WM, Prummel MF. Pathogenesis of Graves' ophthalmopathy—current understanding [editorial]. *J Clin Endocrinol Metab.* 2001;86(2):501–503.

Infectious

Bacterial infections

The causes of bacterial infections of the orbit include bacteremia, trauma, retained surgical hardware, and spread from an adjacent sinus infection. Infection may involve a variety of organisms, including *Haemophilus influenzae, Streptococcus, Staphylococcus aureus, Clostridium, Bacteroides, Klebsiella,* and *Proteus.* Histologically, acute inflammation, necrosis, and abscess formation may be present. Tuberculosis, which rarely involves the orbit, produces a necrotizing granulomatous reaction.

Fungal and parasitic infections

Rhinocerebral or rhino-orbitocerebral zygomycosis (mucormycosis) usually occurs in patients with poorly controlled diabetes mellitus (especially those with ketoacidosis), solid malignancies, or extensive burns; in patients undergoing treatment with corticosteroid agents; or in patients with neutropenia related to hematologic malignancies. Fungal infection of the orbit is caused by adjacent sinus infection. Histologically, inflammation (acute and chronic) is present in a background of necrosis and is often granulomatous. Histiocytes are common. Broad, nonseptated hyphae may be identified with H&E, periodic acid–Schiff (PAS), and Gomori methenamine silver (GMS) stains. Diagnosis is achieved by biopsy of necrotic-appearing tissues in the nasopharynx. These fungi can invade blood vessel walls and produce a thrombosing vasculitis.

Sino-orbital aspergillosis is caused by *Aspergillus* infection of the orbit from the adjacent sinuses and may occur in immunocompromised or otherwise healthy individuals. With slowly progressive and insidious symptoms, sino-orbital aspergillosis is often unrecognized, producing a sclerosing granulomatous disease. *Aspergillus* has often been difficult to culture but may be observed in tissue as septated hyphae with 45° angle branching (Fig 14-5). Despite aggressive surgical therapy and adjunctive therapy with antifungal agents, orbital infections with *Aspergillus* may be fatal if extension into the brain occurs.

Allergic fungal sinusitis is a form of noninvasive fungal disease resulting from an IgE-mediated hypersensitivity reaction in atopic individuals and is caused by several species of fungi. The disease may extend into the orbit and intracranially in some instances.

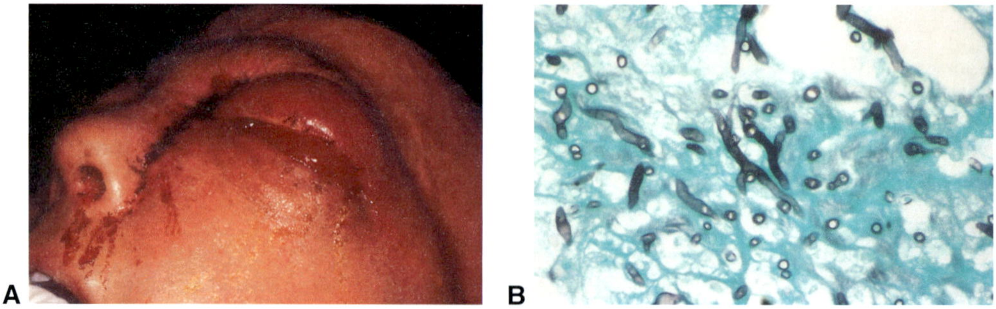

Figure 14-5 *Aspergillus* infections of the orbit generally produce severe, insidious orbital inflammation. **A,** Clinical appearance. **B,** Microscopic section demonstrates the branching fungal hyphae on silver stains. *(Courtesy of Hans E. Grossniklaus, MD.)*

Parasitic infections of the orbit are rare and may be produced by *Echinococcus (orbital hydatid cyst), Taenia solium* (cysticercosis), and *Loa loa* ocular filariasis (loiasis). These infections are mostly seen in patients who come from, or have traveled to, areas where the infections are endemic. Enzyme-linked immunosorbent assay for serum antibodies may be helpful in the diagnosis. See BCSC Section 7, *Orbit, Eyelids, and Lacrimal System.*

Degenerations

Amyloid

Amyloid deposition in the orbit occurs in primary systemic amyloidosis. When it involves the extraocular muscles and nerves, it can produce ophthalmoplegia and ptosis.

See Chapters 5, 6, 10, and 13 in this volume and BCSC Section 8, *External Disease and Cornea.*

Neoplasia

Neoplasms of the orbit may be primary, they may be extensions of locally invasive tumors from adjacent structures, or they may represent metastatic disease. Approximately 60% are benign and 40% malignant, with malignant lesions being more common in adults. The incidence of primary neoplasms is low, with lymphoma being the most common (10%) and hemangioma the next most common (5%). Secondary tumors, either metastatic or extending from adjacent structures, are slightly more common than primary tumors.

In children, approximately 90% of orbital tumors are benign. Benign cystic lesions (epidermoid or simple epithelial cysts) are the most common cystic lesions and represent 50% of orbital lesions in childhood. Rhabdomyosarcoma is the most common orbital malignancy in childhood and represents 3% of all orbital masses. The orbit may be involved secondarily by retinoblastoma, neuroblastoma, or leukemia/lymphoma. See BCSC Section 7, *Orbit, Eyelids, and Lacrimal System,* for additional discussion.

Lacrimal Sac Neoplasia

Lacrimal sac neoplasms are rare, and with endoscopic procedures, a representative biopsy sample may be difficult to achieve. In a study examining 377 nasolacrimal duct specimens obtained during dacryocystorhinostomy (DCR), neoplasms resulting in chronic nasolacrimal duct obstruction occurred in 5% of cases and were unsuspected prior to surgery in 2% of patients.

Anderson NG, Wojno TH, Grossniklaus HE. Clinicopathologic findings from lacrimal sac biopsy specimens obtained during dacryocystorhinostomy. *Ophthal Plast Reconstr Surg.* 2003;19(3):173–176.

Lacrimal Gland Neoplasia

Epithelial lacrimal gland tumors are classified according to the World Health Organization (WHO) epithelial salivary gland classification because the lacrimal gland is a modified salivary gland. The most common types of epithelial lacrimal gland tumors are the pleomorphic adenoma, adenocarcinoma (carcinoma ex pleomorphic adenoma), and adenoid cystic carcinoma.

Weis E, Rootman J, Joly TJ, et al. Epithelial lacrimal gland tumors: pathologic classification and current understanding. *Arch Ophthalmol.* 2009;127(8):1016–1028.

Pleomorphic adenoma

Pleomorphic adenoma (benign mixed tumor) is the most common epithelial tumor of the lacrimal gland. The tumor is pseudoencapsulated and grows slowly by expansion. This progressive expansive growth may indent the bone of the lacrimal fossa, producing excavation of the area. Tumor growth stimulates the periosteum to deposit a thin layer of new bone (cortication). The adjacent orbital bone is not eroded. Typically, the patient experiences no pain. This tumor is more common in men than in women, and the median age at presentation is 35 years.

Histologically, pleomorphic adenoma has a fibrous pseudocapsule with microprojections extending from the capsule surface to the tumor (bosselation) and is composed of a mixture of ductal derived epithelial and stromal elements. The epithelial component may form nests or tubules lined by 2 layers of cells, the outermost layer blending imperceptibly with the stroma (Fig 14-6). The stroma may appear myxoid and may contain heterologous elements, including cartilage and bone. Immunohistochemistry reflects the epithelial and myoepithelial components, both of which are derived from epithelium. It is typically positive for keratin and epithelial membrane antigen in the ductal portions and positive for keratin, actin, myosin, fibronectin, and S-100 in the myoepithelial areas.

Chromosomal translocations are recognized in salivary gland tumors and pleomorphic adenomas. Specifically, translocations involving the *PLGA1* (chromosome 8q12) or *HMGA2* gene have been identified. These genes are involved in growth factor signaling and cell cycle regulation.

Transformation into a malignant mixed tumor may take place in a long-standing pleomorphic adenoma with relatively rapid growth after a period of relative quiescence. Carcinomas, including adenocarcinoma (carcinoma ex pleomorphic adenoma) and adenoid cystic carcinoma, may also arise in recurrent pleomorphic adenomas.

Adenoid cystic carcinoma

As mentioned in the previous section, adenoid cystic carcinoma (ACC) can arise in a pleomorphic adenoma or de novo in the lacrimal gland. The tumor is slightly more common in women than in men, and the median age of presentation is about 40. Unlike pleomorphic adenoma, adenoid cystic carcinoma is not encapsulated; it tends to erode the adjacent bone and invade orbital nerves, accounting for the pain that is a frequent presenting complaint. Grossly, the appearance is grayish white, firm, and nodular. Histologically, a variety of patterns may appear, including the cribriform (Swiss cheese) pattern, which is the most common (Fig 14-7). Other histologic patterns include basaloid (solid), comedo, sclerosing, and tubular. Presence of a basaloid pattern has been associated with a worse prognosis (5-year survival of 20%) compared to tumors without a basaloid component (5-year survival of 70%). Immunohistochemistry is typically positive for S-100, keratin, and actin with areas of epithelial and myoepithelial differentiation. There is a positive correlation between prognosis and protein expression of bcl-2 and bax. Expression of p53 is

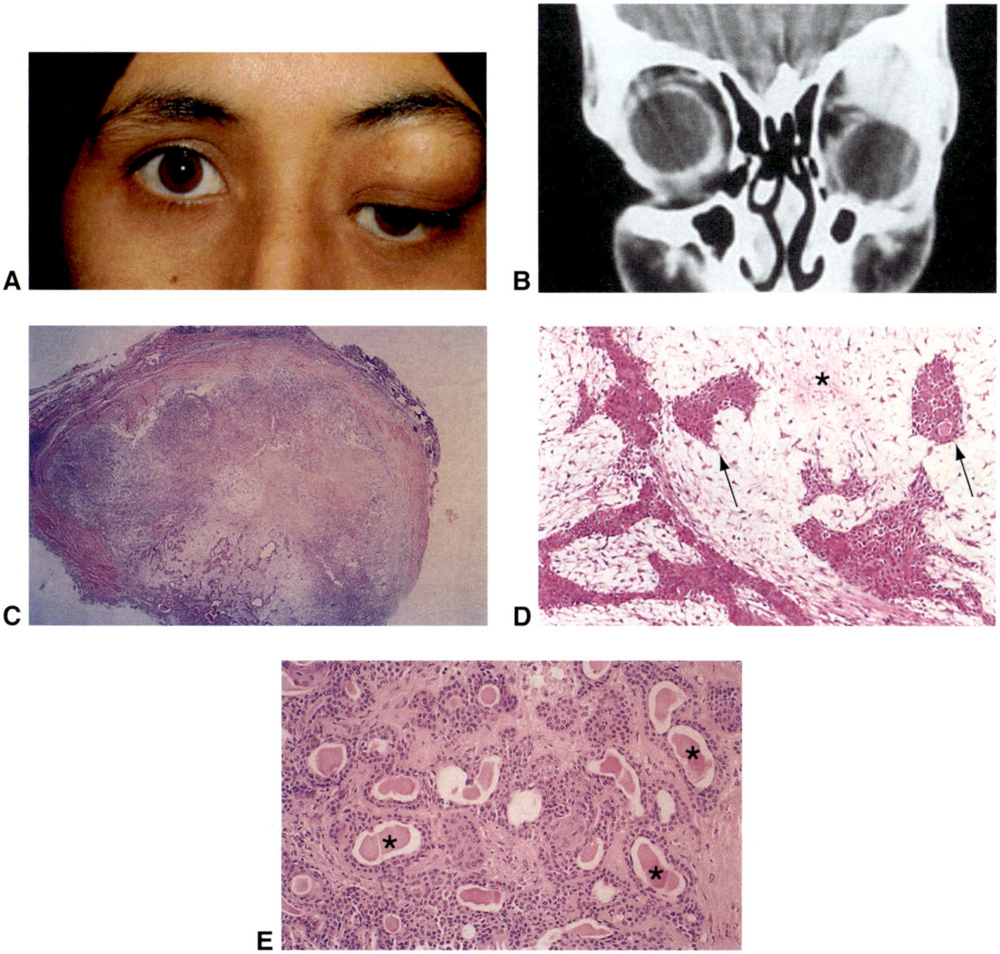

Figure 14-6 Pleomorphic adenoma (benign mixed tumor) of the lacrimal gland. **A,** Clinical appearance. A superotemporal orbital mass is present, causing proptosis and downward displacement of the left globe. **B,** CT scan (coronal view) demonstrating left orbit tumor. **C,** Low power shows the circumscribed nature of this pleomorphic adenoma. **D,** Note both the epithelial *(arrows)* and the mesenchymal *(asterisk)* elements. **E,** Well-differentiated glandular structures (epithelial component) with lumina *(asterisks)*. *(Parts A and B courtesy of Sander Dubovy, MD; parts C–E courtesy of Hans E. Grossniklaus, MD.)*

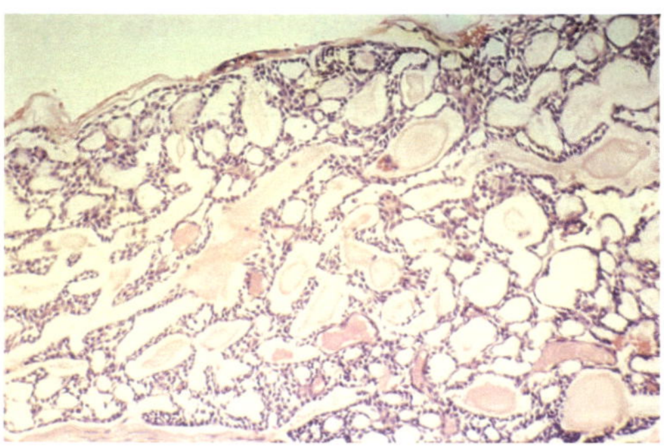

Figure 14-7 Adenoid cystic carcinoma of the lacrimal gland. Note the characteristic cribriform (Swiss cheese) pattern of tumor cells. *(Courtesy of Ben J. Glasgow, MD.)*

associated with a poor prognosis. Genetic microarray analysis has demonstrated loss of 1p36 as an initial event in the pathogenesis of adenoid cystic carcinoma.

Because of the diffuse infiltration of this tumor, exenteration may be recommended, often with removal of adjacent bone. Despite aggressive surgical intervention, the long-term prognosis is poor.

Ahmad SM, Esmaeli B, Williams M, et al. American Joint Committee on Cancer classification predicts outcome of patients with lacrimal gland adenoid cystic carcinoma. *Ophthalmology.* 2009;116(6):1210–1215.

Font RL, Smith SL, Bryan RG. Malignant epithelial tumors of the lacrimal gland: a clinicopathologic study of 21 cases. *Arch Ophthalmol.* 1998;116(5):613–616.

Lymphoproliferative Lesions

Most classifications of lymphoid lesions have been based on lymph node architecture, and such nodal classifications have been difficult to apply to so-called extranodal lymphoid lesions. Because there are no lymph nodes in the orbit, it is problematic to classify these lesions according to the criteria used for lymph nodes. The development of classification schemes for lymphomas is, thus, an ongoing and controversial process. In general, lymphoproliferative lesions are divided into reactive lymphoid hyperplasia (RLH), atypical lymphoid hyperplasia (ALH), and ocular adnexal lymphoma (OAL). OAL is then subtyped according to the WHO Classification of Tumours of Haematopoietic and Lymphoid Tissues. The more recent American Joint Committee on Cancer–International Union Against Cancer TNM-based staging system for OAL defines disease extent and identifies clinical and histomorphologic features of prognostic significance. Data revealing OAL patients' prognosis using these classifications are beginning to emerge. Many lymphoid masses in the orbit that were previously classified as reactive or atypical hyperplasia would now be considered neoplastic under the TNM-based staging system.

Unlike patients with nonspecific orbital inflammation, those with orbital lymphoproliferative lesions present with a gradual, painless progression of proptosis. Every patient with an orbital lymphoproliferative lesion must be investigated for evidence of systemic lymphoma, including examination for lymphadenopathy, a complete blood count (CBC) and differential, and imaging of the thoracic and abdominal viscera. In general, biopsy of an accessible lymph node is preferred over an orbital biopsy because nodal architecture is helpful in diagnosis and the procedure may be safer. A bone marrow biopsy is preferred to an aspirate because it includes bone spicules; the presence of a paratrabecular lymphoid infiltrate may indicate systemic lymphoma. In contrast to most cases of nonspecific orbital inflammation, which are treated with corticosteroids, lymphoproliferative lesions confined to the orbit are treated with radiation.

The ophthalmologist taking a biopsy of an orbital or conjunctival lymphoproliferative lesion should consult with the pathologist to determine the optimal method for handling the tissue. Fresh (unfixed) tissue is preferred for touch preparations, immunohistochemistry, flow cytometry, and gene rearrangement studies. The type of fixative used for permanent sections varies from one laboratory to another. For biopsy of suspected lymphoma, the surgeon should alert the pathologist in advance and may need to perform the procedure near a pathology laboratory. Exposure of the biopsy specimen to air for long periods should be avoided. Tissue samples may be wrapped in saline-moistened gauze and transported on ice. It is very important that the tissue be handled gently; crush artifact can prevent the pathologist from rendering a diagnosis. See also Chapter 4, Table 4-1.

Demirci H, Shields CL, Karatza EC, Shields JA. Orbital lymphoproliferative tumors: analysis of clinical features and systemic involvement in 160 cases. *Ophthalmology.* 2008;115(9):1626–1631, 1631.e1–3.

Swerdlow SH, Campo E, Harris NL, et al. *WHO Classification of Tumours of Haematopoietic and Lymphoid Tissues.* Lyon, France: IARC; 2008.

Reactive lymphoid hyperplasia

Reactive lymphoid hyperplasia is composed of well-differentiated, somewhat pleomorphic lymphocytes, with occasional plasma cells, macrophages, eosinophils, and follicles with germinal centers. Usually, the follicles contain tingible body macrophages (containing apoptotic debris), and there is mitotic activity; they also often have vessels with endothelial hyperplasia.

Atypical lymphoid hyperplasia

Atypical lymphoid hyperplasia is diffuse lymphoid proliferation, generally without reactive germinal centers. It is composed of an admixture of small, mature-appearing lymphocytes and larger lymphoid cells of questionable maturity.

Lymphoma

Lymphomas of the orbit may be a presenting manifestation of systemic lymphomas, or they may arise primarily from the orbit. The incidence of orbital involvement in systemic lymphomas is approximately 1%–2%. Hodgkin disease is exceedingly rare in the orbit, and the majority of primary malignant orbital lymphomas are non-Hodgkin lymphomas. Multinucleated Reed-Sternberg cells are the characteristic histologic finding in Hodgkin disease. Immunohistochemistry is typically positive for CD45, CD15, and CD30. Non-Hodgkin lymphomas constitute one-half of malignancies arising in the orbit and the ocular adnexa (Fig 14-8). They have diffuse architecture and mark immunophenotypically as

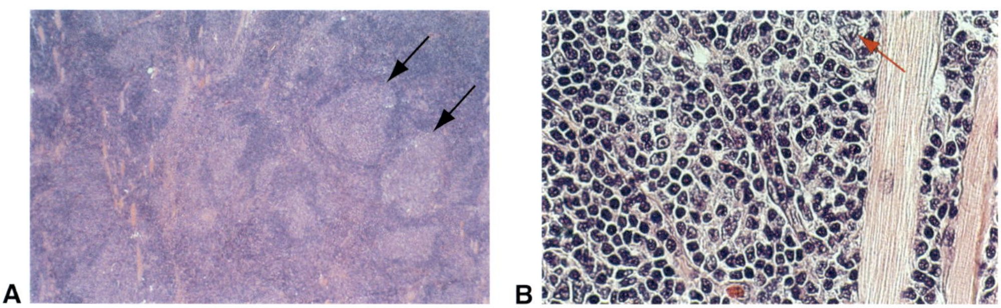

Figure 14-8 Low-grade B-cell lymphoma of the orbit. **A,** Low-power photomicrograph shows a dense lymphoid infiltrate with a vague follicular arrangement. Note poorly defined follicles or germinal centers *(arrows).* **B,** Higher magnification shows small lymphocytes with mild nuclear membrane abnormalities, plasma cells, and atypical lymphocytes with cytoplasmic clearing (monocytoid B cells, *arrow*). *(Courtesy of Ben J. Glasgow, MD.)*

B cells with immunopositivity for CD19 and CD20. In rare instances, T-cell lymphomas of the orbit are found and demonstrate immunopositivity for CD3, CD4, and CD8. See Chapter 5.

Soft-Tissue Tumors

Soft-tissue tumors make up a small subset of human benign and malignant tumors, but they can be life threatening and may pose significant diagnostic and therapeutic challenges. Recognizing the main histologic patterns of soft-tissue tumors, which include round cell, spindle cell, myxoid, epithelioid, pericytomatous, and pleomorphic, is the most important aspect in the diagnosis of these tumors. Immunohistochemistry is also helpful; the characteristic pathologic features and immunohistochemistry staining patterns of soft-tissue tumors can be found on websites such as PathologyOutlines.com (http://www.pathologyoutlines.com/eye.html). Typically, a panel including S-100, CD99, CD34, vimentin, actin, desmin, and CD68 is used for initial differentiation, and the results direct further studies.

Malignant soft-tissue tumors, or sarcomas, can be divided into 2 major genetic groups: (1) sarcomas with specific genetic alterations and usually simple karyotypes, such as reciprocal chromosomal translocations (eg, *FUS-DDIT3* in myxoid liposarcoma) and specific oncogenic mutations (eg, *KIT* mutation in gastrointestinal stromal tumors); and (2) sarcomas with nonspecific genetic alterations and complex unbalanced karyotypes. Some of these genetic abnormalities, including chromosomal numerical changes, translocations, gene amplifications, and large deletions, can be apparent at the cytogenetic level (karyotyping, fluorescence in situ hybridization), while others, such as small deletions, insertions, and point mutations, require molecular genetic techniques (polymerase chain reaction and sequence analysis).

Vascular Tumors

Lymphangiomas occur in children and are characterized by fluctuation in proptosis. Lymphangiomas of the orbit are unencapsulated, diffusely infiltrating tumors that feature lymphatic vascular spaces and lymphoid aggregates in a fibrotic interstitium (Fig 14-9).

Hemangioma in the adult is encapsulated and consists of cavernous spaces *(cavernous hemangioma)* with variably thick, fibrosed walls (Fig 14-10). Vessels may show thrombosis and calcification. Hemangioma in the child is unencapsulated, more cellular, and composed of capillary-sized vessels *(capillary hemangioma)*.

Tumors With Fibrous Differentiation

Fibrous histiocytoma (fibroxanthoma) is one of the most common mesenchymal tumors of the orbit in adults. The median age at presentation is 43 years (with a range of 6 months to 85 years), and the upper nasal orbit is the most common site. Most fibrous histiocytomas are benign. The tumor is composed of an admixture of histiocytes and fibroblasts, some of which form a storiform (matlike or whorly) pattern (Fig 14-11). Immunohistochemistry is typically positive for CD45 and CD68. Although most are benign, intermediate and malignant varieties do exist. Malignant tumors are identified by a high rate of mitotic activity

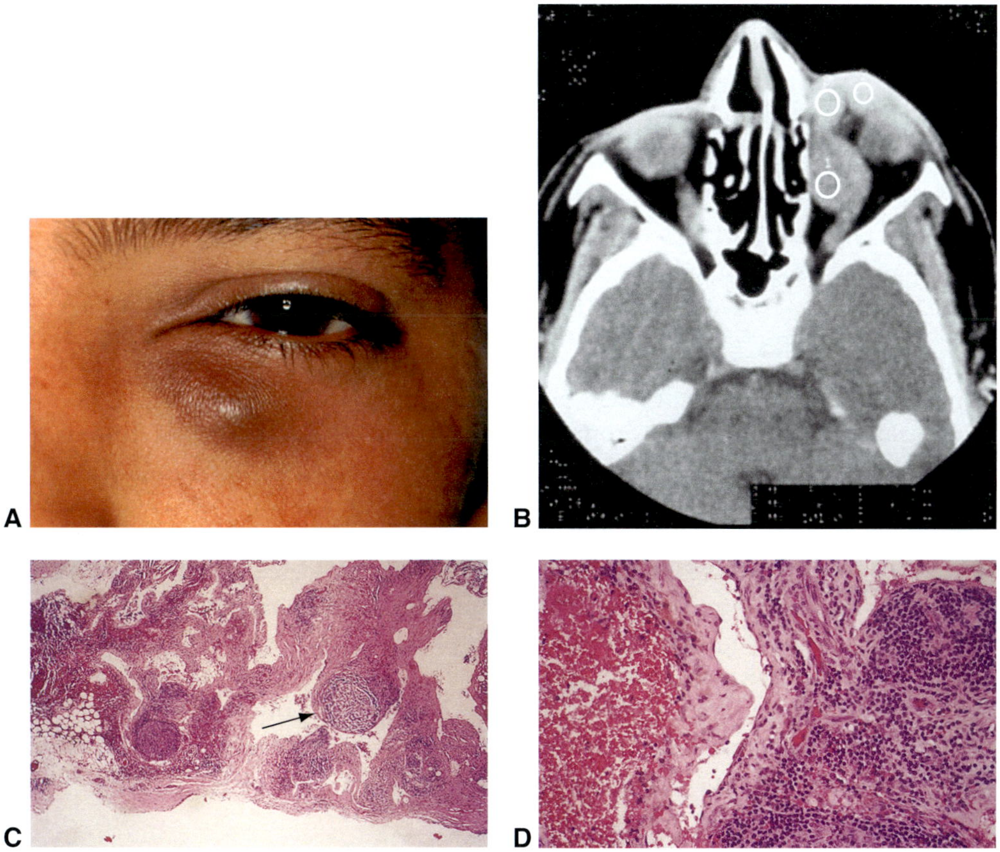

Figure 14-9 Lymphangioma. **A,** Clinical appearance. A young boy with an inferior orbital lesion extending anteriorly and nasally below the left lower eyelid. **B,** CT scan (axial view) showing a multilobulated mass *(white circles)* within the left orbit. **C,** Photomicrograph shows numerous vascular channels and lymphoid follicles *(arrow)* with a fibrotic stroma. **D,** Higher magnification demonstrates the lymphocytes and plasma cells within the fibrous walls. *(Parts A and B courtesy of Sander Dubovy, MD; parts C and D courtesy of Ben J. Glasgow, MD.)*

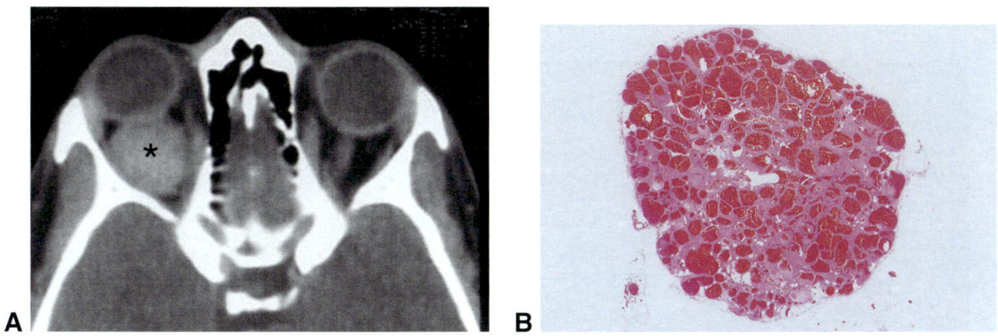

Figure 14-10 Cavernous hemangioma. **A,** CT scan (axial view) showing a well-circumscribed retrobulbar mass *(asterisk)*. **B,** Large spaces of blood are separated by thick septa. *(Part A courtesy of Sander Dubovy, MD; part B courtesy of Hans E. Grossniklaus, MD.)*

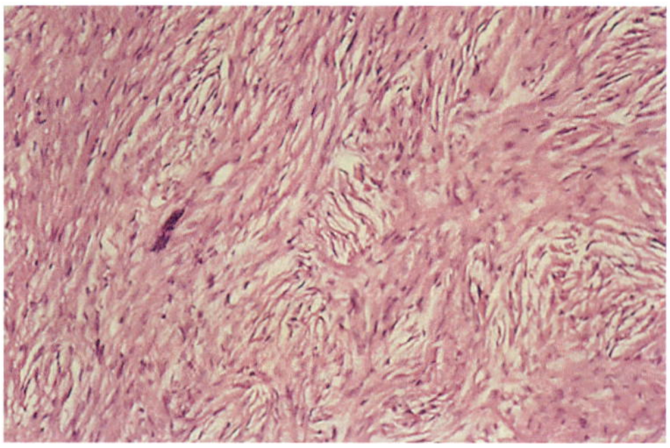

Figure 14-11 Fibrous histiocytoma. This photomicrograph illustrates the storiform (mat-like or whorly) pattern.

(more than 1 mitotic figure per high-power field), nuclear pleomorphism, and necrosis. Other primary tumors of fibrous connective tissue include nodular fasciitis, fibroma, and fibrosarcoma.

Hemangiopericytoma occurs mainly in adults (median age is 42 years) and manifests with proptosis, pain, diplopia, and decreased visual acuity. Histologically, a "staghorn" vascular pattern is displayed with densely packed spindle-shaped cells (Fig 14-12). The reticulin stain is useful in demonstrating tumor cells that are individually wrapped in a network of collagenous material. Hemangiopericytomas include a spectrum of benign, intermediate, and malignant lesions. Features of malignancy include an infiltrating border, anaplasia, mitotic figures, and necrosis. Immunohistochemistry is typically positive for CD34. However, these features may be absent in tumors that eventually metastasize. A solitary fibrous tumor is part of the hemangiopericytoma spectrum.

Tumors With Muscle Differentiation

Rhabdomyosarcoma

Rhabdomyosarcoma is the most common primary malignant orbital tumor of childhood (average age of onset is 7–8 years). Proptosis is often sudden and rapidly progressive; it requires emergency treatment. Reddish discoloration of the eyelids is *not* accompanied by local heat or systemic fever, as it is in cellulitis. Orbital rhabdomyosarcomas have a better prognosis (overall 5-year survival of about 90%) than do their extraorbital counterparts.

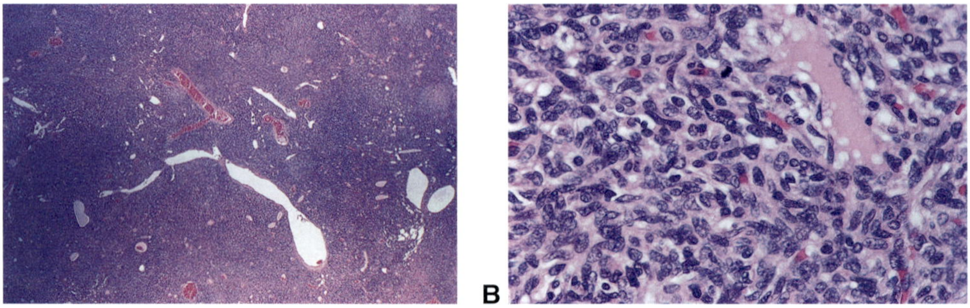

A B

Figure 14-12 Hemangiopericytoma. **A,** Photomicrograph demonstrates a dense, cellular tumor with a characteristic branching vascular pattern. **B,** Higher magnification demonstrates closely packed cells with oval to spindle-shaped, vesicular nuclei. *(Courtesy of Ben J. Glasgow, MD.)*

Rhabdomyosarcomas arise from primitive mesenchymal cells that differentiate toward skeletal muscle. Three histologic types of orbital rhabdomyosarcoma are recognized (Fig 14-13):

1. embryonal (the most common)
2. alveolar
3. pleomorphic

Embryonal rhabdomyosarcoma may develop in the conjunctiva and may present as grapelike submucosal clusters *(botryoid variant)*. Histologically, spindle cells are arranged in a loose syncytium with occasional cells bearing cross-striations, which are found in approximately 60% of embryonal rhabdomyosarcomas. Well-differentiated rhabdomyosarcomas feature numerous cells with striking cross-striations. Immunohistochemical reactivity is typically positive for desmin, muscle-specific actin, vimentin, and, less

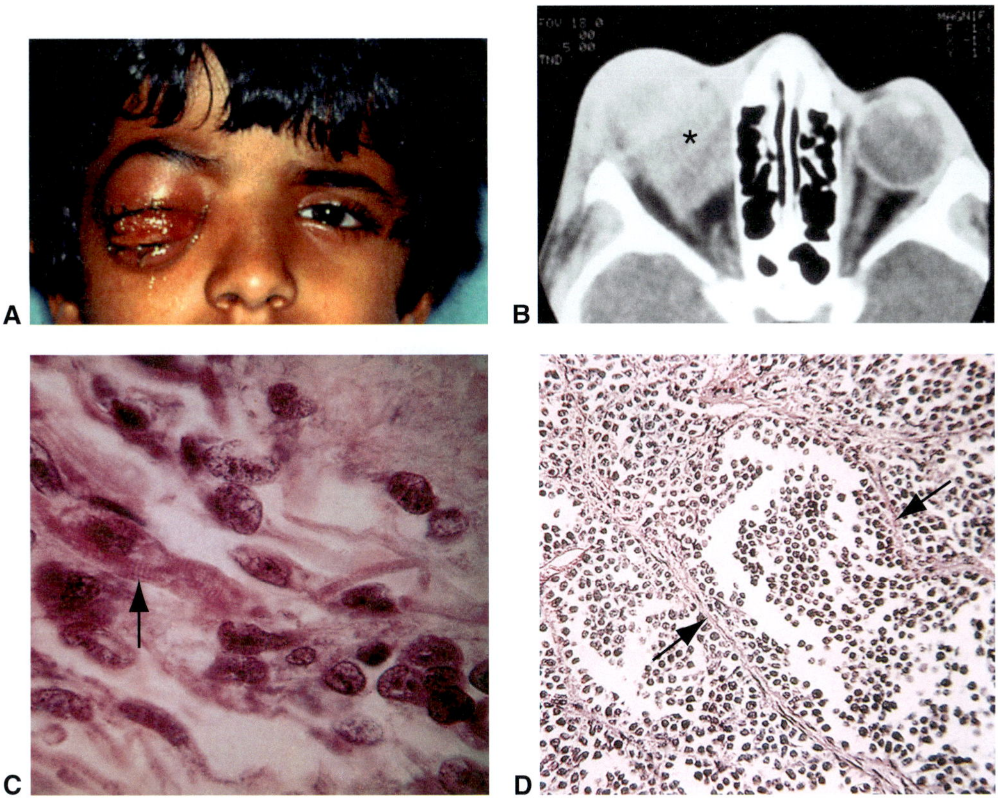

Figure 14-13 Rhabdomyosarcoma. **A,** Child with a large right orbital mass. **B,** CT scan (axial view) showing a large, poorly circumscribed orbital tumor *(asterisk)* and proptosis. **C,** In this embryonal example, cross-striations *(arrow)* representing Z-bands of actin-myosin complexes within the cytoplasm of a tumor cell can be identified. **D,** Poorly cohesive rhabdomyoblasts separated by fibrous septa *(arrows)* into "alveoli" are low-magnification histologic features of the alveolar variant of rhabdomyosarcoma. This variant may have a less favorable natural history than the more common embryonal type. *(Parts A and B courtesy of Sander Dubovy, MD.)*

commonly, myogenin. Electron microscopy is helpful for demonstrating the typical sarcomeric banding pattern, especially in the less-well-differentiated cases of embryonal rhabdomyosarcoma.

Leiomyomas and leiomyosarcomas

Tumors with smooth-muscle differentiation are rare. *Leiomyomas* are benign tumors that typically manifest with slowly progressive proptosis in patients in the fourth and fifth decades of life. Histologically, these spindle cell tumors show blunt-ended, cigar-shaped nuclei and trichrome-positive filamentous cytoplasm. Immunohistochemistry displays smooth-muscle differentiation. *Leiomyosarcomas* are malignant lesions that typically occur in patients in their seventh decade. Histologically, more cellularity, necrosis, nuclear pleomorphism, and mitotic figures appear in leiomyosarcomas than in leiomyomas.

Nerve Sheath Tumors

Neurofibromas are the most common nerve sheath tumor. This slow-growing tumor includes an admixture of endoneural fibroblasts, Schwann cells, and axons. Neurofibromas may be circumscribed but are not encapsulated. The consistency is firm and rubbery. Microscopically, the spindle-shaped cells are arranged in ribbons and cords in a matrix of myxoid tissue and collagen that contains axons. Cytogenetic studies indicate that the most frequent structural rearrangements involve chromosome arm 9p.

Isolated neurofibromas do not necessarily indicate systemic involvement, but the plexiform type of neurofibroma is associated with neurofibromatosis type 1 (NF1) (Fig 14-14). Studies indicate that a limited number of pathways are potentially involved in tumorigenesis of the plexiform neurofibroma. The *CCN1* gene may be a useful diagnostic or prognostic marker and form the basis for novel therapeutic strategies. The CCNs (cysteine-rich proteins) have been shown to have key roles as matricellular proteins, serving as adaptor molecules that connect the cell surface and the extracellular matrix (ECM).

The *neurilemoma* (also called *schwannoma*) arises from Schwann cells. Slow growing and encapsulated, this yellowish tumor may show cysts and areas of hemorrhagic necrosis. It may be solitary or associated with neurofibromatosis. Two histologic patterns appear microscopically: Antoni A spindle cells are arranged in interlacing cords, whorls,

A B
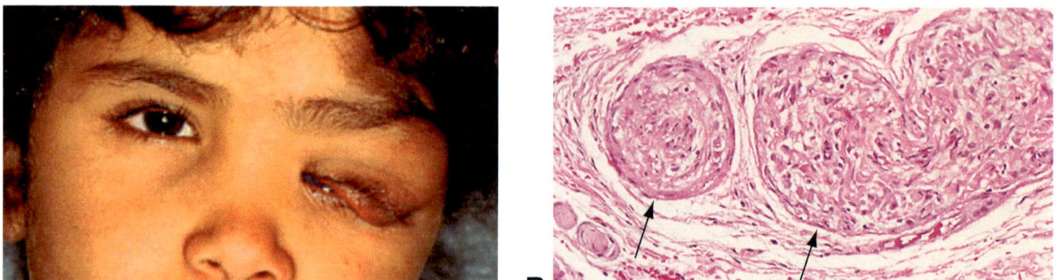

Figure 14-14 Plexiform neurofibroma. **A,** Clinical photograph depicting a typical S-shaped deformity of the upper eyelid. **B,** Note the thickened, tortuous nerves *(arrows)* with proliferation of endoneural fibroblasts and Schwann cells. *(Part A courtesy of Sander Dubovy, MD.)*

or palisades that may form Verocay bodies (collections of fibrils resembling sensory corpuscles). The Antoni B pattern is made up of stellate cells with a mucoid stroma. Vessels are usually prominent and thick-walled, and no axons are present (Fig 14-15). Immunohistochemistry is typically positive for S-100, vimentin, and CD68.

Liu K, DeAngelo P, Mahmet K, Phytides P, Osborne L, Pletcher BA. Cytogenetics of neurofibromas: two case reports and literature review. *Cancer Genet Cytogenet.* 2010;196(1):93–95.

Pasmant E, Ortonne N, Rittié L, et al. Differential expression of CCN1/CYR61, CCN3/NOV, CCN4/WISP1, and CCN5/WISP2 in neurofibromatosis type 1 tumorigenesis. *J Neuropathol Exp Neurol.* 2010;69(1):60–69.

Adipose Tumors

Lipomas are rare in the orbit. Pathologic characteristics include encapsulation and a distinctive lobular appearance. Because lipomas are histologically difficult to distinguish from normal or prolapsed fat, their incidence might have been previously overestimated.

Liposarcomas are malignant tumors that are extremely rare in the orbit. Histologic criteria depend on the type of liposarcoma, but the unifying diagnostic feature is the presence of lipoblasts. These tumors tend to recur before they metastasize.

Bony Lesions of the Orbit

Fibrous dysplasia of bone may be monostotic or polyostotic. When the orbit is affected, the condition is usually monostotic, and the patient often presents during the first 3 decades of life. The tumor may cross suture lines to involve multiple orbital bones. Narrowing of

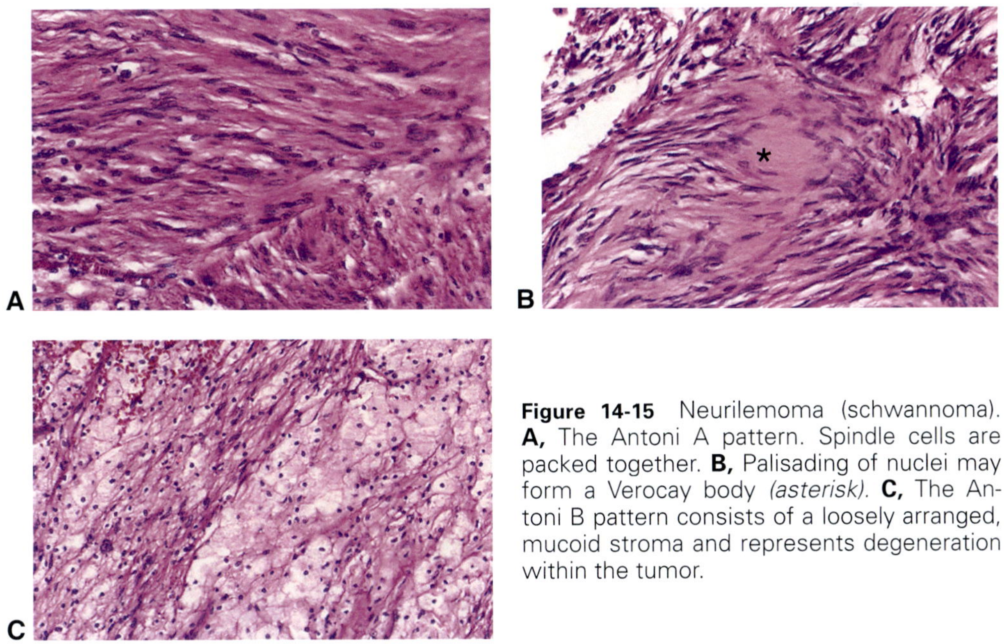

Figure 14-15 Neurilemoma (schwannoma). **A,** The Antoni A pattern. Spindle cells are packed together. **B,** Palisading of nuclei may form a Verocay body *(asterisk).* **C,** The Antoni B pattern consists of a loosely arranged, mucoid stroma and represents degeneration within the tumor.

the optic canal and lacrimal drainage system can occur. Plain radiographic studies show a ground-glass appearance with lytic foci. Cysts containing fluid also appear. As a result of arrest in the maturation of bone, trabeculae are composed of woven bone with a fibrous stroma that is highly vascularized rather than lamellar bone. The bony trabeculae often have a C-shaped appearance (Fig 14-16).

Fibro-osseus dysplasia (juvenile ossifying fibroma), a variant of fibrous dysplasia, is characterized histologically by spicules of bone rimmed by osteoblasts (Fig 14-17). At low magnification, ossifying fibroma may be confused with a psammomatous meningioma.

Osseous and cartilaginous tumors are rare; of these, *osteoma* is the most common. It is slow growing, well circumscribed, and composed of mature bone. Most commonly, an osteoma arises from the frontal sinus. Other primary tumors in this group include

- osteoblastoma
- giant cell tumor
- chondroma
- Ewing sarcoma
- osteogenic sarcoma
- chondrosarcoma

See the appendix for AJCC definitions and staging of orbital sarcomas.

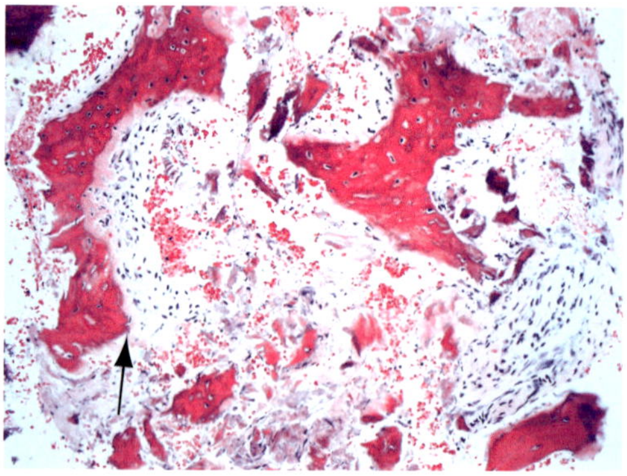

Figure 14-16 Fibrous dysplasia. Bony trabeculae are C-shaped *(arrow),* composed of immature woven bone, and surrounded by a fibrous stroma. *(Courtesy of Tatyana Milman, MD.)*

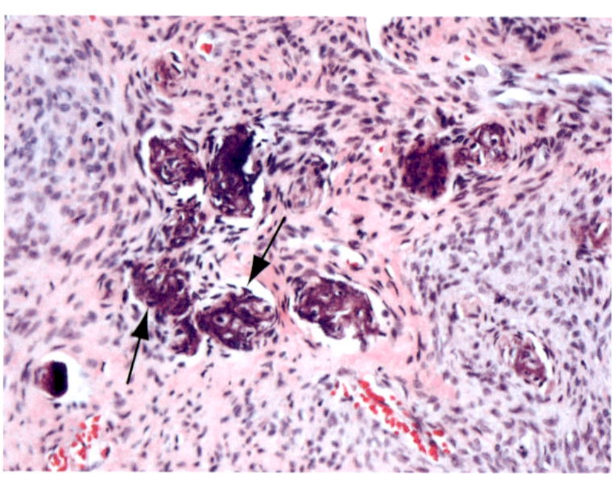

Figure 14-17 Fibro-osseus dysplasia (ossifying fibroma). Spicules of lamellar bone are set in a cellular fibrous stroma. Note the osteoblasts *(arrows)* lining the bony spicules. *(Courtesy of Tatyana Milman, MD.)*

Metastatic Tumors

Secondary orbital tumors are those that invade the orbit by direct extension from adjacent structures, such as sinus, bone, or eye. *Metastatic* tumors are those that spread from a primary site. The most common primary tumor sites with orbital metastasis are the breast in women and the prostate in men. In children, neuroblastoma is the most common primary tumor metastatic to the orbit.

CHAPTER 15

Optic Nerve

Topography

The optic nerve, embryologically derived from the optic stalk, is a continuation of the optic tract; thus, the pathology of the optic nerve reflects that of the central nervous system (CNS). The optic nerve extends from the eye to the optic chiasm and is 35–55 mm in length (intraocular portion, 0.7–1.0 mm; intraorbital portion, 25–30 mm; intracanalicular portion, 4–10 mm; intracranial portion averages 10 mm). Optic nerve axons originate from the retinal ganglion cell layer and have a myelin coat posterior to the lamina cribrosa.

Oligodendrocytes, astrocytes, and microglial cells are glial cells (*glia* = glue). Oligodendrocytes produce and maintain the myelin sheath of the optic nerve. Astrocytes are involved with support and nutrition. Microglial cells (CNS histiocytes) have a phagocytic function.

The meningeal coat that covers the optic nerve includes the dura mater (which merges with the sclera), the cellular arachnoid layer, and the vascular pia mater. The pial vessels extend into the optic nerve and subdivide the nerve fibers into fascicles. The subarachnoid space, which contains cerebrospinal fluid (CSF), ends blindly at the termination of the meninges (Figs 15-1, 15-2). See BCSC Section 2, *Fundamentals and Principles of Ophthalmology,* and Section 5, *Neuro-Ophthalmology,* for additional discussion.

Congenital Anomalies

Numerous congenital defects can involve the optic nerve, including optic nerve hypoplasia, optic nerve head pit, morning glory disc anomaly, Bergmeister papilla, and optic nerve coloboma. These are discussed in BCSC Section 5, *Neuro-Ophthalmology,* and Section 6, *Pediatric Ophthalmology and Strabismus.*

Colobomas

Typical colobomas of the optic nerve head result from defective closure of the embryonic fissure. They are observed inferonasally in the optic nerve head and are associated with colobomatous defects of the retina/choroid, ciliary body, and iris, which may occur at any point along the course of the embryonic fissure (Fig 15-3A).

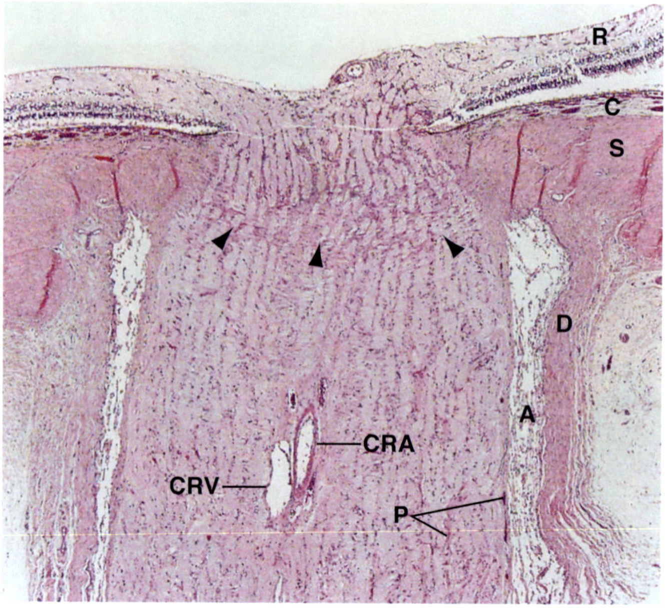

Figure 15-1 Longitudinal section of normal optic nerve. Axons of the retinal ganglion cells *(R)* become axonal fibers of the optic nerve. Optic nerve axons pass through the fenestrations in the lamina cribrosa *(arrowheads)*, which is continuous with the anterior sclera *(S)*. The posterior sclera is continuous with the dura *(D)*. *C* = choroid, *A* = arachnoid, *P* = pia, *CRA* = central retinal artery, *CRV* = central retinal vein. *(Courtesy of Tatyana Milman, MD.)*

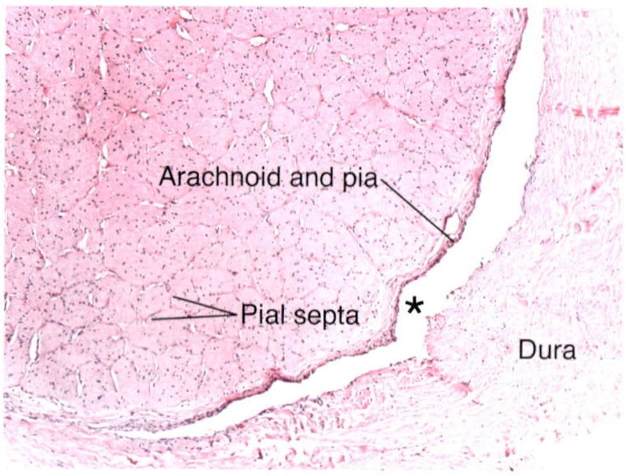

Figure 15-2 Transverse or cross section of the normal optic nerve. The axons of the optic nerve are segregated into fascicles by the delicate fibrovascular pial septa. The nuclei of oligodendrocytes, astrocytes, and microglia are present between the eosinophilic axons. The subdural space *(asterisk)* is relatively narrow in a normal optic nerve. *(Courtesy of Tatyana Milman, MD.)*

Histologically, an optic nerve coloboma consists of a large defect in the optic nerve, involving the retina, retinal pigment epithelium, and choroid. An atrophic and gliotic retina lines the defect. The sclera is ectatic and bowed posteriorly. The wall of the defect may contain adipose tissue and even smooth muscle (Fig 15-3B).

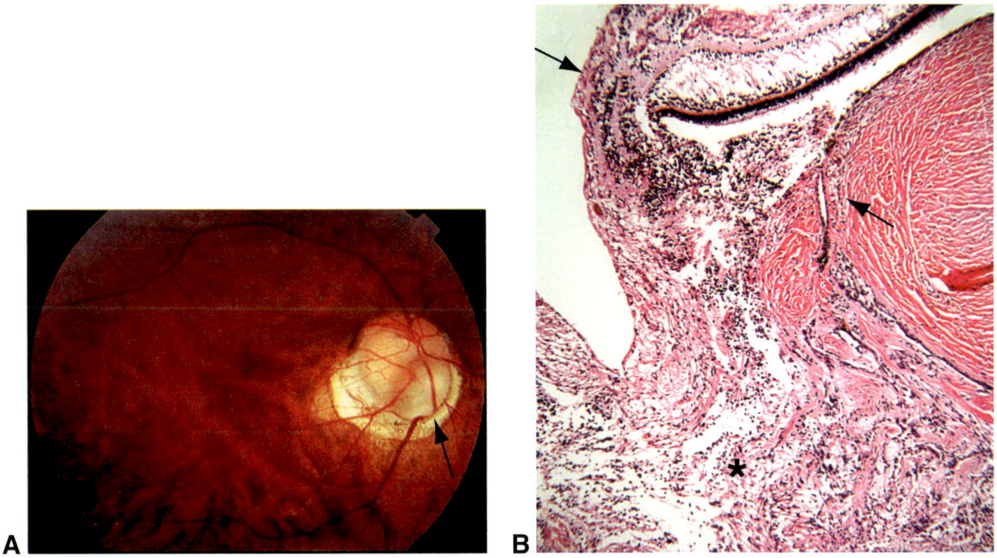

Figure 15-3 Optic nerve coloboma. **A,** Fundus photograph of the right eye shows a colobomatous defect in the inferonasal optic nerve *(arrow).* **B,** The gliotic, disorganized retina *(asterisk)* prolapses into the defect, which is lined by excavated sclera. The normal retina, retinal pigment epithelium, and choroid terminate at the edge of the colobomatous defect *(arrows).* *(Courtesy of Tatyana Milman, MD.)*

Inflammations

Infectious

Infections of the optic nerve may be secondary to *bacterial* or *fungal* infections of adjacent anatomical structures, such as the eye, brain, or sinuses, or they may occur as part of a systemic infection, particularly in an immunosuppressed patient. Fungal infections include mucormycosis, cryptococcosis, and coccidiomycosis. Mucormycosis generally results from contiguous sinus infection. Cryptococcosis results from direct extension of the infection from the CNS and often produces multiple foci of necrosis with little inflammatory reaction (Fig 15-4). Coccidiomycosis produces necrotizing granulomas.

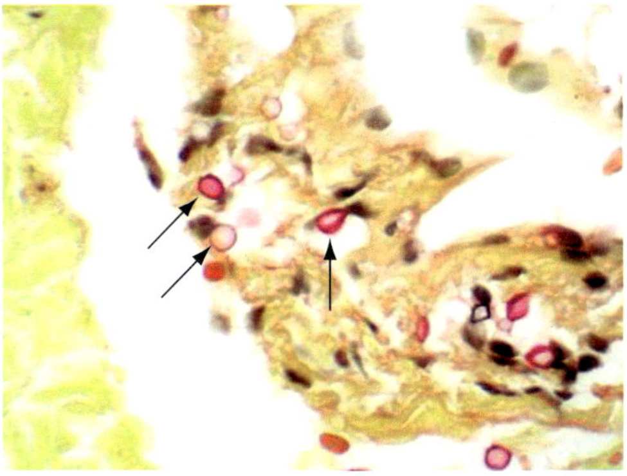

Figure 15-4 Cryptococcosis of the optic nerve in an immunocompromised patient. The dura is infiltrated by cryptococcal organisms *(arrows).* This yeast has a mucopolysaccharide capsule, highlighted with mucicarmine stain. No inflammatory infiltrate is observed. *(Courtesy of Tatyana Milman, MD.)*

Viral infections of the optic nerve are usually associated with other CNS lesions. *Multiple sclerosis* and *acute disseminated encephalomyelitis* are immune-mediated demyelinating diseases with multifactorial etiologies, including infectious causes. The damaged myelin is removed by macrophages (Fig 15-5). Astrocytic proliferation ultimately produces a glial scar, known as a *plaque.*

Noninfectious

Noninfectious inflammatory disorders of the optic nerve include giant cell arteritis and sarcoidosis. Giant cell arteritis can produce granulomatous inflammation in the blood vessel wall and occlusion of the posterior ciliary vessels with liquefactive necrosis of the optic nerve. Superficial temporal artery biopsy is the gold standard for histologic diagnosis of giant cell arteritis (Fig 15-6). The involvement of the vessel wall in giant cell arteritis can be patchy *(skip lesions).* Obtaining a biopsy specimen of adequate length (approximately 2 cm) and performing a careful histologic examination of the specimen can increase the diagnostic yield.

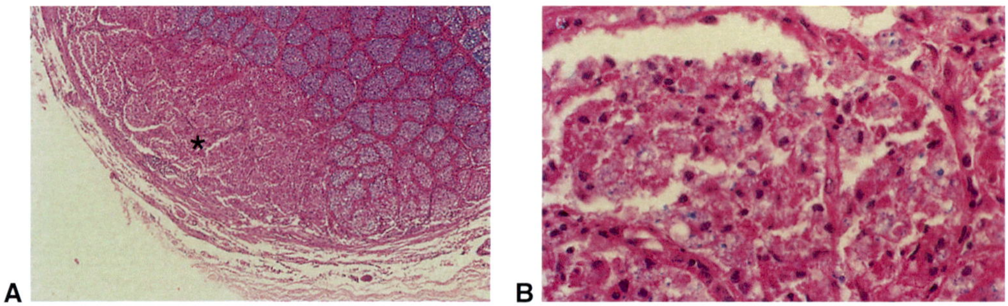

Figure 15-5 Multiple sclerosis, optic nerve. **A,** Luxol fast blue stain, counterstained with H&E. The blue-staining area indicates normal myelin. Note the absence of myelin in the lower left corner of the optic nerve *(asterisk),* corresponding to a focal lesion. **B,** Higher magnification. The blue material (myelin) is engulfed by macrophages.

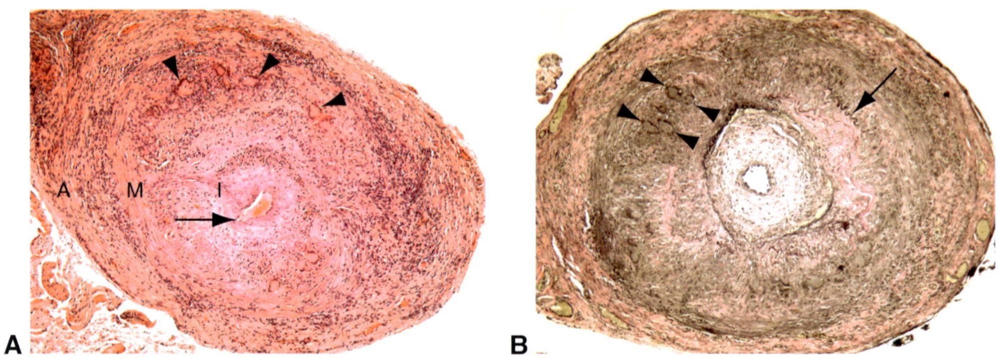

Figure 15-6 Giant cell arteritis, superficial temporal artery. **A,** Vascular lumen *(arrow)* is narrowed by concentric intimal hyperplasia. Prominent transmural inflammatory infiltrate with numerous multinucleated giant cells *(arrowheads)* is observed. **B,** Elastic stain highlights the diffuse loss of the internal elastic lamina. A short segment of remaining internal elastic lamina is marked with an arrow. Giant cells *(arrowheads)* are noted at the level of the internal elastic lamina. *I* = intima, *M* = media, *A* = adventitia. *(Courtesy of Tatyana Milman, MD.)*

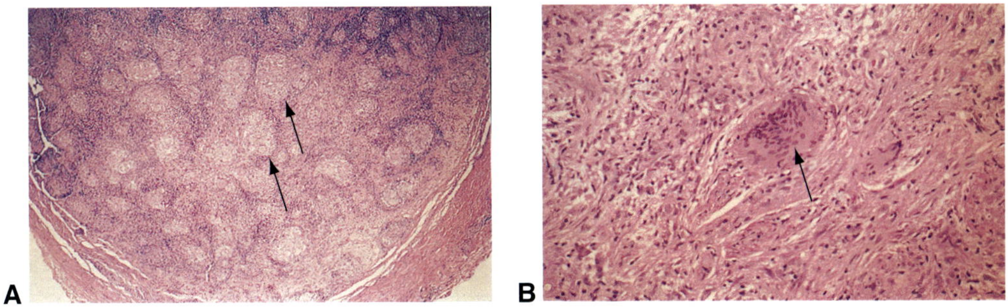

Figure 15-7 Sarcoidosis. **A,** Low-magnification photomicrograph of the optic nerve with discrete noncaseating granulomas *(arrows)*. **B,** Higher magnification shows multinucleated giant cells *(arrow)* in the granulomas. *(Courtesy of Hans E. Grossniklaus, MD.)*

Sarcoidosis of the optic nerve is often associated with retinal, vitreal, and uveitic lesions (Fig 15-7; see also Chapter 12, Fig 12-8). Unlike the characteristic noncaseating granulomas in the eye, optic nerve lesions may feature necrosis.

Degenerations

Optic Atrophy

Injury to the retinal ganglion cells and to the axons of the peripheral optic nerve (that portion of the nerve near the retina) results in axonal swelling. This swelling manifests clinically as optic disc edema (Fig 15-8). Axonal swelling and loss of retinal ganglion cells are followed by retrograde degeneration of axons *(ascending atrophy, Wallerian degeneration)* toward the lateral geniculate body. Pathologic processes within the cranial cavity or

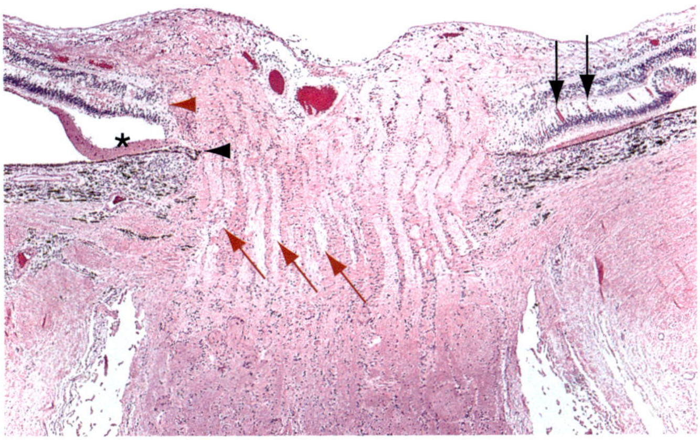

Figure 15-8 Optic disc edema. Swollen prelaminar axons demonstrate vacuolar alteration *(red arrows)* and displace the retina laterally *(red arrowhead)* from its normal termination just above the end of the Bruch membrane *(black arrowhead)*. Juxtapapillary serous intraretinal fluid/hard exudates *(black arrows)* and serous subretinal fluid *(asterisk)* are also observed. *(Courtesy of Tatyana Milman, MD.)*

orbit result in *descending atrophy* toward the retinal ganglion cells (see BCSC Section 5, *Neuro-Ophthalmology*).

Axonal degeneration is accompanied by loss of myelin and oligodendrocytes. The optic nerve shrinks despite the proliferation of astrocytes and of fibroconnective tissue in the pial septa (Fig 15-9).

Cavernous optic atrophy of Schnabel is characterized microscopically by large cystic spaces that are posterior to the lamina cribrosa and contain mucopolysaccharide material, which stains with alcian blue stain (Fig 15-10). Although the changes associated with cavernous optic atrophy were initially observed in glaucomatous eyes after acute intraocular pressure elevation, the condition has been increasingly identified in nonglaucomatous elderly patients with generalized arteriosclerotic disease. The mucopolysaccharide was originally thought to be vitreous, forced by increased intraocular pressure into the ischemic necrosis–induced cavernous spaces, but it is more likely produced in situ, within the atrophic spaces of the optic nerve.

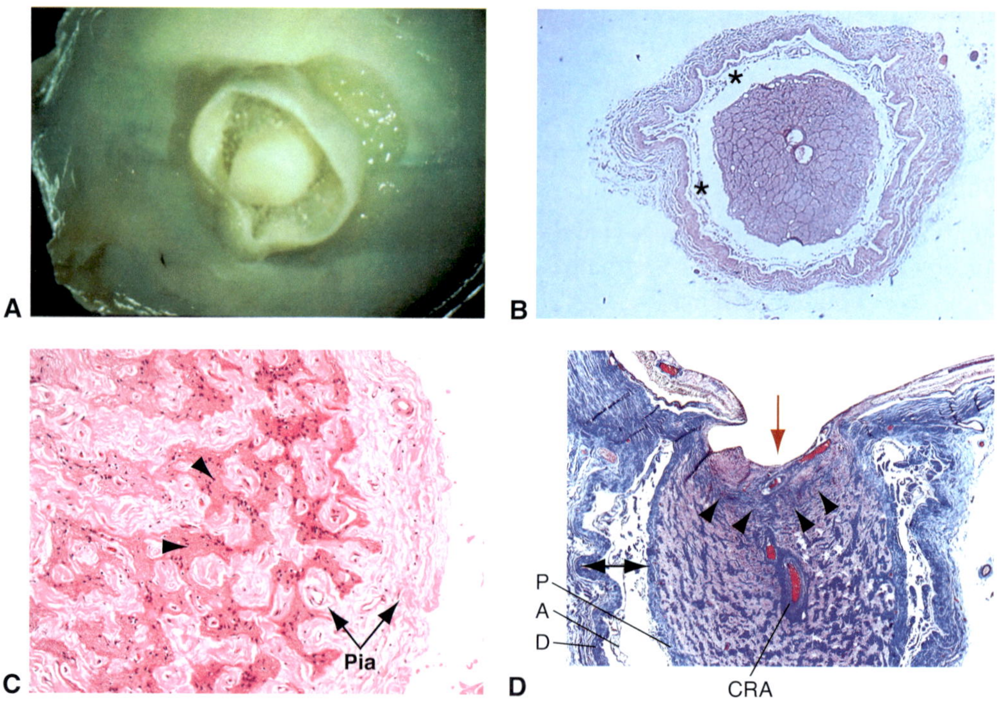

Figure 15-9 Atrophic optic nerve. **A,** Gross appearance of atrophic optic nerve. **B,** Low-magnification photomicrograph. Note the widened subdural space *(asterisks)*. **C,** High magnification. Transverse or cross section of atrophic nerve shows loss of axons *(arrowheads)*, accompanied by glial proliferation and widening of fibrovascular pial septa *(arrows)*. **D,** Glaucomatous optic atrophy. Masson trichrome stains the collagen of the sclera, lamina cribrosa, and meninges dark blue and the axonal fascicles pink. The optic nerve demonstrates advanced cupping *(red arrow)*, accompanied by posterior bowing of the lamina cribrosa *(arrowheads)*. Axonal atrophy and thickening of pial septa are present. The intermeningeal space is widened due to severe optic nerve atrophy *(double-ended arrow)*. *CRA* = central retinal artery, *P* = pia, *A* = arachnoid, *D* = dura. *(Part A courtesy of Debra J. Shetlar, MD; parts C and D courtesy of Tatyana Milman, MD.)*

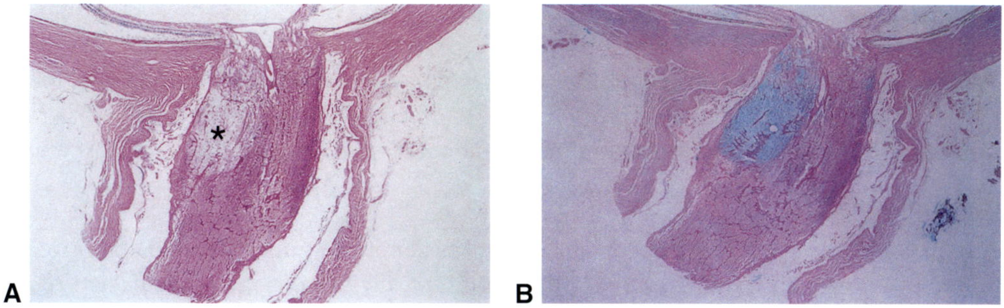

Figure 15-10 Cavernous optic atrophy of Schnabel. **A,** Photomicrograph shows cystic atrophy *(asterisk)* within the optic nerve. **B,** The cystic space is filled with alcian blue–staining material. *(Courtesy of Hans E. Grossniklaus, MD.)*

Giarelli L, Falconieri G, Cameron JD, Pheley AM. Schnabel cavernous degeneration: a vascular change of the aging eye. *Arch Pathol Lab Med.* 2003;127(10):1314–1319.

Drusen

Drusen of the optic disc are calcific, usually bilateral deposits embedded within the parenchyma of small, crowded optic discs with abnormal vasculature. When superficial, optic disc drusen appear as refractile, rounded, pale yellow or white deposits. Deeper drusen may be mistaken for papilledema (pseudopapilledema). Optic disc drusen can be associated with angioid streaks, papillitis, optic atrophy, chronic glaucoma, and vascular occlusions, but they are more commonly observed in otherwise normal eyes and are occasionally dominantly inherited.

Evidence suggests that abnormal axonal metabolism leads to mitochondrial calcification and drusen formation. Histologically, optic disc drusen appear as basophilic, calcified acellular deposits that contain mucopolysaccharides, amino acids, DNA, RNA, and iron. Most disc drusen are located anterior to the lamina cribrosa and posterior to Bruch membrane (lamina choroidalis portion of the intraocular optic nerve) (Fig 15-11). See also BCSC Section 5, *Neuro-Ophthalmology,* and Section 6, *Pediatric Ophthalmology and Strabismus.*

Lam BL, Morais CG Jr, Pasol J. Drusen of the optic disc. *Curr Neurol Neurosci Rep.* 2008;8(5): 404–408.

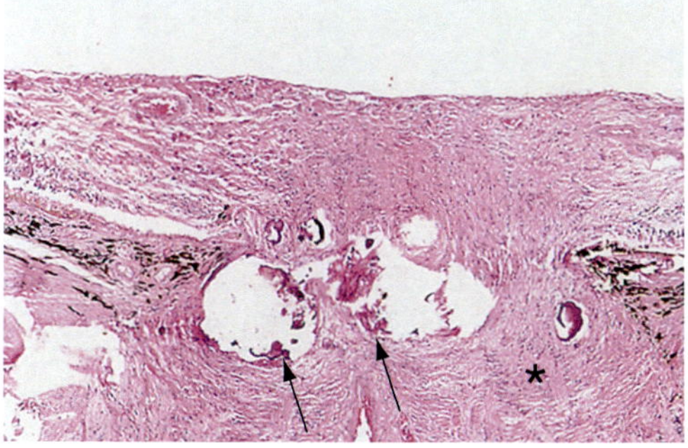

Figure 15-11 Histologically, drusen of the optic nerve head appear as discrete basophilic zones of calcification *(arrows)* just anterior to the lamina cribrosa *(asterisk).* The cystic spaces in the optic nerve head are histologic sectioning artifacts.

Neoplasia

Tumors may affect the optic nerve head (eg, melanocytoma, peripapillary choroidal melanoma, retinal pigment epithelial proliferation, and hemangioma) or the retrobulbar portion of the optic nerve (eg, glioma and meningioma).

Melanocytoma

A melanocytoma is a benign, deeply pigmented melanocytic tumor situated eccentrically on the optic disc. It may be slightly elevated and typically extends into the adjacent retina as well as posteriorly into the optic nerve. Slow growth can occur, but malignant transformation is rare.

Histologically, melanocytoma is a magnocellular nevus, composed of closely packed, maximally pigmented, plump, polyhedral melanocytes. The dense pigment obscures nuclear detail, so that bleached preparations are necessary to demonstrate bland cytologic features: abundant cytoplasm, small nuclei with finely dispersed chromatin, and small and regular nucleoli. Necrosis and melanophagic infiltration within melanocytoma can be observed but are not indicative of aggressive behavior (Fig 15-12). See also Chapter 17.

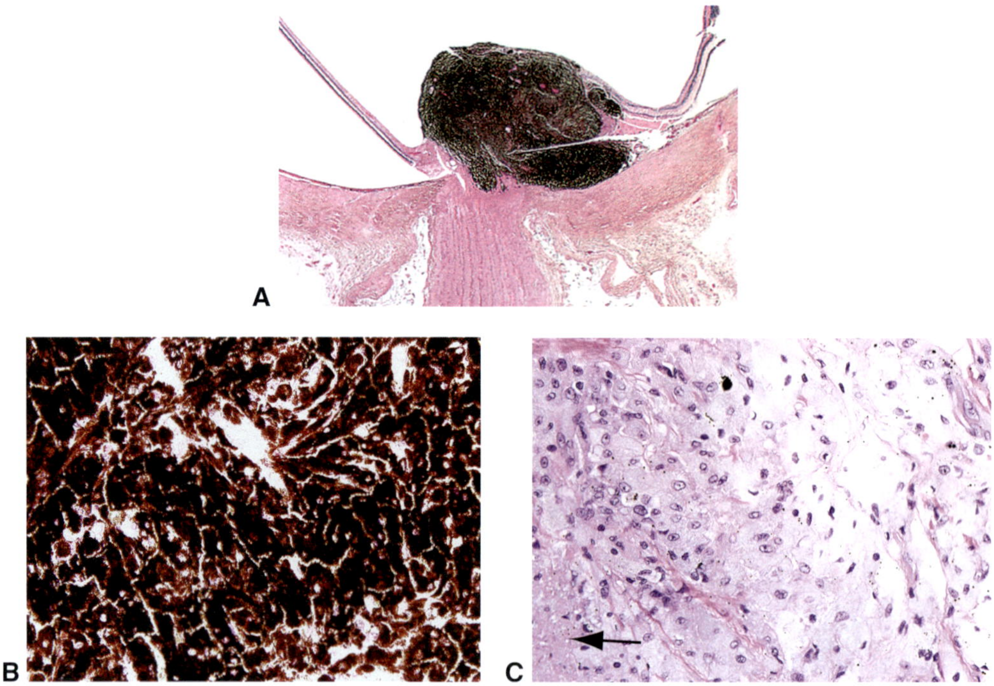

Figure 15-12 Melanocytoma of the optic nerve. **A,** Low-power photomicrograph of melanocytoma shows a dome-shaped, jet-black mass involving the prelaminar optic nerve. The juxtapapillary choroid and retina are also involved by this tumor. **B,** Higher magnification shows darkly pigmented polyhedral melanocytes with dense intracytoplasmic pigment, obscuring the nuclear detail. **C,** Bleached preparation displays the bland nuclear morphology of melanocytoma cells. An area of necrosis within the tumor is also observed *(arrow). (Courtesy of Tatyana Milman, MD.)*

Glioma

A glioma (astrocytoma) may arise in any part of the visual pathway, including the optic disc and optic nerve. Optic nerve gliomas are frequently associated with neurofibromatosis (NF1). The tumors most commonly present in the first decade of life and are low-grade *juvenile pilocytic astrocytomas.*

Histology of juvenile pilocytic astrocytomas shows proliferation of spindle-shaped astrocytes with delicate, hairlike (pilocytic) cytoplasmic processes that expand the optic nerve parenchyma. Enlarged, deeply eosinophilic filaments, representing degenerating cell processes known as *Rosenthal fibers,* may be found in these low-grade tumors (Fig 15-13). Foci of microcystic degeneration and calcification may occur, and the pial septae are thickened. The meninges show a reactive hyperplasia and infiltration by astrocytes. The dura mater remains intact, so the nerve demonstrates fusiform or sausage-shaped enlargement.

High-grade tumors *(grade 4 astrocytomas, glioblastoma multiforme, malignant gliomas)* rarely involve the optic nerve. When this does occur, the optic nerve is usually involved secondarily from a brain tumor. *Primary malignant gliomas* of the anterior visual pathways occur primarily in adults and are characterized histologically by nuclear pleomorphism, high mitotic activity, necrosis, and hemorrhage. See also BCSC Section 5, *Neuro-Ophthalmology,* and Section 7, *Orbit, Eyelids, and Lacrimal System.*

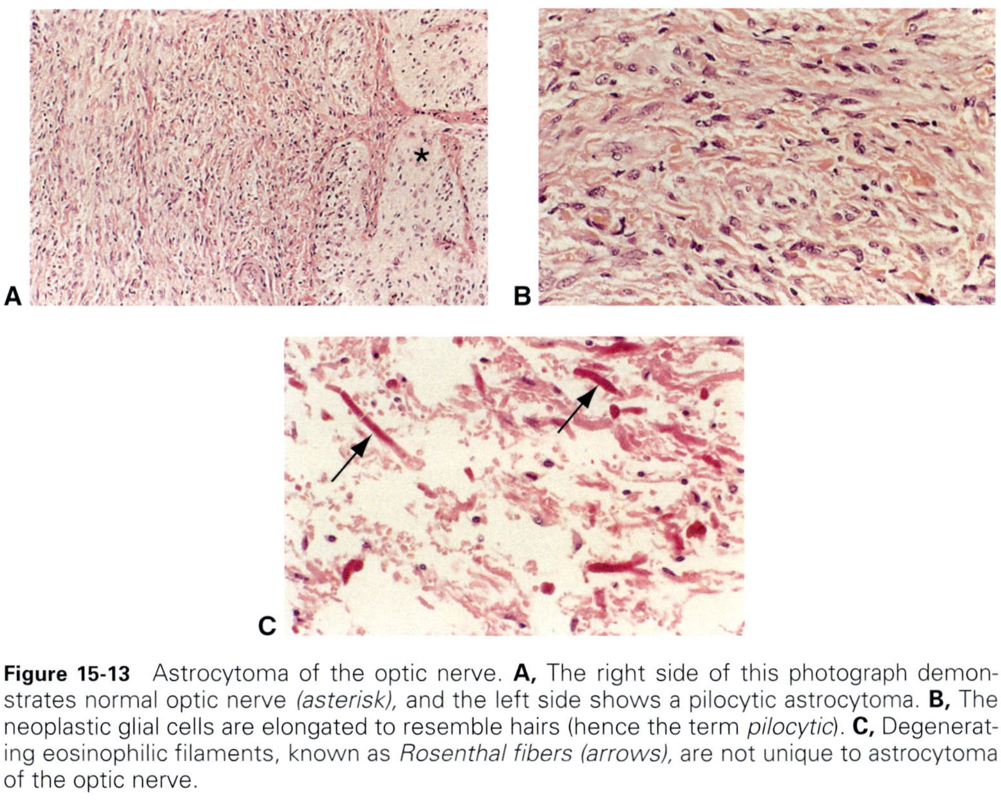

Figure 15-13 Astrocytoma of the optic nerve. **A,** The right side of this photograph demonstrates normal optic nerve *(asterisk),* and the left side shows a pilocytic astrocytoma. **B,** The neoplastic glial cells are elongated to resemble hairs (hence the term *pilocytic*). **C,** Degenerating eosinophilic filaments, known as *Rosenthal fibers (arrows),* are not unique to astrocytoma of the optic nerve.

Meningioma

Primary optic nerve sheath meningiomas arise from the arachnoid sheath of the optic nerve. They are less frequent than *secondary orbital meningiomas,* which extend into the orbit from an intracranial primary site. Although meningioma may, in rare instances, be associated with neurofibromatosis in the younger age group, it is a less frequent hallmark of NF1 than is optic nerve glioma. Primary optic nerve meningiomas may invade the nerve and the eye and may extend through the dura mater to invade muscle (Figs 15-14, 15-15).

Histologically, the tumor (primary or secondary) is usually of the *meningothelial* type, composed of plump cells with indistinct cytoplasmic margins (syncytial growth pattern) arranged in whorls (see Fig 15-14C). *Psammoma bodies,* extracellular rounded calcifications surrounded by a cluster of meningioma cells, tend to be sparse. See BCSC Section 5, *Neuro-Ophthalmology,* and Section 7, *Orbit, Eyelids, and Lacrimal System.*

Miller NR. Primary tumours of the optic nerve and its sheath. *Eye.* 2004;18(11):1026–1037.

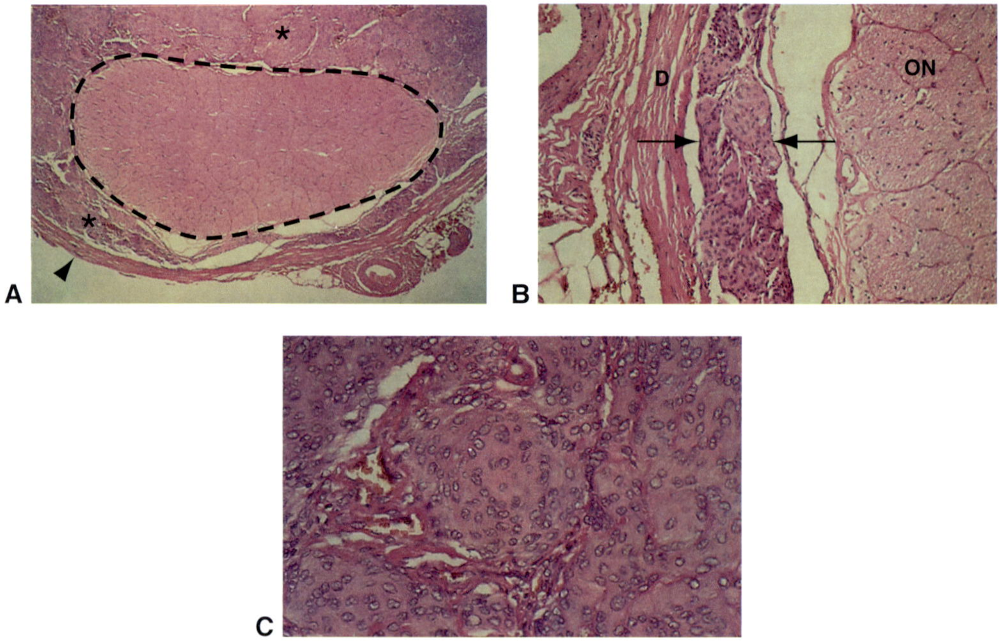

Figure 15-14 Optic nerve meningioma. **A,** This meningioma *(asterisks)* has grown circumferentially around the optic nerve *(outlined by dashed line)* and has compressed the nerve (arrowhead = dura mater). **B,** Meningioma *(between arrows)* of the optic nerve *(ON)* originates from the arachnoid. *D* = dura mater. **C,** Note the whorls of tumor cells, characteristic of the meningothelial type of meningioma, the most common histologic variant arising from the optic nerve.

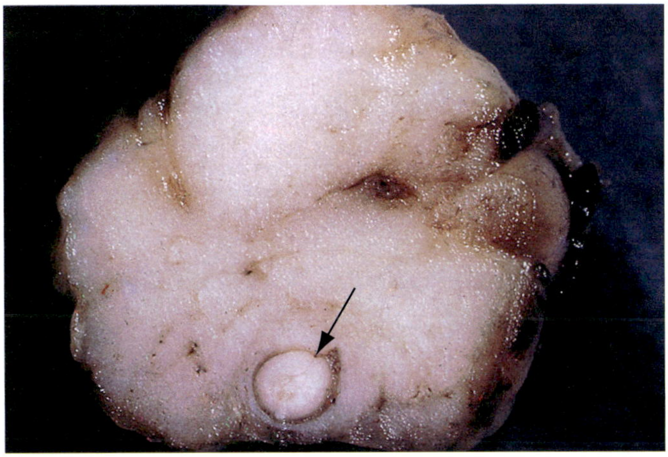

Figure 15-15 Optic nerve meningioma. The shaggy border of this gross specimen emphasizes the tendency of the perioptic meningioma to invade surrounding orbital tissues. Note the size of the optic nerve *(arrow)* in relation to the tumor.

PART II

Intraocular Tumors: Clinical Aspects

CHAPTER 16

Introduction to Part II

Intraocular tumors constitute a broad spectrum of benign and malignant lesions that can lead to loss of vision and loss of life. Effective management of these lesions depends on accurate diagnosis. In most cases, experienced ophthalmologists diagnose intraocular neoplasms by clinical examination and ancillary diagnostic tests. In the past 2 decades, significant advances have been made in the management of intraocular tumors and in understanding their biology.

Important information concerning the most common primary intraocular malignant tumor in adults, choroidal melanoma, was gathered in the Collaborative Ocular Melanoma Study (COMS). The COMS incorporated both randomized clinical trials for patients with medium and large choroidal melanomas and an observational study for patients with small choroidal melanomas. The COMS reported outcomes for enucleation versus brachytherapy for the treatment of medium tumors and for enucleation alone versus pre-enucleation external-beam radiotherapy for large melanomas. Survival data from the large, medium, and small treatment arms of the COMS are available. In addition to the study's primary objectives, the COMS has provided data regarding local tumor failure rates after iodine 125 brachytherapy as well as visual acuity outcomes following this globe-conserving treatment. These findings have shifted the primary treatment of choroidal melanoma from enucleation toward globe-conserving brachytherapy (see Chapter 17).

In recent years, there have been several other advances in the management of choroidal melanoma. Researchers have identified key cytogenetic aberrations, specifically monosomy 3 and isochromosome 8p, in choroidal melanoma that lead to metastatic disease. Fine-needle aspiration biopsy (FNAB, discussed in greater detail in Chapter 4) at the time of treatment can now confirm the diagnosis and yield important prognostic information for the patient. FNAB can also be used to confirm the presence of a choroidal metastasis.

Retinoblastoma is the most common primary intraocular malignant tumor in children. The predisposing gene for retinoblastoma has been isolated, cloned, and sequenced. As with the treatment of choroidal melanoma, treatment of retinoblastoma is undergoing a transition toward globe-conserving therapy, with a renewed interest in combined-modality therapy focused particularly on systemic chemotherapy coupled with focal therapy. The trend away from primary external-beam radiotherapy and toward chemotherapy has been fueled by our growing understanding of the former's potential risk for increasing the incidence of secondary malignancies in children who have a germline mutation of the retinoblastoma gene. Advances in our understanding of the molecular genetics of retinoblastoma continue to enhance our ability to screen for and treat this pediatric ocular malignancy (see Chapter 19).

CHAPTER 17

Melanocytic Tumors

Introduction

Intraocular melanocytic tumors arise from the uveal melanocytes in the iris, ciliary body, and choroid. In contrast to melanocytic tumors of the skin and mucosal membranes, which develop in ectodermal tissue and usually spread through the lymphatics, uveal melanocytic tumors arise in mesodermal tissue and typically disseminate hematogenously, if there is metastatic spread.

There are 2 groups of melanocytic tumors of the uvea: the benign nevi and the melanomas. Pigmented intraocular tumors that originate in the pigmented epithelium of the iris, ciliary body, and retina constitute another group of melanocytic tumors. These rare tumors are discussed separately at the end of this chapter. See also Chapter 12.

Iris Nevus

An iris nevus generally appears as a darkly pigmented lesion of the iris stroma with minimal distortion of the iris architecture (Fig 17-1). The true prevalence of iris nevi remains

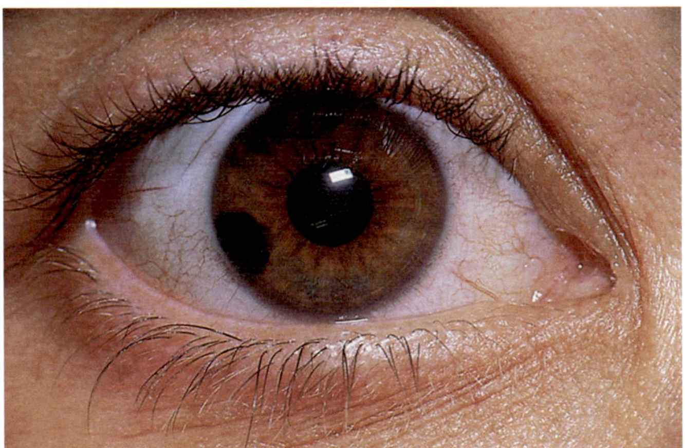

Figure 17-1 Iris nevus, clinical appearance. The lesion is only slightly raised from the iris surface, and lesion color is homogeneous brown.

uncertain because many of these lesions produce no symptoms and are recognized incidentally during routine ophthalmic examination. Iris nevi may present in 2 forms:

- *circumscribed iris nevus:* typically nodular, involving a discrete portion of the iris
- *diffuse iris nevus:* may involve an entire sector or, rarely, the entire iris

In some cases, the lesion causes slight ectropion iridis and sectoral cataract. The incidence of iris nevi may be higher in the eyes of patients with neurofibromatosis.

Iris nevi are best evaluated by slit-lamp biomicroscopy coupled with gonioscopic evaluation of the angle structures. Specific attention should be given to lesions involving the angle structures to rule out a previously unrecognized ciliary body tumor. The most important possibility in the differential diagnosis of iris nevi is iris melanoma. When iris melanoma is included within the differential diagnosis, close observation with scheduled serial follow-up examinations is indicated. Clinical evaluation of suspicious iris nevi should include slit-lamp photography and high-frequency ultrasound biomicroscopy. Iris nevi usually require no treatment once they are diagnosed, but, when suspected, they should be followed closely and photographed to evaluate for growth.

Nevus of the Ciliary Body or Choroid

Nevi of the ciliary body are occasionally incidental findings in histopathologic examination of globes that are enucleated for other reasons. Choroidal nevi may occur in up to 10% of the population. In most cases, they have no clinical symptoms and are recognized on routine ophthalmic examination. The typical choroidal nevus appears ophthalmoscopically as a flat or minimally elevated, pigmented (gray-brown) choroidal lesion with indistinct margins (Fig 17-2). Some nevi are amelanotic and may be less apparent. Choroidal nevi may be associated with overlying RPE disturbance, drusen, serous detachment, choroidal neovascular membranes, and orange pigment; and they may produce visual field defects. On fluorescein angiography, choroidal nevi may either hypofluoresce or hyperfluoresce, depending on the associated findings. Ocular and oculodermal melanocytosis may predispose to uveal malignancy, with an estimated lifetime risk of 1 in 400 in the white population. Choroidal nevi are distinguished from choroidal melanomas by clinical evaluation and ancillary testing. No single clinical factor is pathognomonic for benign versus malignant choroidal melanocytic lesions. The differential diagnosis for pigmented lesions in the ocular fundus most commonly includes the following:

- choroidal nevus
- choroidal melanoma
- atypical disciform scar associated with age-related macular degeneration (AMD)
- suprachoroidal hemorrhage
- RPE hyperplasia
- congenital hypertrophy of the retinal pigment epithelium (CHRPE)
- choroidal hemangioma with RPE hyperpigmentation
- melanocytoma
- metastatic carcinoma with RPE hyperpigmentation
- choroidal osteoma

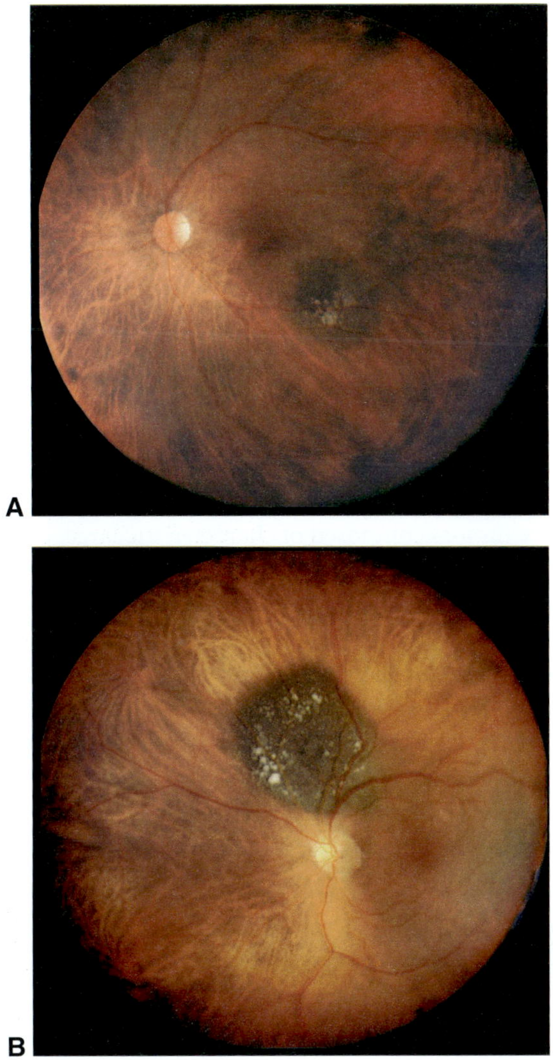

Figure 17-2 Choroidal nevi, clinical appearance. **A,** Choroidal nevus with overlying drusen, under the lower temporal retinovascular arcade. **B,** Medium-sized choroidal nevus with overlying drusen, superior to the optic nerve head. *(Courtesy of Jacob Pe'er, MD.)*

Virtually all choroidal melanocytic tumors thicker than 3 mm are melanomas, and virtually all choroidal melanocytic lesions thinner than 1 mm are nevi. Many lesions 1–2 mm in thickness (apical height) may be benign, although the risk of malignancy increases with height. It is difficult to classify with certainty tumors that are 1–2 mm in thickness. Flat lesions with a basal diameter of 10 mm or less are almost always benign. The risk of malignancy increases for lesions that are larger than 6 mm in basal diameter.

Clinical risk factors for enlargement of choroidal melanocytic lesions have been well characterized and include

- subjective clinical symptoms such as metamorphopsia, photopsia, visual field loss
- presence of orange pigmentation

- associated subretinal fluid
- larger size at presentation
- juxtapapillary location
- absence of drusen or RPE changes
- hot spots on fluorescein photography
- homogeneous, low internal reflectivity on ultrasonography

If definite enlargement is documented, malignant change should be suspected.

The recommended management of choroidal nevi is photographic documentation for lesions less than 1 mm in thickness and photographic and ultrasonographic documentation for lesions greater than 1 mm in thickness, coupled with regular, periodic reassessment for signs of growth.

Melanocytoma of the Iris, Ciliary Body, or Choroid

Melanocytomas are rare tumors composed of characteristic large, polyhedral-shaped cells with small nuclei and cytoplasm filled with melanin granules (see Chapter 15, Fig 15-12). Cells from iris melanocytomas may seed to the anterior chamber angle, causing glaucoma. Melanocytomas of the ciliary body are usually not seen clinically because of their peripheral location. In some cases, extrascleral extension of the tumor along an emissary canal appears as a darkly pigmented, fixed subconjunctival mass. Melanocytomas of the choroid appear as elevated, pigmented tumors, simulating a nevus or melanoma. Melanocytomas have been reported to undergo malignant change in some instances. When a melanocytoma is suspected, photographic and echographic studies are appropriate. If growth is documented, the lesion should be treated as a malignancy.

Shields CL, Furuta M, Berman EL, et al. Choroidal nevus transformation into melanoma: analysis of 2514 consecutive cases. *Arch Ophthalmol.* 2009;127(8):981–987.

Shields JA, Shields CL, Eagle RC Jr. Melanocytoma (hyperpigmented magnocellular nevus) of the uveal tract: the 34th G. Victor Simpson lecture. *Retina.* 2007;27(6):730–739.

Iris Melanoma

Iris melanomas account for 3%–10% of all uveal melanomas. Small melanomas of the iris may be impossible to differentiate clinically from benign iris nevi and other simulating lesions. The following conditions may be included in a differential diagnosis of iris melanoma:

- iris nevus
- primary iris cyst (pigment epithelial and stromal)
- iridocorneal endothelial syndrome
- iris foreign body
- peripheral anterior synechiae
- metastatic carcinoma to the iris

- aphakic iris cyst
- iris atrophy, miscellaneous
- pigment epithelial hyperplasia or migration
- juvenile xanthogranuloma
- retained lens material simulating iris nodule

Signs suggesting malignancy include extensive ectropion iridis, prominent vascularity, sectoral cataract, secondary glaucoma, seeding of the peripheral angle structures, extrascleral extension, lesion size, and documented progressive growth. Iris melanomas range in appearance from amelanotic to dark brown lesions, and three-quarters of them involve the inferior iris (Fig 17-3). In rare instances, they assume a diffuse growth pattern, producing a syndrome of unilateral acquired hyperchromic heterochromia and secondary glaucoma. Clinical evaluation is identical to that for iris nevi. The differential diagnosis of iris nodules is listed in Table 17-1; Figure 17-4 illustrates the various iris nodules. See also Figure 12-11 in Chapter 12.

Advances in high-frequency ultrasonography allow for excellent characterization of tumor size and anatomical relationship to normal ocular structures (Fig 17-5). Fluorescein

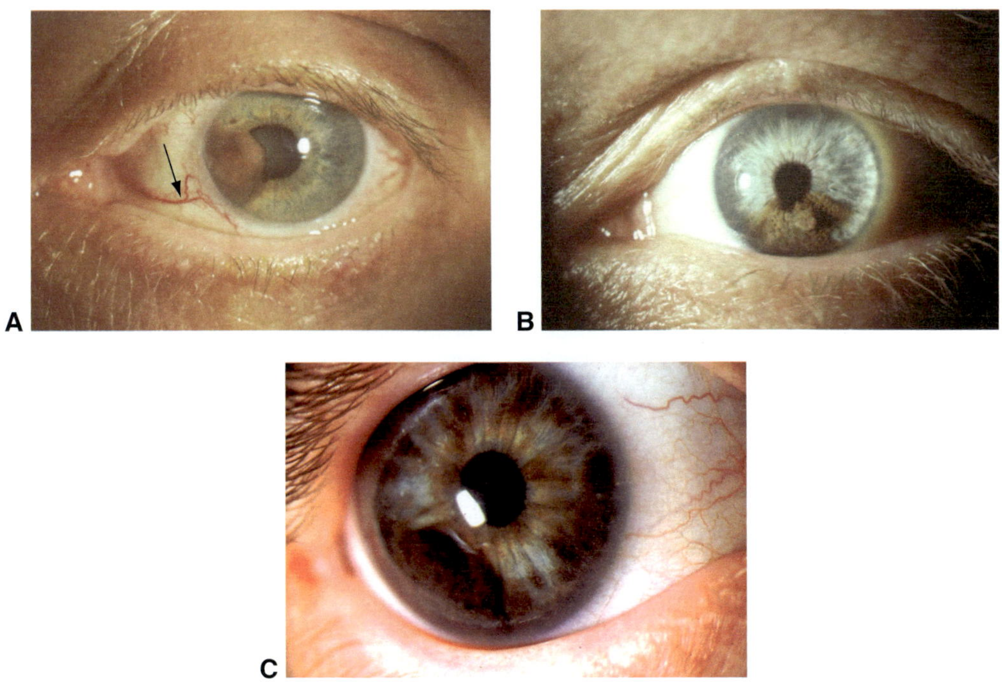

Figure 17-3 Iris melanoma, clinical appearance. **A,** Mildly pigmented iris melanoma on the nasal side, involving also the anterior chamber angle. A sentinel vessel *(arrow)* is present. **B,** Melanoma in the lower part of the iris. **C,** Melanoma in the lower temporal area, spreading to other parts of the iris. *(Courtesy of Jacob Pe'er, MD.)*

Table 17-1 Differential Diagnostic Features of Iris Nodules (alphabetical list)

Lesion	Features
Brushfield spots (Down syndrome) (Fig 17-4A)	Elevated white to light yellow spots in periphery of iris,10–20 per eye. Prevalence in Down syndrome is 85%; otherwise, ≈25%. Histologically, the spots are areas of relatively normal iris stroma surrounded by a ring of mild iris hypoplasia. Anterior border layer slightly increased in density.
Epithelial invasion, serous cyst, solid or pearl cyst, implantation membrane	Each follows surgery or injury. Appears as serous or solid cysts in continuity with the wound or as implantation cysts or membranes on the anterior iris surface.
Foreign body, retained	Usually becomes secondarily pigmented and may be associated with chronic iridocyclitis and peripheral anterior synechiae.
Fungal endophthalmitis	Irregular yellow-white mass on iris. May be accompanied by hypopyon or only mild inflammatory signs.
Iridocyclitis	The iris nodules of classic granulomatous anterior uveitis occur either superficially or deeply within the iris. Koeppe nodules occur at the pupillary border, and Busacca nodules lie on the anterior iris surface. Microscopically, they are composed of large and small mononuclear cells.
Iris freckle (Fig 17-4B)	Stationary, lightly to darkly pigmented flat areas on anterior iris surface composed of anterior border layer melanocytes containing increased pigmentation without increased number of melanocytes.
Iris nevus (see Fig 17-1)	Discrete mass(es) or nodule(s) on anterior iris surface and in the iris stroma. Variable pigmentation. Composed of benign nevus cells. Increased incidence of iris nevi in patients with neurofibromatosis.
Iris nevus syndrome (Cogan-Reese)	Acquired diffuse nevus of iris associated with unilateral glaucoma, heterochromia, peripheral anterior synechiae, and extension of endothelium and Descemet membrane over trabecular meshwork. Obliteration of normal iris architecture. (See ICE syndrome, Chapter 7.)
Iris pigment epithelial cysts (Fig 17-4C)	Cysts encompassing both layers of neuroepithelium. Produce a localized elevation of stroma and may be pigmented. May transilluminate. May be better seen after dilation. B-scan ultrasonography of value in diagnosis.
Iris pigment epithelial proliferation	Congenital or acquired (trauma or surgery) plaques of pigment epithelium displaying a black, velvety appearance.
Juvenile xanthogranuloma	Yellowish to gray, poorly demarcated iris lesions associated with raised orange skin lesion(s) (single or multiple) appearing in the first year of life. May be associated with spontaneous hyphema and secondary glaucoma. Histologically, there is a diffuse granulomatous infiltrate with lipid-containing histiocytes and Touton giant cells. The lesions regress spontaneously. May also be found in ciliary body, anterior choroid, episclera, cornea, eyelids, and orbit.
Leiomyoma	May be well localized and even pedunculated, often diffuse and flat, and usually lightly pigmented. Electron microscopy may be helpful in differentiating leiomyoma from amelanotic spindle cell melanoma.

Table 17-1 *(continued)*

Lesion	Features
Leukemia (Fig 17-4D)	Very rare nodular or diffuse milky lesions with intense hyperemia. Often, the iris loses its architecture, becomes thickened, and develops heterochromia. Pseudohypopyon is common.
Lisch nodules (neurofibromatosis) (Fig 17-4E)	One of the diagnostic criteria for neurofibromatosis. Multiple lesions varying from tan to dark brown and about the size of a pinhead. May be flat or project from the surface. Histologically, they are composed of collections of nevus cells.
Melanocytosis, congenital ocular and oculodermal	Generally unilateral with diffuse uveal nevus causing heterochromia iridis associated with blue or slate gray patches of sclera and episclera. In oculodermal melanocytosis, eyelid and brow are also involved. Malignant potential exists.
Melanoma (see Fig 17-3)	Occurs as nodular or flat growths, usually in the periphery, especially inferiorly or inferotemporally. Variably pigmented, often with satellite pigmentation and pigmentation in the anterior chamber angle and nutrient vessels. Pupil may dilate irregularly, and elevated IOP may be present.
Metastatic carcinoma	Gelatinous to white vascularized nodules on the iris surface and in the anterior chamber angle. May be associated with anterior uveitis, hyphema, rubeosis, and glaucoma.
Retinoblastoma	White foci on the anterior iris surface or in the anterior chamber angle, or a pseudohypopyon.
Tapioca melanoma	Tapioca-like nodules lying over a portion or all of the iris. May be translucent to lightly pigmented. Often associated with unilateral glaucoma.

angiography may document intrinsic vascularity, although this finding is of limited value in establishing a differential diagnosis. In rare instances, biopsy may be considered when the management of the lesion is in question. In most cases, when growth or severe glaucoma occurs, diagnostic and therapeutic excisional treatment is indicated. Brachytherapy using custom-designed plaques may be used in selected cases. Specifically designed proton-beam radiotherapy has also been reported for iris melanoma. The prognosis for most patients with iris melanoma is excellent, with a lower mortality rate (1%–4%) than that for ciliary body and choroidal melanomas, possibly because the biological behavior of most of these iris tumors appears distinctly different from that of ciliary body or choroidal melanoma. Anterior chamber angle invasion increases the risk of metastasis.

Henderson E, Margo CE. Iris melanoma. *Arch Pathol Lab Med.* 2008;132(2):268–272.

Jakobiec FA, Silbert G. Are most iris "melanomas" really nevi? A clinicopathologic study of 189 lesions. *Arch Ophthalmol.* 1981;99(12):2117–2132.

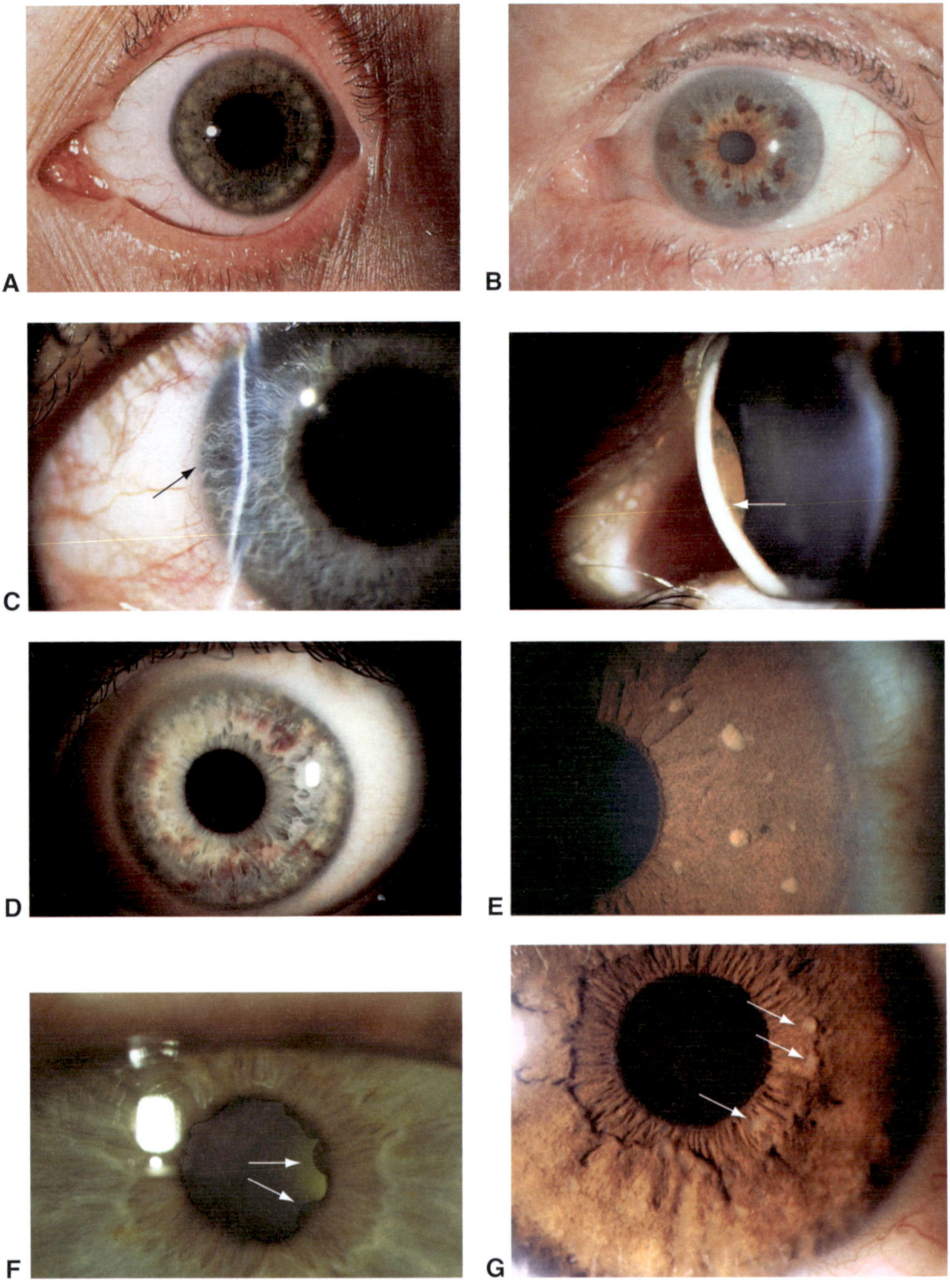

Figure 17-4 Iris nodules. **A,** Brushfield spots in Down syndrome. **B,** Iris freckles. **C,** Pigment epithelial cyst. Before dilation *(left),* the iris stroma is bowed forward *(arrow)* in the area of the cyst, which is invisible posteriorly. After dilation *(right),* the cyst of the posterior iris epithelium can be seen *(arrow)* with eye adduction. **D,** Leukemic infiltration of the iris. Note color variation, prominent vascularity, and stromal thickening. **E,** Multiple Lisch nodules in neurofibromatosis. **F,** Koeppe nodules at pupil margin *(arrows)* in sarcoidosis. **G,** Busacca nodules in mid-iris *(arrows)* in sarcoidosis. *(Part A courtesy of W.R. Green, MD; parts B and E courtesy of Timothy G. Murray, MD; parts F and G courtesy of R. Christopher Walton, MD.)*

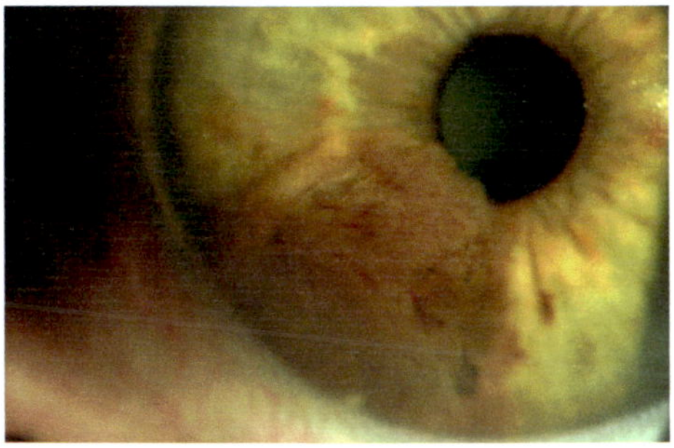

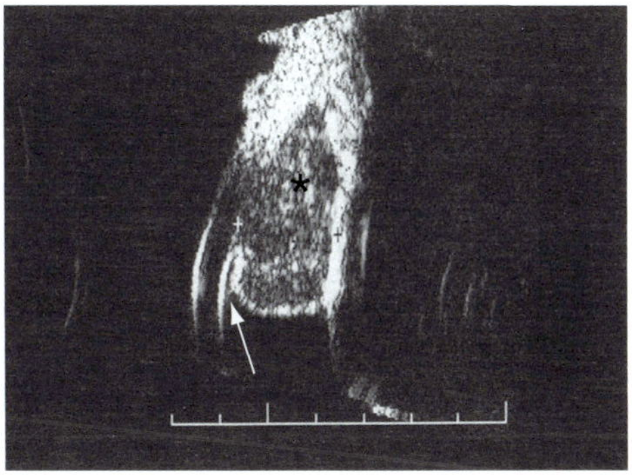

Figure 17-5 **A,** Iris melanoma, clinical appearance. **B,** This high-frequency ultrasonogram shows a melanoma mass *(asterisk)* occupying the iris stroma and anterior chamber angle and abutting the posterior corneal surface *(arrow)*. *(Part A courtesy of Matthew W. Wilson, MD; part B courtesy of Jacob Pe'er, MD.)*

Melanoma of the Ciliary Body or Choroid

Ciliary body and choroidal melanomas are the most common primary intraocular malignancies in adults. The incidence in the United States is approximately 6–7 cases per million. The tumor, extremely rare in children, primarily affects patients in their 50s and early 60s; it has a predilection for lightly pigmented individuals. Risk factors have not been conclusively identified but may include

- light-colored complexion (white skin, blue eyes, blond hair)
- ocular melanocytic conditions such as ocular and oculodermal melanocytosis
- genetic predisposition (dysplastic nevus syndrome; *BAP1* mutation)

Ciliary body melanomas can be asymptomatic in the early stages. Because of their location behind the iris, ciliary body melanomas may be rather large by the time they are detected. Patients who have symptoms most commonly note vision loss, photopsias, or visual field alterations. Ciliary body melanomas are not usually visible unless the pupil is widely dilated (Fig 17-6A). Some erode through the iris root into the anterior chamber and eventually become visible on external examination or with gonioscopy. In rare cases, tumors extend directly through the sclera in the ciliary region, producing a dark epibulbar mass. The initial sign of a ciliary body melanoma may be dilated episcleral sentinel vessels in the quadrant of the tumor (Fig 17-6B). The tumor may eventually become quite large, producing a sectoral or diffuse cataract, subluxated lens (Fig 17-6C), secondary glaucoma, retinal detachment, and even iris neovascularization. In rare instances, a ciliary body melanoma assumes a diffuse growth pattern that extends 180°–360° around the ciliary body. This type of melanoma is called a *ring melanoma* (see Chapter 12, Fig 12-18).

The typical *choroidal melanoma* is a pigmented, elevated, dome-shaped subretinal mass (Fig 17-7A, B). The degree of pigmentation ranges from totally amelanotic to dark brown. With time, many tumors erupt through the Bruch membrane to assume a mushroom-like shape (Fig 17-7C, D). Prominent clumps of orange pigment at the RPE level may appear over the surface of the tumor, and serous detachment of the neurosensory retina is common. If an extensive retinal detachment develops, anterior displacement

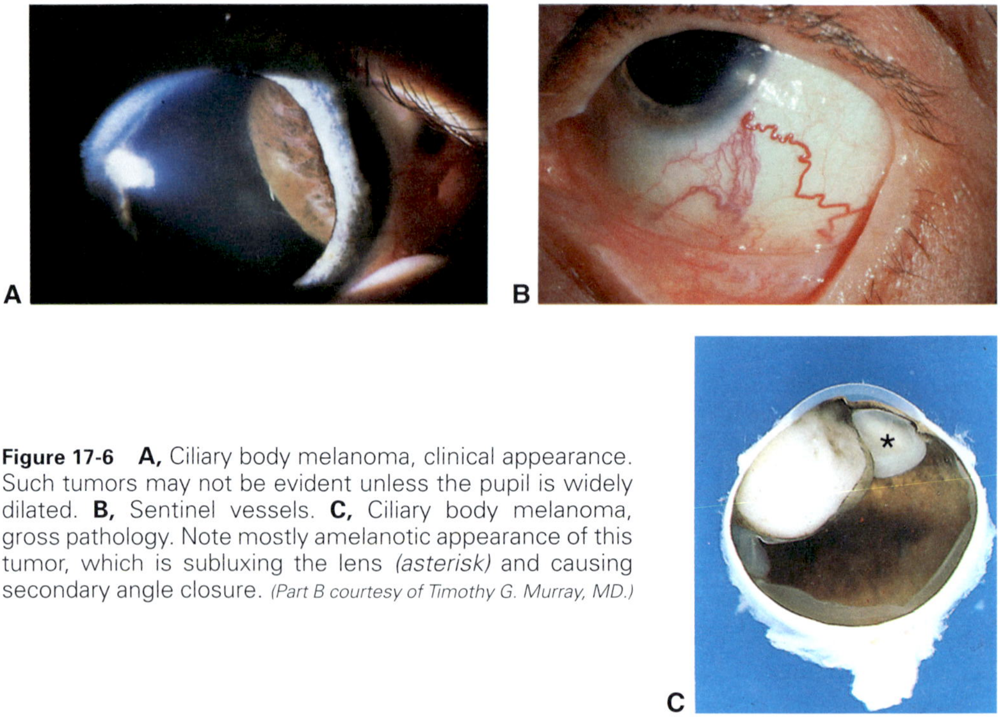

Figure 17-6 **A,** Ciliary body melanoma, clinical appearance. Such tumors may not be evident unless the pupil is widely dilated. **B,** Sentinel vessels. **C,** Ciliary body melanoma, gross pathology. Note mostly amelanotic appearance of this tumor, which is subluxing the lens *(asterisk)* and causing secondary angle closure. *(Part B courtesy of Timothy G. Murray, MD.)*

of the lens–iris diaphragm and secondary angle-closure glaucoma occasionally occur. Neovascularization of the iris may also appear in such eyes, and there may be spontaneous hemorrhage into the subretinal space. Vitreous hemorrhage is usually seen only in cases when the melanoma has erupted through the Bruch membrane and the retina.

Diagnostic Evaluation

Clinical evaluation of all suspected posterior uveal melanomas of the ciliary body and the choroid should include a history, ophthalmoscopic evaluation, and ancillary testing to definitively establish the diagnosis. When used appropriately, the tests described here enable accurate diagnosis of melanocytic tumors in almost all cases. Atypical lesions may be characterized by several other testing modalities, such as fine-needle aspiration biopsy; or, when appropriate, lesions may be observed for characteristic changes in clinical behavior that will establish a correct diagnosis.

Indirect ophthalmoscopic viewing of the tumor remains the gold standard. It is the single most important diagnostic technique for evaluating patients with intraocular tumors, as it provides stereopsis and a wide field of view and facilitates visualization of the peripheral fundus, particularly when performed with scleral depression. Indirect ophthalmoscopy allows for clinical assessment of tumor basal dimension and apical height. However, it is not useful in eyes with opaque media, which require other diagnostic methods, such as ultrasonography, computed tomography (CT), and/or magnetic resonance imaging (MRI).

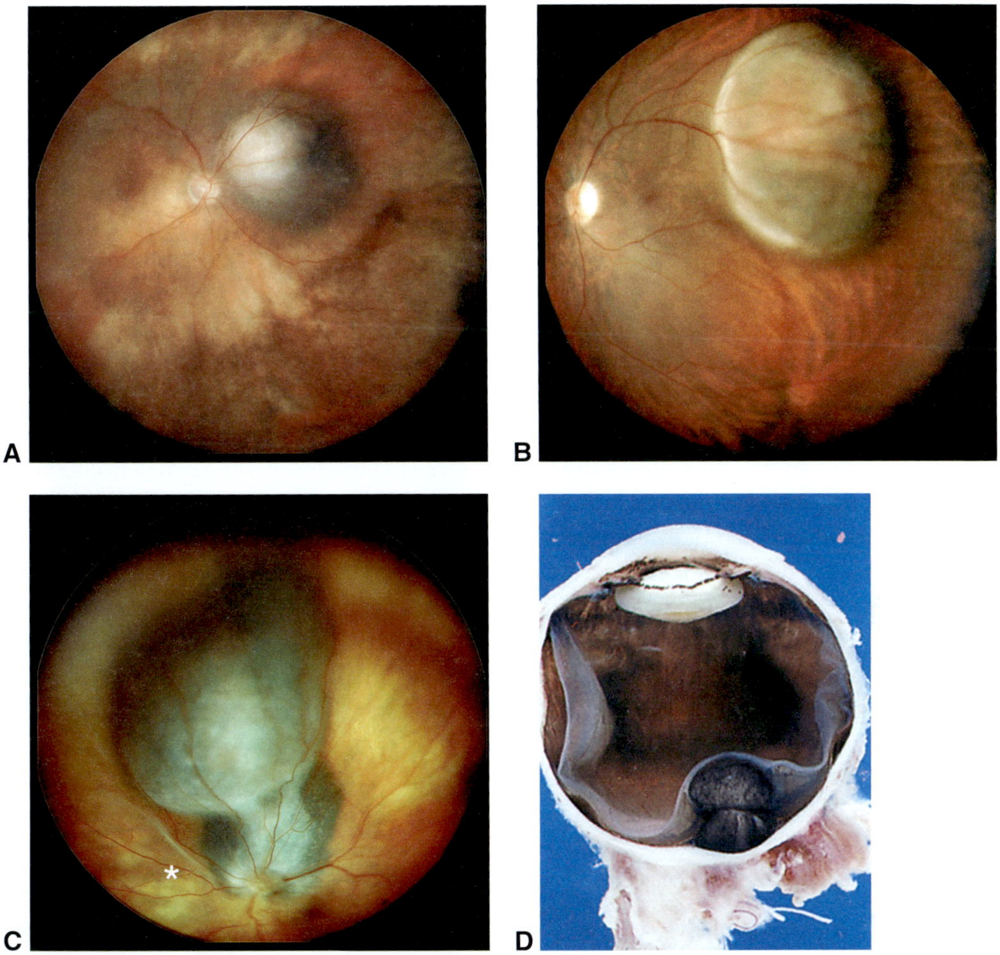

Figure 17-7 Choroidal melanoma. **A,** Small choroidal melanoma touching the nasal border of the optic nerve head. **B,** Medium-sized choroidal melanoma temporal to the macula. **C,** A large choroidal melanoma surrounding the optic nerve head and extending upward to the ora serrata. Note the retinal detachment in the lower half of the retina *(asterisk).* **D,** Gross pathology. Note the mushroom-shaped cross section of this darkly pigmented tumor and the associated retinal detachment. *(Parts A–C courtesy of Jacob Pe'er, MD.)*

Slit-lamp biomicroscopy used in combination with *gonioscopy* offers the best method for establishing the presence and extent of anterior involvement of ciliary body tumors. The use of high-frequency ultrasound biomicroscopy enables excellent visualization of anterior ocular structures and is a significant adjunct to slit-lamp photography for the evaluation and documentation of anterior segment pathology.

In addition, the presence of sectoral cataract, secondary angle involvement, or sentinel vessel formation may be a clue to the diagnosis of ciliary body tumor. Hruby, Goldmann, and other wide-field fundus lenses can be used with the slit lamp to evaluate lesions of the posterior fundus under high magnification. High-magnification fundus evaluation can delineate neurosensory retinal detachment, orange pigmentation, rupture of Bruch membrane, intraretinal tumor invasion, and vitreous involvement. Fundus biomicroscopy with the 3-mirror contact lens is useful in assessing lesions of the peripheral fundus.

Ultrasonography is the most important ancillary tool for evaluating ciliary body and choroidal melanomas (Fig 17-8). It also remains the ancillary test of choice for detection of orbital extension associated with intraocular malignancy. Standardized A-scan ultrasonography provides an accurate assessment of the internal reflectivity and vascularity of a lesion, as well as a measurement of its thickness. Serial examination with A-scan ultrasonography can be used to document growth or regression of an intraocular tumor.

A-scan ultrasonography usually demonstrates a solid tumor pattern with high-amplitude initial echoes and low-amplitude internal reflections (low internal reflectivity). Spontaneous vascular pulsations can also be demonstrated in most cases. B-scan examination provides information about the relative size (height and basal diameters), general shape, and position of intraocular tumors. Occasionally, cross-sectional tumor shape and associated retinal detachment can be detected more easily by ultrasonography than by ophthalmoscopy. B-scan ultrasonography usually shows a dome- or mushroom-shaped choroidal mass with a highly reflective anterior border, acoustic hollowness, choroidal excavation, and occasional orbital shadowing. B-scan ultrasonography can be used to detect intraocular tumors in eyes with either clear or opaque media.

Ultrasonography for ciliary body melanomas is more difficult to interpret because the peripheral location of these tumors makes the test technically more demanding to perform. High-frequency ultrasonography is not limited by the technical difficulties associated with standard B-scan testing and enables excellent imaging of the anterior segment and ciliary body.

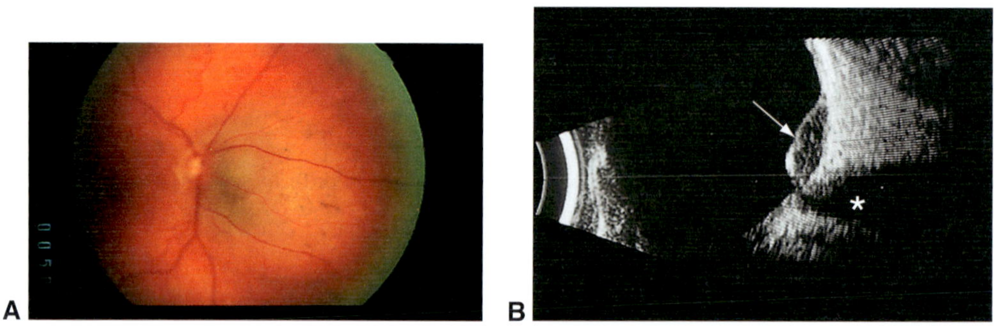

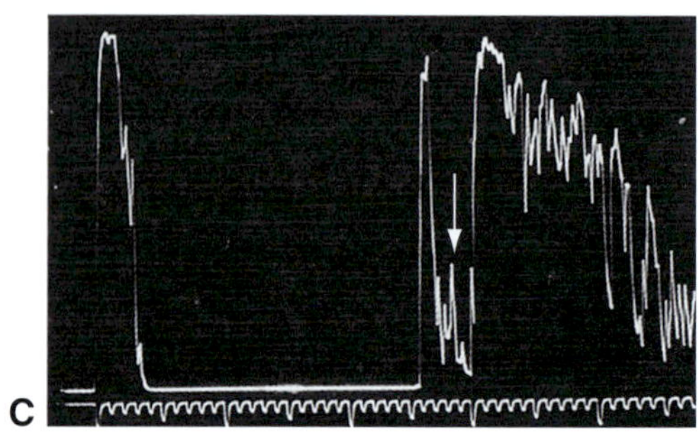

Figure 17-8 **A,** Peripapillary choroidal melanoma. **B,** The peripapillary tumor *(arrow)* is seen nasal to the optic nerve *(asterisk)*. B-scan ultrasonography is used primarily to show the tumor location and its topography. **C,** The A-scan ultrasonogram shows characteristic low internal reflectivity *(arrow)*.

Although ultrasonography is generally considered highly reliable in the differential diagnosis of posterior uveal melanoma, it may be difficult or impossible to differentiate a necrotic melanoma from a small subretinal hematoma or a metastatic carcinoma. Advances in 3-dimensional ultrasound imaging may allow for better evaluation of tumor volume, and advances in high-resolution imaging may be able to determine tumor microvasculature patterns predictive of tumor biology (see Chapter 12).

Transillumination may be helpful in evaluating suspected ciliary body or anterior choroidal melanomas. It is valuable in assessing the degree of pigmentation within a lesion and in determining basal diameters of anterior tumors. The shadow of a tumor is visible with a transilluminating light source, preferably a high-intensity fiber-optic device, placed either on the surface of the topically anesthetized eye in a quadrant opposite the lesion or directly on the cornea with a smooth, dark, specially designed corneal cap (Fig 17-9). Fiber-optic transillumination is used during surgery for radioactive applicator insertion to locate the uveal melanoma and delineate its borders.

Fundus photography is valuable for documenting the ophthalmoscopic appearance of choroidal melanoma and for identifying interval changes in the basal size of a lesion in follow-up examinations. Wide-angle fundus photographs (60°–180°) of intraocular tumors can reveal the full extent of most lesions and can document the relationship between lesions and other intraocular structures. The relative positions of retinal blood vessels can be helpful markers of changes in the size of a lesion. Wide-angle fundus cameras enable accurate measurement of the basal diameter of a choroidal melanoma as well as changes in its size, using intrinsic scales. No patterns of *fluorescein angiography* are pathognomonic for choroidal melanoma.

Although *CT* and *MRI* are not widely used in the assessment of uncomplicated intraocular melanocytic tumors, these modalities are useful in identifying tumors in eyes with opaque media and in determining extrascleral extension and involvement of other organs. MRI may be helpful in differentiating atypical vascular lesions from melanocytic tumors.

Differential Diagnosis

The most common lesions that should be considered in the differential diagnosis of posterior uveal melanoma include suspicious choroidal nevi, disciform macular and extramacular lesions, congenital hypertrophy of the RPE (CHRPE), choroidal hemangioma (see Chapter 18), melanocytoma, hemorrhagic detachment of the choroid or RPE, metastatic

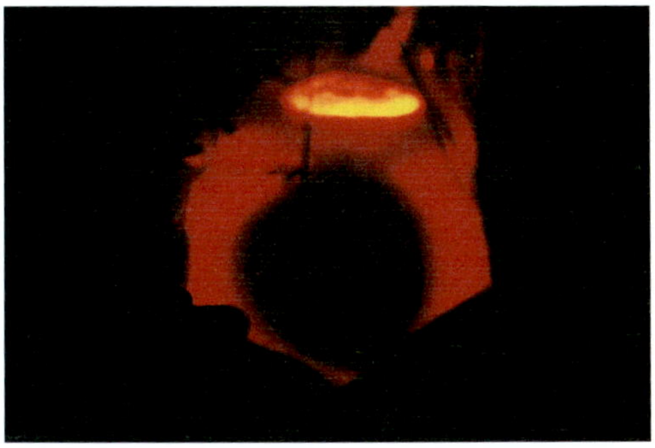

Figure 17-9 Transillumination (TI) of the eye shows the shadow of a choroidal melanoma (decreased TI through the tumor). This technique may be used to mark the tumor base to ensure accurate placement of the radioactive plaque.

Table 17-2 Differential Diagnosis of Amelanotic Choroidal Mass

Amelanotic melanoma
Choroidal metastasis
Choroidal hemangioma
Choroidal osteoma
Sclerochoroidal calcification
Age-related macular or extramacular degeneration
Choroidal detachment
Posterior scleritis
Chorioretinal granuloma
Neurilemoma
Leiomyoma

Modified from Shields JA, Shields CL. Differential diagnosis of posterior uveal melanoma. In: Shields JA, Shields CL. *Intraocular Tumors: A Text and Atlas.* Philadelphia: Saunders; 1992:137–153.

carcinoma (see Chapter 20) or melanoma, and choroidal osteoma. Table 17-2 offers a more complete list to be considered in cases with *amelanotic* choroidal masses.

Choroidal nevus has been discussed previously, but it should be reemphasized that no single clinical characteristic is pathognomonic of choroidal melanoma. Diagnostic accuracy is associated with clinical experience and outstanding ancillary testing facilities. Evaluation and management of these complex cases within regional ocular oncology referral centers appears to enhance patient outcome.

Age-related macular degeneration (AMD) may present with extramacular or macular subretinal neovascularization and fibrosis accompanied by varying degrees and patterns of pigmentation. Hemorrhage, a common finding associated with disciform lesions, is not commonly seen with melanomas unless the tumor extends through the Bruch membrane. Clinical evaluation of the fellow eye is important in documenting the presence of degenerative changes in AMD. Fluorescein angiography results are virtually pathognomonic, revealing early hypofluorescence secondary to blockage from the hemorrhage, often followed by late hyperfluorescence in the distribution of the choroidal neovascular membrane. Ultrasonographic testing may reveal increased heterogeneity and a lack of intrinsic vascularity on standardized A-scan. Serial observation will document involutional alterations of the evolving disciform lesion.

CHRPE is a well-defined, flat, darkly pigmented lesion ranging in size from 1 mm to greater than 10 mm in diameter. Patients are asymptomatic, and the lesion is noted during ophthalmic examination, typically in patients in their teens or twenties. In younger patients, CHRPE often appears homogeneously black; in older individuals, foci of depigmentation (lacunae) often develop (Fig 17-10). The histology is identical to a condition known as *grouped pigmentation of the retina,* or *bear tracks* (Fig 17-11).

The presence of multiple patches of congenital hypertrophy in family members of patients who have Gardner syndrome, a familial polyposis, appears to be a marker for the development of colon carcinoma. Fundus findings enable the ophthalmologist to help the gastroenterologist determine the recommended frequency of colon carcinoma screening in family members (see Chapter 11).

Melanocytoma (magnocellular nevus) of the optic disc typically appears as a dark brown to black epipapillary lesion, often with fibrillar margins as a result of extension into

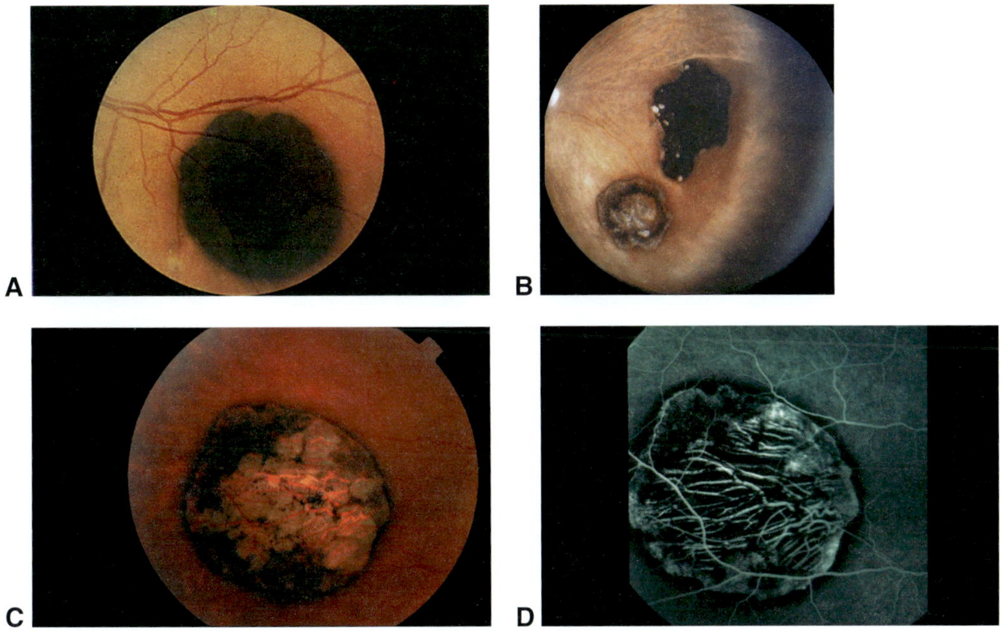

Figure 17-10 Congenital hypertrophy of the RPE (CHRPE). Examples of varying clinical appearances. **A,** CHRPE. Note the homogeneous black color and well-defined margins of the nummular lesion. **B,** Two lesions of CHRPE in the nasal periphery of the fundus. **C, D,** Color fundus photograph and corresponding fluorescein angiogram of a large CHRPE. Note focal loss of RPE architecture and pigmentation (lacunae) in part C and visible choroidal vasculature in part D. *(Part B courtesy of Jacob Pe'er, MD; parts C and D courtesy of Timothy G. Murray, MD.)*

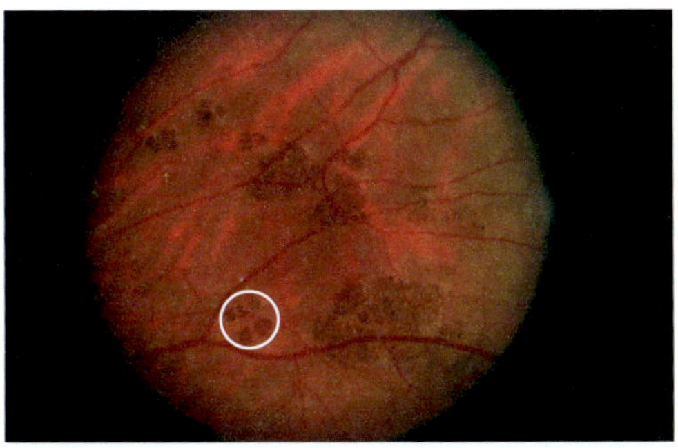

Figure 17-11 Bear tracks. Grouped pigmentation of the retina/RPE represents a forme fruste of CHRPE. Note the distinct bear track configuration *(circle)* and increased pigmentation.

the nerve fiber layer (Fig 17-12; see also Chapter 15, Fig 15-12). It is usually located eccentrically over the optic disc and may be elevated. It is important to differentiate this lesion from melanoma, because a melanocytoma has minimal malignant potential. Studies have shown that about one-third of optic disc melanocytomas have a peripapillary nevus component and that 10% of cases will show minimal but definite growth over a 5-year period. In addition, these lesions can produce an afferent pupillary defect and a variety of visual field abnormalities, ranging from an enlarged blind spot to extensive nerve fiber layer defects.

Suprachoroidal detachments present in 2 forms: *hemorrhagic* and *serous*. These lesions are often associated with hypotony and may present in the immediate period after

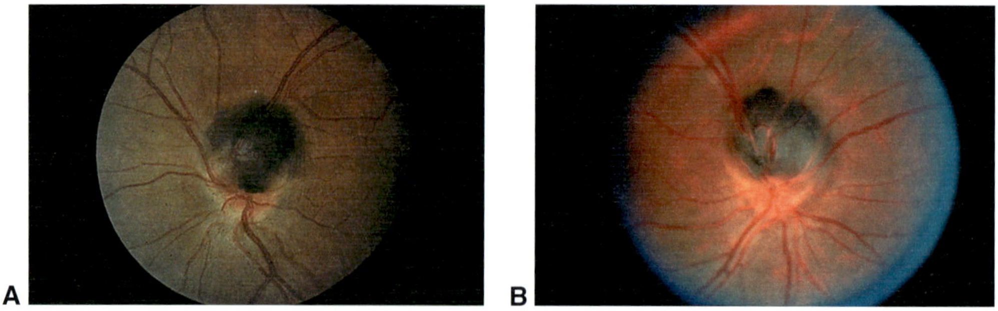

Figure 17-12 Melanocytoma of the optic disc. Note varying clinical appearance in these 2 examples based on degree of choroidal pigmentation: lesion in **(A)** darkly pigmented fundus and **(B)** lightly pigmented fundus. *(Part B courtesy of Timothy G. Murray, MD.)*

ophthalmic surgery. Clinically, hemorrhagic detachments are often dome-shaped, they involve multiple quadrants, and they are associated with breakthrough vitreous bleeding. A- and B-scan ultrasonography readings may closely resemble those of melanoma but show an absence of intrinsic vascularity and an evolution of the hemorrhage over time. Observational management is indicated in most cases. MRI with gadolinium enhancement may be of benefit in selected cases to document characteristic alterations.

Choroidal osteomas are benign bony tumors that typically arise from the juxtapapillary choroid in adolescent to young adult patients (more commonly in women than men) and are bilateral in 20%–25% of cases. The characteristic lesion appears yellow to orange, and it has well-defined margins (Fig 17-13). Ultrasonography reveals a high-amplitude echo corresponding to the plate of bone and loss of the normal orbital echoes behind the lesion. These tumors can also be seen on CT; their hallmark is calcification. Choroidal osteomas typically enlarge slowly over many years. If these lesions involve the macula, vision is generally impaired. Subretinal neovascularization is a common complication of macular choroidal osteomas. The etiology of these lesions is unknown, but chronic low-grade choroidal inflammation has been suspected in some cases (see Chapter 12).

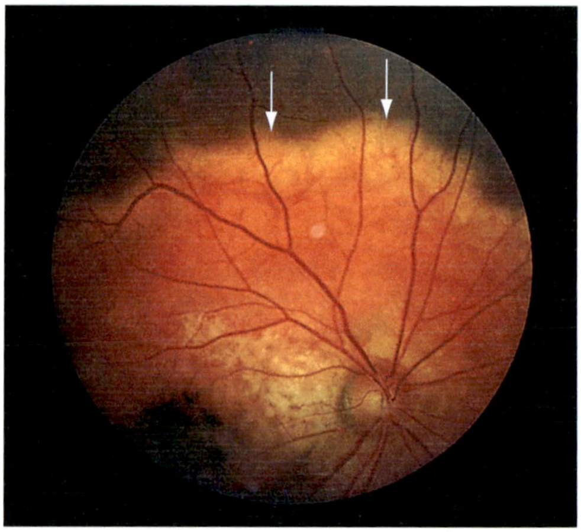

Figure 17-13 Choroidal osteoma, clinical appearance. Note the yellow-orange color, well-defined pseudopod-like margins *(arrows),* and characteristic spotted pigmentation on the surface of this circumpapillary tumor.

Classification

Melanomas of the ciliary body and choroid have been categorized by size in a number of different ways. Although a size classification based on tumor volume is logical, no simple and reliable method for assessing tumor volume is available. The common practice of estimating tumor volume by multiplying maximal basal diameter, minimal basal diameter, and thickness yields a crude assessment of actual tumor size. The Collaborative Ocular Melanoma Study (COMS) classified posterior uveal melanomas as small, medium, or large based on thickness and basal diameter. Recently revised, evidence-based staging developed by the American Joint Committee on Cancer (AJCC) defines small (T1), medium-sized (T2), large (T3), and very large (T4) ciliochoroidal melanomas by tumor height, basal diameter, and extension to the ciliary body and extrasclerally. See the AJCC staging forms in the appendix, pages 337–341.

Metastatic Evaluation

In a study by Kujala and colleagues, the incidence of metastatic uveal melanoma was observed to be as high as 50% at 25 years after treatment for choroidal melanoma. The COMS reported an incidence of metastatic disease of 25% at 5 years after initial treatment and 34% at 10 years. Nevertheless, clinically evident metastatic disease at the time of initial presentation can be detected in less than 2% of patients. Currently, it is hypothesized that many patients have undetectable micrometastatic disease at the time of their primary treatment. Despite the great accuracy that has been achieved in diagnosing uveal melanoma, mortality owing to this tumor has not changed significantly for many years. In general, survival with metastatic uveal melanoma is poor, with a median survival of less than 12 months, although early detection and prompt treatment of liver metastases can increase survival time significantly.

The liver is the predominant organ involved in metastatic uveal melanoma. Liver involvement also tends to be the first manifestation of metastatic disease. In the presence of liver involvement, lung, bone, and skin are other sites that may be affected. An assessment of metastatic disease patterns in the COMS revealed liver involvement in at least 90% of patients, lung involvement in 25%, bone involvement in nearly 20%, and skin and subcutaneous tissue involvement in approximately 10%. In cases that were autopsied, liver involvement was found in 100% and lung involvement in 50% of the patients with metastatic disease.

All patients require metastatic evaluation prior to definitive treatment of the intraocular melanoma (Table 17-3). The purpose of this evaluation is twofold:

1. To determine whether the patient has any other medical conditions that contraindicate surgical treatment or need to be ameliorated before surgery. For example, in one small series, 15% of the patients had a second malignancy at the time of presentation or during the course of a 10-year follow-up; the COMS found preexisting independent primary cancers in approximately 10% of patients. If there is any question whether the lesion in the eye is a metastatic tumor, this possibility must be ruled out with a thorough medical evaluation directed at determining the site of primary malignancy.
2. To rule out the possibility of detectable metastatic melanoma from the eye. Only rarely is metastatic disease from uveal melanoma detectable at the time of initial

Table 17-3 Clinical Evaluation of Metastatic Uveal Melanoma

- Liver imaging—ultrasonography in routine evaluation
- Liver function tests
- Chest x-ray

If any of the above are abnormal:

- Triphasic liver CT
- CT-PET of the abdomen/chest
- MRI of the abdomen/chest

presentation. If metastatic disease is clinically present during the pretreatment evaluation of the eye tumor, enucleation is inappropriate unless the eye is painful.

To detect metastatic disease of uveal melanoma at an early stage, metastatic evaluation should be performed on all patients on a yearly follow-up basis, and some centers will do so every 6 months. Metastatic evaluation should include a comprehensive physical examination. Liver imaging studies are probably the most important component of the metastatic evaluation. Ultrasonography of the abdomen is usually sufficient, but when a suspicion of metastatic disease is raised, triphasic CT, MRI, or PET-CT is usually recommended in order to evaluate the extent of the disease.

Liver function tests are usually performed; however, in recent years, they have become less reliable in the evaluation of liver metastases, because of the common use of cholesterol-lowering statins, which may alter liver enzyme levels. Chest x-ray is also usually performed, although its yield was found to be low. Recently, research has been performed in several centers investigating possible blood markers for early detection of metastatic uveal melanoma.

A liver or other organ site biopsy may be confirmatory of metastatic disease and is appropriate before the institution of any treatment for metastatic disease.

The interval between the diagnosis of primary uveal melanoma and its metastasis depends on various clinical, histopathologic, cytogenetic, and molecular genetic factors. It varies from 1–2 years to over 15–20 years. When metastatic disease is diagnosed early enough, before developing miliary spread, the options for treatment of the metastasis, mainly liver metastasis, include surgical resection; chemotherapy, including intra-arterial hepatic chemotherapy and chemoembolization; and immunotherapy.

Kaiserman I, Amer R, Pe'er J. Liver function tests in metastatic uveal melanoma. *Am J Ophthalmol.* 2004;137(2):236–243.

Treatment

Management of posterior uveal melanomas has long been the subject of considerable controversy. Two factors lie at the heart of this controversy:

1. the limited amount of data on the natural history of untreated patients with posterior uveal melanoma

2. the lack of groups of patients matched for known and for unknown risk factors and managed by different therapeutic techniques to assess the comparative effectiveness of those treatments

In 1882, Fuchs wrote that all intraocular melanomas were treated by enucleation and the only untreated cases were in the "older literature." Currently, both surgical and radiotherapeutic management are used for intraocular melanoma. The COMS has reported randomized, prospectively administered treatment outcomes for patients with medium and large choroidal melanomas. The methods of patient management in use at this time depend on several factors:

- size, location, and extent of the tumor
- visual status of the affected eye and of the fellow eye
- age and general health of the patient

Observation

In certain instances, serial observation without treatment of an intraocular tumor is indicated. Most types of benign retinal and choroidal tumors, such as choroidal nevi, choroidal osteoma, and hyperplasia of the RPE, can be managed with observation. Growth of small melanocytic lesions of the posterior uvea that are 1 mm or less in thickness can be documented periodically by fundus photography and ultrasonography. Significant controversy persists regarding the management of small choroidal melanomas.

Lesions greater than 1 mm in thickness, with documented growth, should be considered for definitive treatment. Observation of active larger tumors may be appropriate in elderly and systemically ill patients who are not candidates for any sort of therapeutic intervention.

Enucleation

Historically, enucleation has been the gold standard in the treatment of malignant intraocular tumors. Although some authors in the past hypothesized that surgical manipulation of eyes containing melanoma leads to tumor dissemination and increased mortality, this hypothesis is no longer accepted, and enucleation remains appropriate for some medium-sized (T2), many large (T3), and most very large (T4) choroidal melanomas. The COMS compared the application of pre-enucleation external-beam radiation therapy followed by enucleation with enucleation alone for patients with large choroidal melanomas and found no statistically significant survival difference in 5-year mortality rates. Enucleation remains one of the most common primary treatments for choroidal melanoma.

Brachytherapy (radioactive plaque)

The application of a radioactive plaque to the sclera overlying an intraocular tumor is probably the most common method of treating uveal melanoma. It allows the delivery of a high dose of radiation to the tumor and a relatively low dose to the surrounding normal structures of the eye. The technique has been available since the 1950s. Although various isotopes have been used (eg, strontium 90, iridium 192, and palladium 103), the most common today are iodine 125 and ruthenium 106. Cobalt 60 plaques, which were the main source for brachytherapy in the past, are rarely used today. In the United States, ^{125}I is the isotope most frequently used in the treatment of ciliary body and choroidal melanomas. Advances in intraoperative localization, especially the use of ultrasound, have increased local tumor control rates to as high as 95%. In most patients, the tumor decreases in size (Fig 17-14); in others, the result is total flattening of the tumor with scar formation or no change in tumor size, although clinical and ultrasound changes can be seen. Regrowth is diagnosed in only about 10% of the treated tumors. Late radiation complications, especially optic neuropathy and retinopathy, are visually limiting in as many as 50% of patients undergoing treatment. Radiation complications appear dose-dependent, and they increase for tumors involving, or adjacent to, the macula or optic nerve.

Charged-particle radiation

High-linear-energy transfer radiation with charged particles (protons and helium ions) has been used effectively in managing ciliary body and choroidal melanomas. The technique requires surgical attachment of tantalum clips to the sclera to mark the basal margins of the tumor prior to the first radiation fraction. The charged-particle beams deliver a more homogeneous dose of radiation energy to a tumor than does a radioactive plaque, and the lateral spread of radiation energy from such beams is less extensive (Bragg peak effect). Local tumor control rates of up to 98% have been reported. The response is similar to that seen after brachytherapy.

Unfortunately, charged-particle radiation often delivers a higher dose to anterior segment structures. Radiation complications, most commonly anterior, lead to uncontrolled neovascular glaucoma in 10% of treated eyes and vision loss in approximately 50%.

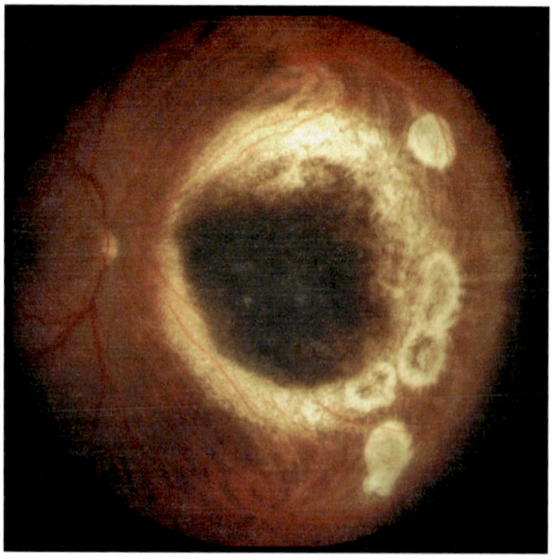

A

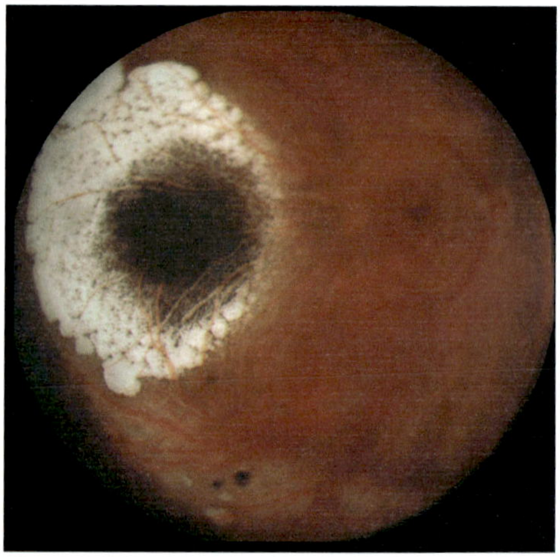

B

Figure 17-14 Choroidal melanoma treated by radioactive brachytherapy. **A,** Mildly elevated remnants of melanoma surrounded by atrophic chorioretinal scarring, nasal to the optic nerve head. **B,** Flat remnants of melanoma pigmentation surrounded by chorioretinal scarring located temporal to the macula. *(Courtesy of Jacob Pe'er, MD.)*

External-beam radiation

Conventional external-beam radiation therapy is ineffective as a single-modality treatment for melanoma. Pre-enucleation external-beam radiotherapy combined with enucleation appears to limit orbital recurrence in large melanomas and showed a non–statistically significant reduction in 5-year and 10-year mortality in the COMS large-tumor trial. In recent years, several centers have used fractionated stereotactic radiotherapy and gamma knife radiosurgery, reporting results comparable to those of other irradiation methods.

Cataract may develop following all types of radiotherapy. Surgical removal of radiation-induced cataract is indicated if the intraocular tumor is nonviable and the patient appears to have visual limitations attributable to the cataract. No increase in mortality after cataract extraction has been documented.

Alternative treatments

Photoablation and hyperthermia Laser photocoagulation has played a limited role in the treatment of melanocytic tumors. Reports of focal/grid laser treatment to eradicate active subretinal fluid in choroidal melanoma have documented a propensity for accelerated tumor growth with rupture of the Bruch membrane. Advances in the delivery of hyperthermia (heat) using transpupillary thermotherapy (TTT) have been reported. Direct diode laser treatment using long duration, large spot size, and relatively low-energy laser has been associated with a reduction in tumor volume. Some reports have suggested that TTT is associated with an increased rate of local tumor recurrence compared with brachytherapy.

Cryotherapy Although cryotherapy using a triple freeze-thaw technique has been tried in the treatment of small choroidal melanomas, it is not considered standard therapy and is not currently undergoing further evaluation for efficacy.

Transscleral diathermy Diathermy is *contraindicated* in the treatment of malignant intraocular tumors because the induced scleral damage may provide a route for extrascleral extension of tumor cells.

Surgical excision of tumor Surgical excision has been performed successfully in many eyes with malignant and benign intraocular tumors. Concerns regarding surgical excision include the inability to evaluate tumor margins for residual disease and the high incidence of pathologically recognized scleral, retinal, and vitreous involvement in medium and large choroidal melanomas. When this treatment is used, the surgical techniques are generally quite difficult, requiring an experienced surgeon. In some centers, local excision of uveal melanoma has been coupled with globe-conserving radiotherapy, such as brachytherapy.

Chemotherapy Currently, chemotherapy is not effective in the treatment of primary or metastatic uveal melanoma. Various regimens have been used, however, for palliative treatment of patients with metastatic disease.

Immunotherapy Immunotherapy uses systemic cytokines, immunomodulatory agents, or local vaccine therapy to try to activate a tumor-directed T-cell immune response. This treatment may be appropriate for uveal melanoma, because primary tumors arise in an immune-privileged organ and may express antigens to which the host is not sensitized. Currently, however, immunotherapy for primary uveal melanoma is not available, and immunotherapy for metastatic disease is still under investigation.

Exenteration Exenteration, traditionally advocated for patients with extrascleral extension of a posterior uveal melanoma, is rarely employed today. The current trend is toward more conservative treatment for these patients, with enucleation plus a limited tenonectomy. The addition of local radiotherapy appears to achieve survival outcomes similar to those of exenteration.

Bergman L, Nilsson B, Lundell G, Lundell M, Seregard S. Ruthenium brachytherapy for uveal melanoma, 1979–2003: survival and functional outcomes in the Swedish population. *Ophthalmology.* 2005;112(5):834–840.

Damato B, Jones AG. Uveal melanoma: resection techniques. *Ophthalmol Clin North Am.* 2005;18(1):119–128.

Diener-West M, Earle JD, Fine SL, et al. The COMS randomized trial of iodine 125 brachytherapy for choroidal melanoma, III: initial mortality findings. COMS report no. 18. *Arch Ophthalmol.* 2001;119(7):969–982.

Hawkins BS; Collaborative Ocular Melanoma Study Group. The Collaborative Ocular Melanoma Study (COMS) randomized trial of pre-enucleation radiation of large choroidal melanoma: IV. Ten-year mortality findings and prognostic factors. COMS report no. 24. *Am J Ophthalmol.* 2004;138(6):936–951.

Prognosis and Prognostic Factors

According to an analysis of 5403 patients with a choroidal and ciliary body melanoma of known tumor size, ciliary body involvement, and extraocular extension, 10-year survival estimates for AJCC stages I, IIA to IIB, and IIIA to IIIC were 88%, 80%, 67%, 45%, 27%, 10%, respectively (see the AJCC staging forms in the appendix, pages 337–341). Retrospective analysis of patients with melanoma suggests that clinical risk factors for mortality are

- larger tumor size at time of treatment
- tumor growth
- anterior tumor location (eg, ciliary body)
- extraocular extension
- older age
- tumor regrowth after globe-conserving therapy
- rapid decrease in tumor size after globe-conserving therapy
- juxtapapillary tumors

Histologic and molecular features associated with a higher rate of metastases include

- epithelioid cells
- high mitotic index and high cell proliferation indices
- extracellular matrix patterns (loops, networks of loops, and parallel with cross-linking)
- mean diameter of the 10 largest nucleoli

- tumor-infiltrating lymphocytes
- monosomy 3, trisomy 8
- *BAP1* mutation, wild type *E1F1AX* and *SF3B1*
- gene expression profiling (class 1B and class 2)

A more in-depth discussion is provided in Chapter 12.

Harbour JW, Chao DL. A molecular revolution in uveal melanoma: implications for patient care and targeted therapy. *Ophthalmology.* 2014;121(6):1281–1288.

Kujala E, Damato B, Coupland SE, et al. Staging of ciliary body and choroidal melanomas based on anatomic extent. *J Clin Oncol.* 2013;31(22):2825–2831.

Sisley K, Rennie IG, Parsons MA, et al. Abnormalities of chromosomes 3 and 8 in posterior uveal melanoma correlate with prognosis. *Genes Chromosomes Cancer.* 1997;19(1):22–28.

Collaborative Ocular Melanoma Study (COMS)

Survival data from the COMS have been reported for the randomized clinical trials of large and medium choroidal melanoma and for the observational study of small choroidal melanoma. These results provide the framework for patient discussions concerning treatment-related long-term survival, rates of globe conservation with ^{125}I brachytherapy, and predictors of small-tumor growth.

- COMS Large Choroidal Melanoma Trial
  - evaluated 1003 patients with choroidal melanomas greater than 16 mm in basal diameter and/or greater than 10 mm in apical height
  - compared enucleation alone with enucleation preceded by external-beam radiotherapy
  - reported no statistically significant difference in 5-year and 10-year survival rates between cohorts (approximately 60% and 40%, respectively)
  - concluded that adjunctive radiotherapy did not improve overall survival
  - established the appropriateness of primary enucleation alone in managing large choroidal melanomas that are not amenable to globe-conserving therapy
- COMS Medium Choroidal Melanoma Trial
  - evaluated 1317 patients with choroidal melanomas ranging in size from 6 mm to 16 mm in basal diameter and/or 2.5 mm to 10 mm in apical height
  - compared standardized enucleation and ^{125}I brachytherapy
  - all-cause mortality at 5 years and 10 years: no significant difference between cohorts (approximately 20% and 35%, respectively)
  - histologically confirmed metastases at 5 years and 10 years found in approximately 10% and 18% of patients, respectively, in both cohorts
  - secondary finding in enucleated eyes:
    —only 2/660 enucleated eyes misdiagnosed as having a choroidal melanoma
  - secondary findings in patients undergoing brachytherapy:
    —10% local tumor recurrence at 5 years
    —13% risk of enucleation after brachytherapy at 5 years

—local tumor recurrence weakly associated with a reduced survival
—decline in visual acuity to 20/200 in approximately 40% of patients at 3 years
—quadrupling of the visual angle (6 lines of visual loss) in approximately 50% of patients at 3 years

- COMS Small Choroidal Tumor Trial
  - observational study of 204 patients with tumors measuring 4.0–8.0 mm in basal diameter and/or 1.0–2.4 mm in apical height
  - melanoma-specific mortality 1% at 5 years
  - clinical growth factors included
    —greater initial thickness and basal diameter
    —presence of orange pigmentation
    —absence of drusen and/or retinal pigment epithelial changes
    —presence of tumor pinpoint hyperfluorescence on angiography

Detailed findings of the COMS can be found at www.jhu.edu/wctb/coms.

Pigmented Epithelial Tumors of the Uvea and Retina

Adenoma and Adenocarcinoma

Benign adenomas of the nonpigmented and pigmented ciliary epithelium may appear indistinguishable clinically from melanomas arising in the ciliary body. Benign adenomas of the RPE are very rare. These lesions occur as oval, deeply melanotic tumors arising abruptly from the RPE. Adenomas rarely enlarge and seldom undergo malignant change. Adenocarcinomas of the RPE are also very rare; only a few cases have been reported in the literature. Although these lesions have malignant features histologically, their metastatic potential appears to be minimal.

Fuchs adenoma (pseudoadenomatous hyperplasia) is usually an incidental finding at autopsy and rarely becomes apparent clinically. It appears as a glistening, white, irregular tumor arising from a ciliary crest. Histologically, it consists of benign proliferation of the nonpigmented ciliary epithelium with accumulation of basement membrane–like material.

Acquired Hyperplasia

Hyperplasia of the pigmented ciliary epithelium or the RPE usually occurs in response to trauma, inflammation, or other ocular insults. Ciliary body lesions, because of their location, often do not become evident clinically. Occasionally, however, they may reach a large size and simulate a ciliary body melanoma. Posteriorly located lesions may be more commonly recognized and can lead to diagnostic uncertainty. In the early management of these atypical lesions, observation is often appropriate to document stability of the lesion. Adenomatous hyperplasia, which has been reported only rarely, may clinically mimic a choroidal melanoma.

Combined Hamartoma

Combined hamartoma of the RPE and retina is a rare disorder that occurs most frequently at the disc margin. Typically, it appears as a darkly pigmented, minimally elevated lesion with retinal traction and tortuous retinal vessels (Fig 17-15). Glial cells within this lesion may contract, producing the traction lines seen clinically in the retina. Exudative complications associated with the vascular component of the lesion may be observed. This lesion has been mistaken for melanoma because of its dark pigmentation and slight elevation. In rare cases, a combined hamartoma may be situated in the peripheral fundus.

Shields CL, Thangappan A, Hartzell K, Valente P, Pirondini C, Shields JA. Combined hamartoma of the retina and retinal pigment epithelium in 77 consecutive patients' visual outcome based on macular versus extramacular tumor location. *Ophthalmology.* 2008;115(12):2246–2252.

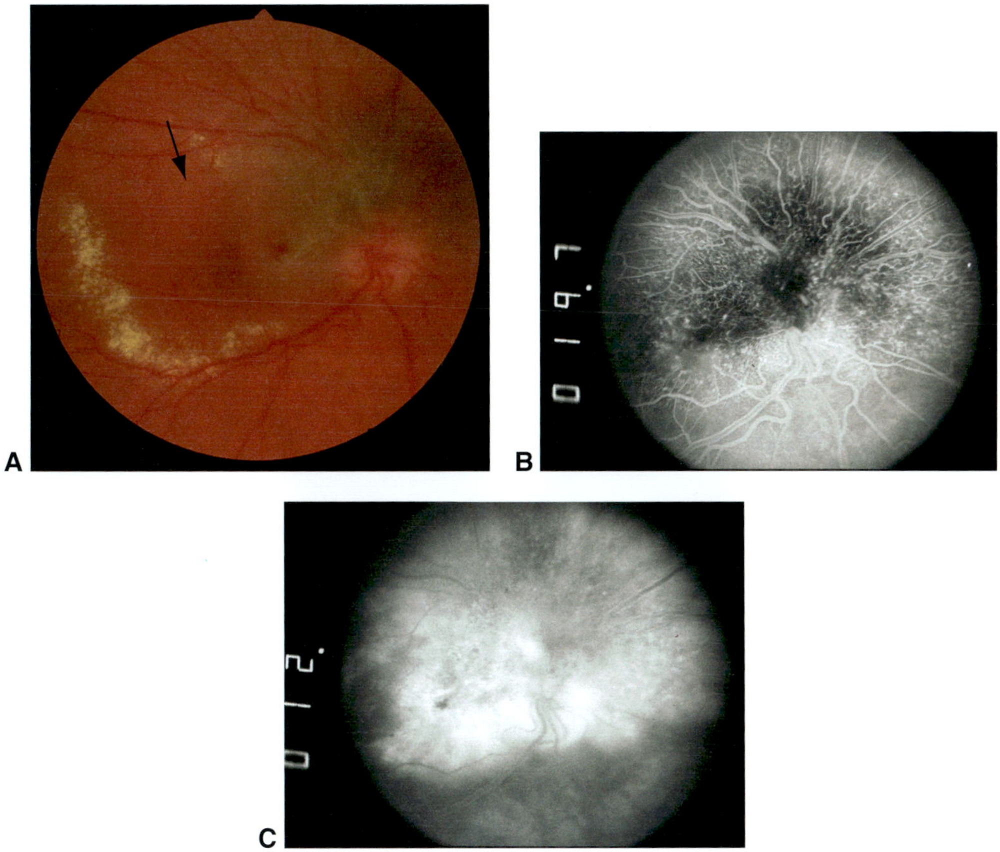

Figure 17-15 Peripapillary combined hamartoma of the retina and RPE. **A,** Fundus photograph showing obscuration of the retinal vessels in superior aspect of the optic disc, pigmentation, retinal striae *(arrow)*, and hard exudates. **B,** Fluorescein angiogram (19.7 sec) showing the vascular component of this lesion composed of small capillary-like telangiectatic vessels. Note the relative hypofluorescence superior to the optic disc due to the RPE component of this lesion. **C,** Late fluorescein angiogram (12 min) showing diffuse late fluorescein leakage in the distribution of the lesion. *(Courtesy of Robert H. Rosa, Jr, MD.)*

CHAPTER 18
Angiomatous Tumors

Hemangiomas

Choroidal Hemangiomas

Hemangiomas of the choroid occur in 2 specific forms: circumscribed and diffuse. The *circumscribed choroidal hemangioma* is a benign vascular tumor that typically occurs in patients with no systemic disorders. It generally appears as a red or orange tumor located in the postequatorial zone of the fundus, often in the macular area (Fig 18-1). Such tumors commonly produce a secondary retinal detachment that extends into the foveal region, resulting in blurred vision, metamorphopsia, and micropsia. These tumors characteristically affect the overlying retinal pigment epithelium (RPE) and cause cystoid degeneration of the outer retinal layers.

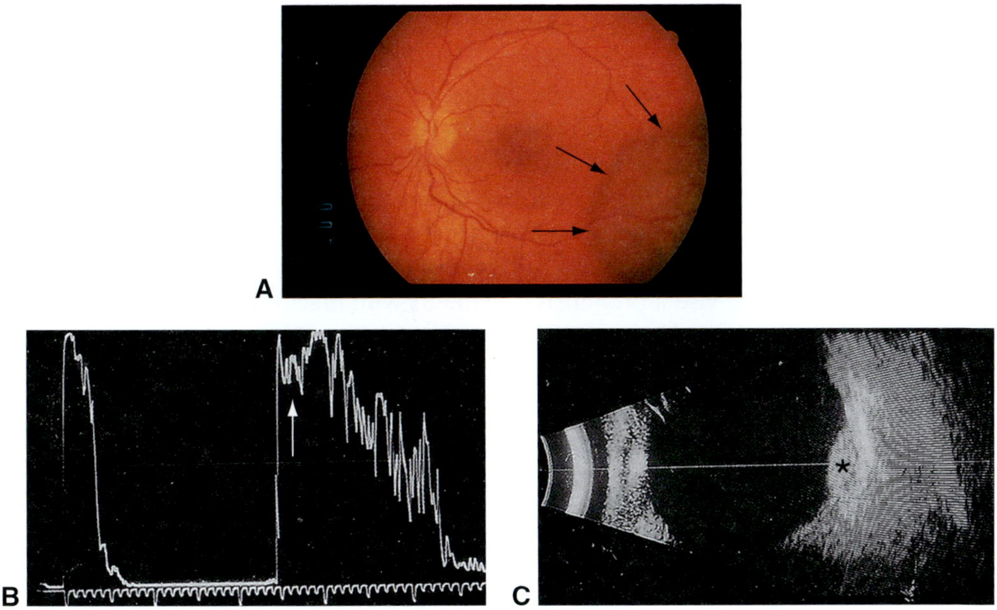

Figure 18-1 **A,** Circumscribed choroidal hemangioma *(arrows).* **B,** A-scan ultrasound study shows characteristic high internal reflectivity *(arrow).* **C,** B-scan ultrasound study shows a highly reflective tumor *(asterisk).*

The principal entities in the differential diagnosis of circumscribed choroidal hemangioma include

- amelanotic choroidal melanoma
- choroidal osteoma
- metastatic carcinoma to the choroid
- granuloma of the choroid

The *diffuse choroidal hemangioma* is generally seen in patients with Sturge-Weber syndrome (encephalofacial angiomatosis). This choroidal tumor produces diffuse reddish orange thickening of the entire fundus, resulting in an ophthalmoscopic pattern commonly referred to as *tomato ketchup fundus* (Fig 18-2). Retinal detachment and glaucoma often occur in eyes with this lesion. See also Chapter 12 in this volume, BCSC Section 12, *Retina and Vitreous,* and BCSC Section 6, *Pediatric Ophthalmology and Strabismus.*

Ancillary diagnostic studies may be of considerable help in evaluating choroidal hemangiomas. Fluorescein angiography reveals the large choroidal vessels in the prearterial or arterial phases with late staining of the tumor and the overlying cystoid retina. Ultrasonography is helpful in differentiating choroidal hemangiomas from amelanotic melanomas and other simulating lesions. A-scan ultrasonography generally shows a high-amplitude initial echo and high-amplitude broad internal echoes (high internal reflectivity; see Fig 18-1B). B-scan ultrasonography demonstrates localized or diffuse choroidal thickening with prominent internal reflections (acoustic heterogeneity) without choroidal excavation or orbital shadowing (see Fig 18-1C). Radiographic studies, particularly CT scanning, can be helpful in differentiating a choroidal hemangioma from a choroidal osteoma.

Asymptomatic choroidal hemangiomas require no treatment. The most common complication of both circumscribed and diffuse choroidal hemangiomas is serous detachment of the retina involving the fovea, with resultant vision loss. Traditionally, circumscribed choroidal hemangiomas have been managed by laser photocoagulation. The surface of the tumor is treated lightly with laser photocoagulation to create chorioretinal adhesions that prevent further accumulation of subretinal fluid. If the retinal detachment is extensive, photocoagulation is often unsuccessful. Recurrent detachments are common, and the long-term visual prognosis in patients with macular detachment or edema is guarded. Laser photocoagulation has recently been replaced by photodynamic therapy (PDT) as the primary treatment for symptomatic circumscribed choroidal hemangioma.

PDT involves an intravenous infusion of verteporfin (6 mg/m^2), which is followed by an application of diode laser (689 nm) 15 minutes later at a light dose of 50 J/cm^2 for a duration of 83 seconds. Most authors have reported resolution of the subretinal fluid, improvement in visual acuity, and regression of the lesion with this treatment.

Radiation, in the forms of brachytherapy, charged-particle, and external beam, has been used to treat choroidal hemangiomas. Brachytherapy and charged-particle therapy have been used to treat patients with circumscribed choroidal hemangioma, and external-beam radiotherapy (low dose, fractionated) has been used to treat patients with diffuse choroidal hemangioma. Each modality has been reported to cause involution of the

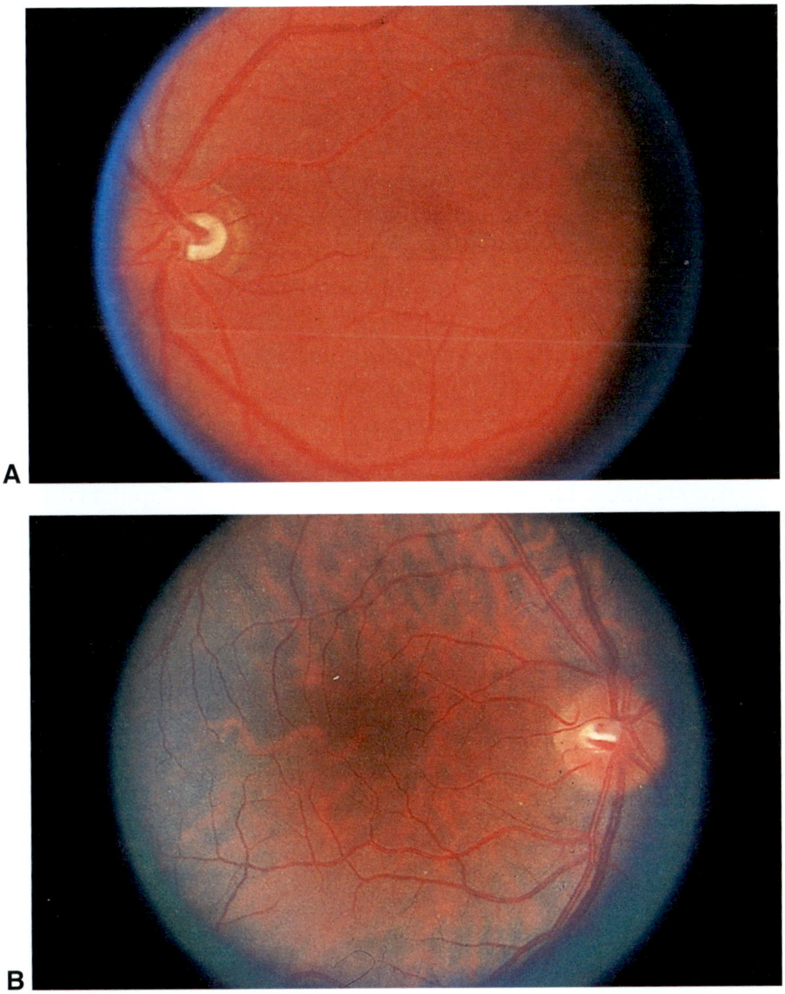

Figure 18-2 Choroidal hemangioma, diffuse type, clinical appearance. The saturated red color of the affected fundus **(A)** contrasts markedly with the color of the unaffected fundus **(B)** of the same patient.

hemangiomas, with subsequent resolution of the associated serous retinal detachment. Complications from the radiation and the serous retinal detachment may limit vision in patients who are irradiated.

To date, little data have been published to support the use of vascular endothelial growth factor (VEGF) inhibitors in the treatment of choroidal hemangiomas.

Boixadera A, García-Arumí J, Martínez-Castillo V, et al. Prospective clinical trial evaluating the efficacy of photodynamic therapy for symptomatic circumscribed choroidal hemangioma. *Ophthalmology.* 2009;116(1):100–105.

Retinal Angiomas

Capillary hemangioblastoma

Retinal capillary hemangioblastoma (angiomatosis retinae, previously known as *retinal capillary hemangioma*) is a rare autosomal dominant condition with a reported incidence of 1 in 40,000. Typically, patients are diagnosed in the second to third decades of life, although retinal lesions may be present at birth. The retinal capillary hemangioblastoma appears as a red to orange tumor arising within the retina with large-caliber, tortuous afferent and efferent retinal blood vessels (Fig 18-3). Associated yellow-white retinal and subretinal exudates that have a predilection for foveal involvement may appear. Exudative detachments often occur in eyes with hemangioblastomas. Atypical variations include hemangiomas arising from the optic disc, which may appear as encapsulated lesions with or without pseudopapilledema, and in the retinal periphery, where vitreous traction may elevate the tumor from the surface of the retina, giving the appearance of a free-floating vitreous mass. Fluorescein angiography of retinal capillary hemangioblastomas demonstrates a rapid arteriovenous transit, with immediate filling of the feeding arteriole, subsequent filling of the numerous fine blood vessels that constitute the tumor, and drainage by the dilated venule. Massive leakage of dye into the tumor and vitreous can occur.

When a capillary hemangioblastoma of the retina occurs as a solitary finding, the condition is generally known as *von Hippel disease.* This condition is familial in about 20% of cases and bilateral in about 50%. The lesions may be multiple in 1 or both eyes. If retinal capillary hemangiomatosis is associated with a cerebellar hemangioblastoma, the term *von Hippel–Lindau syndrome* is applied. The gene for von Hippel–Lindau syndrome has been isolated on chromosome 3. A number of other tumors and cysts may occur in patients with von Hippel–Lindau syndrome. The most important of these lesions are cerebellar hemangioblastomas, renal cell carcinomas, and pheochromocytomas. Genetic screening now allows for subtyping of patients with von Hippel–Lindau to determine the

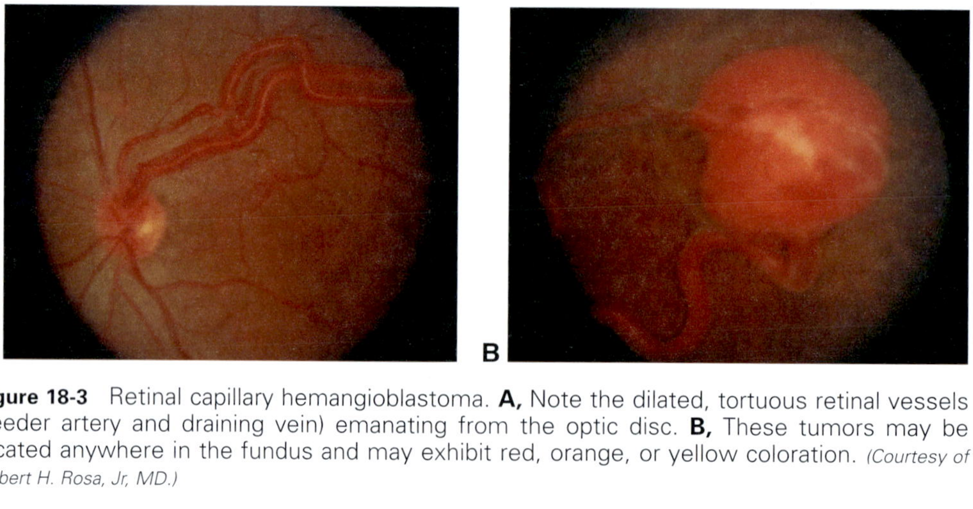

A B

Figure 18-3 Retinal capillary hemangioblastoma. **A,** Note the dilated, tortuous retinal vessels (feeder artery and draining vein) emanating from the optic disc. **B,** These tumors may be located anywhere in the fundus and may exhibit red, orange, or yellow coloration. *(Courtesy of Robert H. Rosa, Jr, MD.)*

risk for systemic manifestations of the disease. When this diagnosis is suspected, appropriate genetic consultation and screening are critical for long-term follow-up of ocular manifestations and the associated systemic complications. Screening for systemic vascular anomalies (eg, cerebellar hemangioblastomas) and malignancies (eg, renal cell carcinoma) may reduce mortality, while aggressive screening for and early treatment of retinal hemangioblastomas may reduce late complications of exudative detachment and improve long-term visual outcomes.

The treatment of retinal capillary hemangioblastomas includes photocoagulation for smaller lesions, cryotherapy for larger and more peripheral lesions, and scleral buckling with cryotherapy or penetrating diathermy for extremely large lesions with extensive retinal detachment. External-beam and charged-particle radiotherapy have also been used. More recently, PDT has been used successfully to treat retinal capillary hemangioblastomas. Standard verteporfin dosing coupled with both standard and modified photodynamic protocols resulted in fibrosis of the hemangiomas with secondary retinal traction and improved visual acuity in recent studies.

Recent case reports have suggested the utility of targeted antiangiogenic therapy in the management of retinal capillary hemangioblastomas. The efficacy of antiangiogenic agents in the treatment of these vascular lesions is of compelling interest to von Hippel–Lindau patients, who have a lifelong risk of developing retinal angiomas. Both systemic and intravitreal VEGF inhibitors have been used. Reports to date suggest that the principal efficacy of VEGF inhibitors is in reducing macular edema. The impact on the actual size of the hemangiomas has been variable. Thus, the visual prognosis remains guarded for patients with large retinal lesions.

Cavernous hemangioma

Cavernous hemangioma of the retina is an uncommon lesion that resembles a cluster of grapes (Fig 18-4). Lesions may also occur on the optic disc. Cavernous hemangiomas may be associated with similar skin and central nervous system lesions. Patients with intracranial lesions may have seizures. In contrast to Coats disease and retinal capillary hemangioblastomas, cavernous hemangiomas are generally not associated with exudation, and treatment is therefore rarely required. However, small hemorrhages as well as areas of gliosis and fibrosis may appear on the surface of the lesion. Within the vascular spaces of the cavernous hemangioma, plasma–erythrocyte separation may appear that can best be demonstrated on fluorescein angiography. Fluorescein angiography is virtually diagnostic of cavernous hemangiomas of the retina. In contrast to a retinal capillary hemangioblastoma, a retinal cavernous hemangioma fills very slowly, and the fluorescein often pools in the upper part of the vascular space, while the cellular elements (erythrocytes) pool in the lower part. The fluorescein remains in the vascular spaces for an extended period. Cavernous hemangiomas generally show no leakage of fluorescein into the vitreous.

Histologically, a cavernous retinal hemangioma consists of dilated, thin-walled vascular channels. The dilated vessels may protrude upward beneath the internal limiting membrane, and associated gliosis and hemorrhage may be seen.

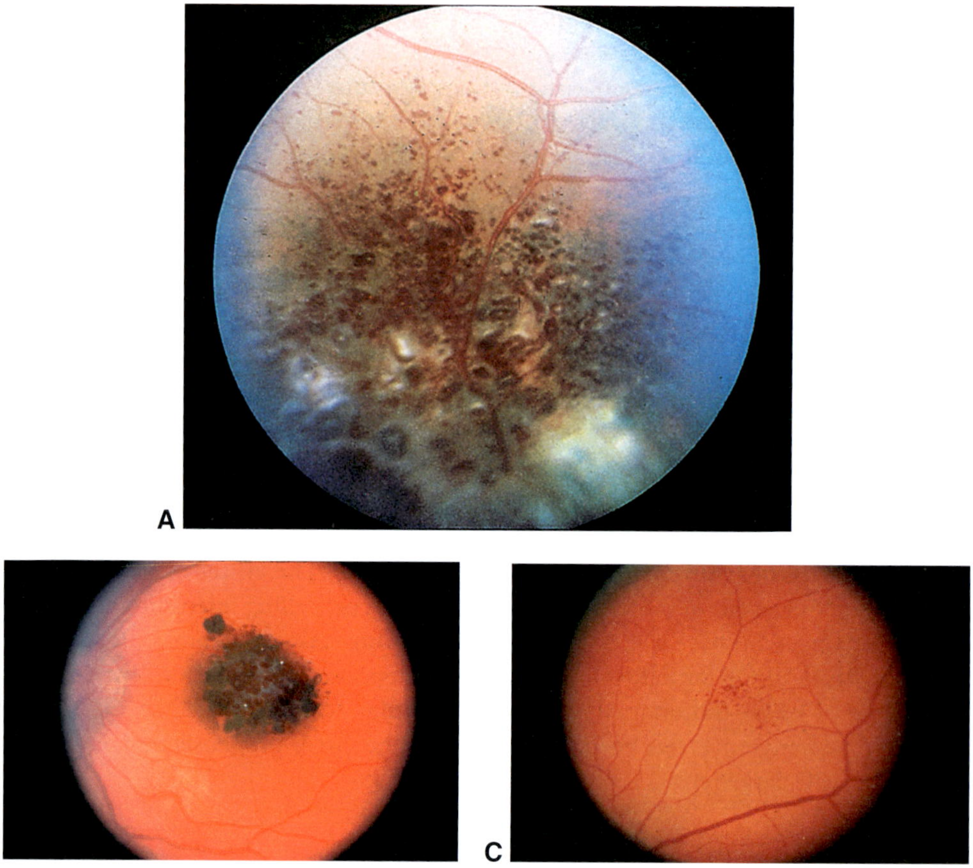

A

B

C

Figure 18-4 Retinal cavernous hemangioma. **A,** Note multiple tiny vascular saccules and associated white fibrovascular tissue. **B,** Note clumped vascular saccules (grape cluster configuration). **C,** When lesions are small, findings may be subtle. *(Part B courtesy of Timothy G. Murray, MD.)*

Arteriovenous Malformation

Congenital retinal arteriovenous malformation (racemose hemangioma) is an anomalous artery-to-vein anastomosis ranging from a small, localized vascular communication near the optic disc or in the periphery to a prominent tangle of large, tortuous blood vessels throughout most of the fundus (Fig 18-5). *Racemose* refers to the clustered or bunched nature of the vessels. When associated with an arteriovenous malformation of the midbrain region, this condition is generally referred to as *Wyburn-Mason syndrome* (see BCSC Section 5, *Neuro-Ophthalmology,* and Section 6, *Pediatric Ophthalmology and Strabismus*). Associated similar arteriovenous malformations may appear in the orbit and mandible.

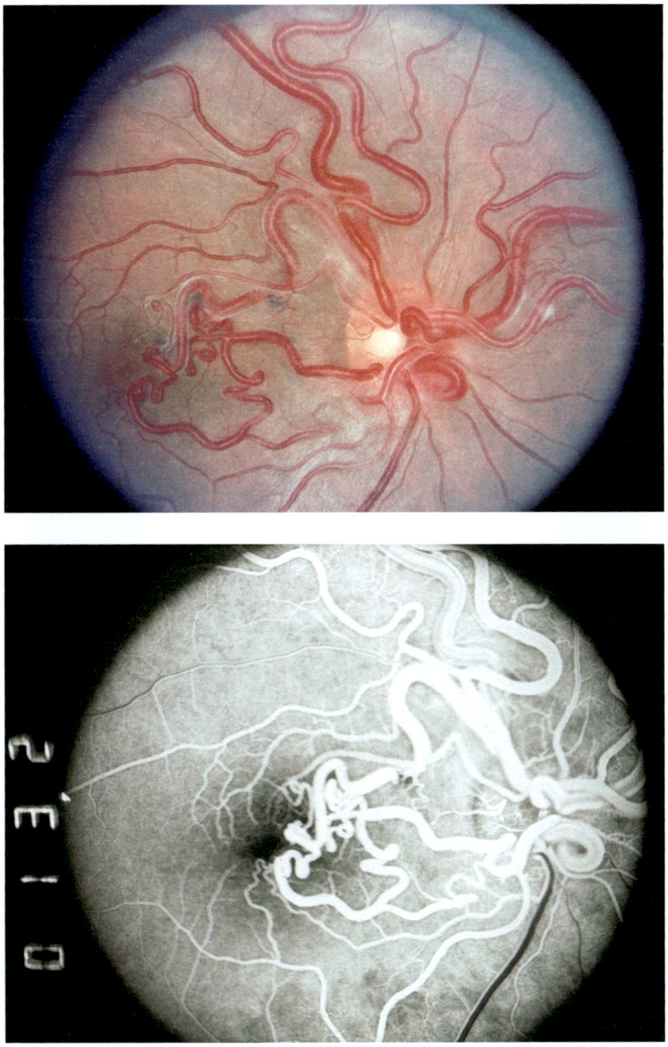

A

B

Figure 18-5 Retinal arteriovenous malformation. **A,** Clinical appearance. **B,** Fluorescein angiogram showing absence of a capillary bed between the afferent and efferent arms of this retinal arteriovenous communication. Note the absence of fluorescein leakage, which is characteristic of this lesion. *(Courtesy of Robert H. Rosa, Jr, MD.)*

CHAPTER 19

Retinoblastoma

Retinoblastoma is the most common primary intraocular malignant tumor of childhood, second only to uveal melanoma as the most common primary intraocular malignant tumor in all age groups (Table 19-1). The frequency of retinoblastoma ranges from 1 in 14,000 to 1 in 20,000 live births, depending on the country. It is estimated that 250–300 new cases occur in the United States each year. There is no sexual predilection, and the tumor occurs bilaterally in 30%–40% of cases. Approximately 90% of cases are diagnosed in patients younger than 3 years. The mean age at diagnosis depends on family history and the laterality of the disease:

- patients with a known family history of retinoblastoma—4 months
- patients with bilateral disease—12 months
- patients with unilateral disease—24 months

Geographic variation in the incidence of the disease has been noted. In Mexico, 6.8 cases per million population have been reported compared to 4 cases per million in the United States. In Central America, there has been an increased incidence in recent years. The highest incidence of the disease has been noted in Africa and India.

Genetic Counseling

Retinoblastoma is caused by a mutation in the *RB1* tumor suppressor gene located on the long arm of chromosome 13 at locus 14 (13q14). Both copies of the *RB1* gene must be mutated in order for a tumor to form. If a patient has bilateral retinoblastoma, there is approximately a 98% chance that it represents a germline mutation. Only about 5% of

Table 19-1 Epidemiology of Retinoblastoma

Most common primary intraocular cancer of childhood
Third most common intraocular cancer overall after melanoma and metastasis
Incidence is 1/14,000–1/20,000 live births
90% of cases present before 3 years of age
Occurs equally in males and females
Occurs equally in right and left eyes
No racial predilection
60%–70% unilateral (mean age at diagnosis, 24 months)
30%–40% bilateral (mean age at diagnosis, 12 months)

retinoblastoma patients have a family history of retinoblastoma. The children of a retinoblastoma survivor who has the hereditary form of retinoblastoma have a 45% chance of being affected (50% chance of inheriting and 90% chance of penetrance). In these cases, the child inherits an abnormal gene from the affected parent. This abnormal gene coupled with somatic mutations in the remaining normal *RB1* allele leads to the development of multiple tumors in 1 or both eyes.

Sporadic cases constitute approximately 95% of all retinoblastomas. Of these, 60% of patients have unilateral disease with no germline mutations. The remaining patients have new germline mutations and will develop multiple tumors. It should be noted that approximately 15% of the sporadic unilateral patients are carriers of a germline *RB1* mutation. Unless there are multiple tumors in the affected eye, these patients cannot be distinguished from children without a germline mutation. Children with unilateral retinoblastoma and a germline mutation, much like their counterparts with bilateral retinoblastoma, are more likely to present at an earlier age. Commercial laboratories are available to test the blood of all retinoblastoma patients for germline mutations. Methods of genetic testing used in retinoblastoma screening include gene sequencing via quantitative polymerase chain reaction (PCR), karyotyping, fluorescent in situ hybridization (FISH), multiplex ligation-dependent probe amplification (MLPA), and RNA analysis. There is approximately a 95% chance of finding a new mutation if one exists.

Genetic counseling for retinoblastoma can be very complex (Fig 19-1). A bilateral retinoblastoma survivor has a 45% chance of having an affected child, whereas a unilateral survivor has a 7% chance of having an affected child. Normal parents of a child with bilateral involvement have less than a 5% risk of having another child with retinoblastoma.

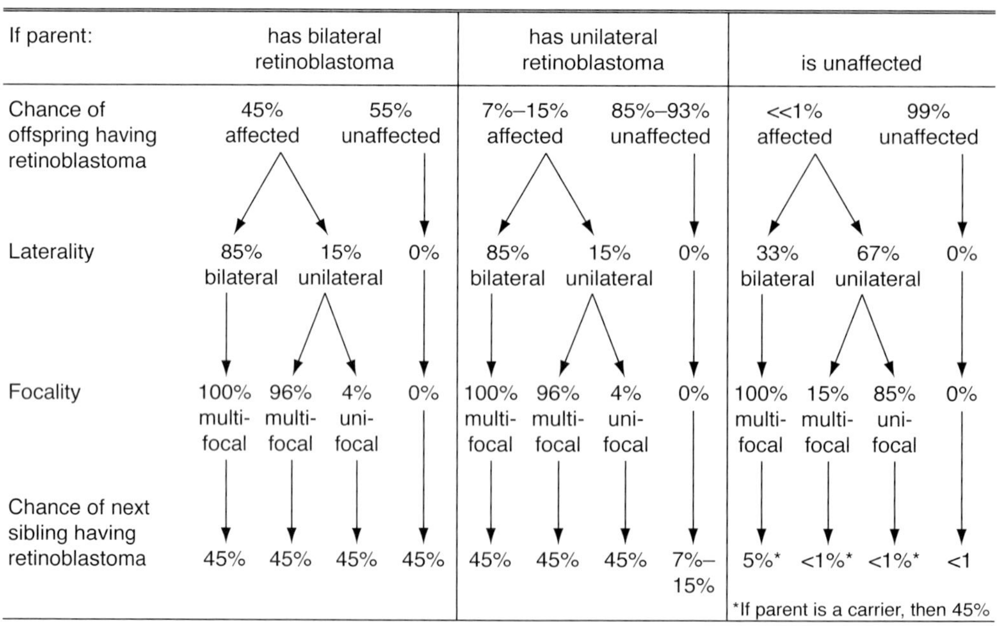

Figure 19-1 Genetic counseling for retinoblastoma. *(Chart created by David H. Abramson, MD.)*

If 2 or more siblings are affected, the chance that another child will be affected increases to 45%. See also Chapter 11 in this volume and BCSC Section 6, *Pediatric Ophthalmology and Strabismus.*

Abramson DH, Mendelsohn ME, Servodidio CA, Tretter T, Gombos DS. Familial retinoblastoma: where and when? *Acta Ophthalmol Scand.* 1998;76(3):334–338.

Gallie BL, Dunn JM, Chan HS, Hamel PA, Phillips RA. The genetics of retinoblastoma: relevance to the patient. *Pediatr Clin North Am.* 1991;38(2):299–315.

Murphree AL. Molecular genetics of retinoblastoma. *Ophthalmol Clin North Am.* 1995;8: 155–166.

Diagnostic Evaluation

Retinoblastoma is a clinical diagnosis. Fine-needle aspiration biopsy (FNAB) should be undertaken only with extreme caution and only by an experienced ocular oncologist, because of the risk of systemic dissemination of tumor.

Clinical Examination

The presenting signs and symptoms of retinoblastoma are determined by the extent and location of tumor at the time of diagnosis. In the United States, the most common presenting signs of retinoblastoma are leukocoria (white pupillary reflex), strabismus, and ocular inflammation (Table 19-2; Fig 19-2). Other presenting features, such as iris heterochromia, spontaneous hyphema, and orbital cellulitis or inflammation are uncommon. In rare instances, a small lesion may be found on routine examination. Visual complaints are infrequent because most patients are preschool-aged children.

The diagnosis of retinoblastoma can generally be suspected on the basis of an office examination with documented visual acuity. An examination under anesthesia (EUA) is needed in all patients suspected of having retinoblastoma to permit a complete assessment of the extent of ocular disease prior to treatment (Fig 19-3). The intraocular pressure and

Table 19-2 Presenting Signs of Retinoblastoma

Among Patients <5 Years of Age	Among Patients ≥5 Years of Age
Leukocoria (≈60%)	Leukocoria (35%)
Strabismus (≈20%)	Decreased vision (35%)
Ocular inflammation (≈5%)	Strabismus (15%)
Hypopyon	Floaters (5%)
Hyphema	Pain (5%)
Iris heterochromia	
Spontaneous globe perforation	
Proptosis	
Cataract	
Glaucoma	
Nystagmus	
Tearing	
Anisocoria	

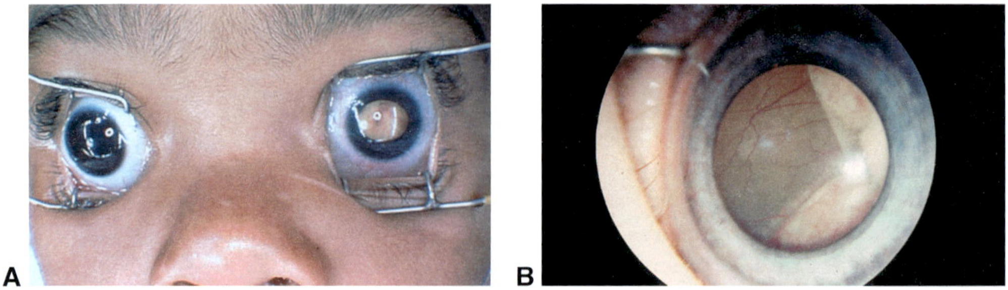

Figure 19-2 Retinoblastoma. **A,** Clinical appearance shows leukocoria and strabismus associated with advanced intraocular tumor. **B,** High magnification. Note large retrolental tumor and secondary total exudative retinal detachment. *(Courtesy of Timothy G. Murray, MD.)*

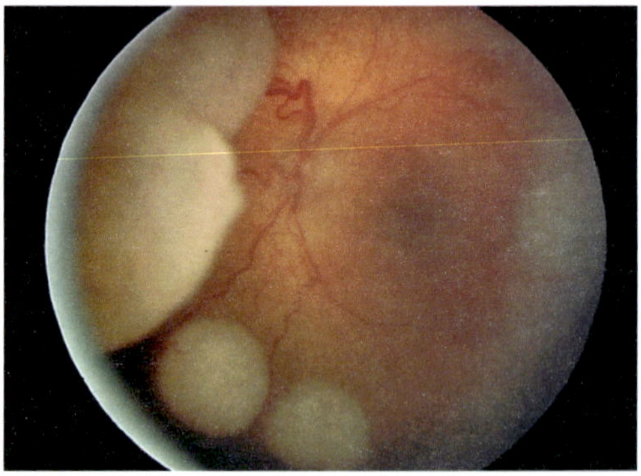

Figure 19-3 Retinoblastoma. Multiple tumor foci in an eye of a patient with a germline *RB1* mutation. *(Courtesy of Matthew W. Wilson, MD.)*

corneal diameter of both eyes should be measured intraoperatively. The location of all tumors in each eye should be clearly documented. Retinoblastoma begins as a translucent, gray to white intraretinal tumor, fed and drained by dilated, tortuous retinal vessels (Fig 19-4). As the tumor grows, foci of calcification develop, giving the characteristic chalky white appearance. Exophytic tumors grow beneath the retina and may have an associated serous retinal detachment (Fig 19-5). As the tumor grows, the retinal detachment may become extensive, obscuring visualization of the tumor (Fig 19-6). Endophytic tumors grow on the retinal surface into the vitreous cavity. Blood vessels may be difficult

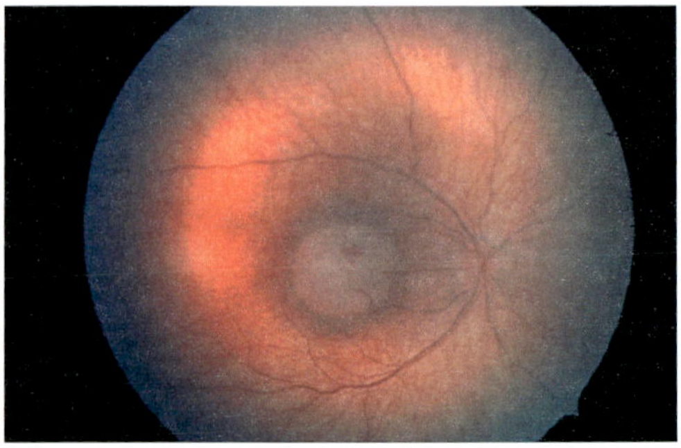

Figure 19-4 Retinoblastoma, clinical appearance. Small, discrete white tumor supplied by dilated retinal blood vessels. *(Courtesy of Timothy G. Murray, MD.)*

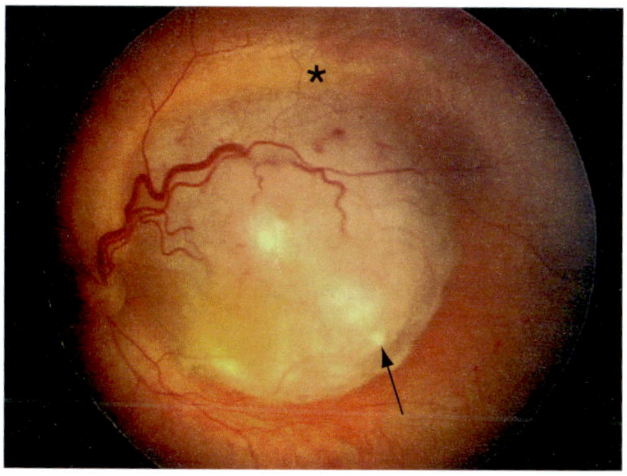

Figure 19-5 Retinoblastoma. Note the dilated retinal blood vessels, foci of calcification *(arrow)*, and cuff of subretinal fluid *(asterisk)*. *(Courtesy of Matthew W. Wilson, MD.)*

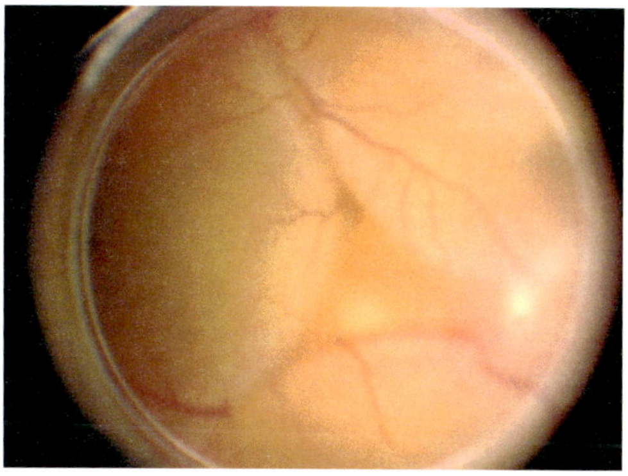

Figure 19-6 Retinoblastoma. Complete exudative detachment obscures tumor visualization. Note normal-appearing retinal vessels as opposed to those found in Coats disease. *(Courtesy of Matthew W. Wilson, MD.)*

to discern in endophytic tumors. Endophytic tumors are more apt to give rise to vitreous seeds (Fig 19-7). Cells shed from retinoblastoma remain viable in the vitreous and subretinal space and may eventually give rise to tumor implants throughout the eye. Vitreous seeds may also enter the anterior chamber, where they can aggregate on the iris to form nodules or settle inferiorly to form a pseudohypopyon (Fig 19-8). Secondary glaucoma and rubeosis iridis occur in approximately 50% of such cases. A rare variant of retinoblastoma is the *diffuse infiltrating retinoblastoma,* which is detected at a later age (>5 years) and is typically unilateral. Diffuse infiltrating retinoblastoma presents a diagnostic dilemma, as the retina may be difficult to see through the dense vitreous cells. This variant is often mistaken for an intermediate uveitis of unknown etiology.

Ultrasonography can be helpful in the diagnosis of retinoblastoma by demonstrating characteristic calcifications within the tumor. Although these calcifications can also be seen on CT scan, MRI has become the preferred diagnostic modality for evaluating

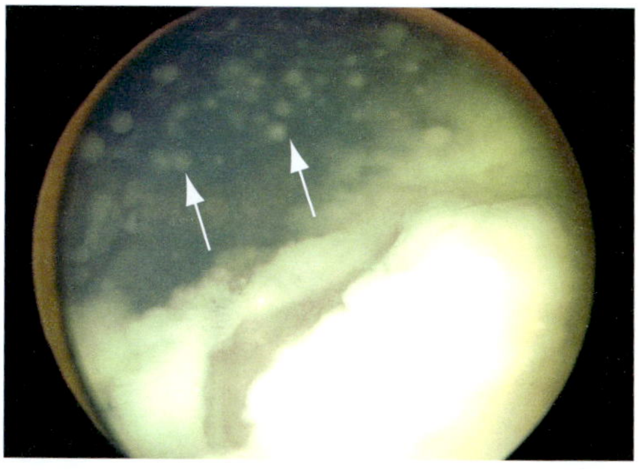

Figure 19-7 Retinoblastoma. Large endophytic tumor with extensive vitreous seeding *(arrows)*. *(Courtesy of Matthew W. Wilson, MD.)*

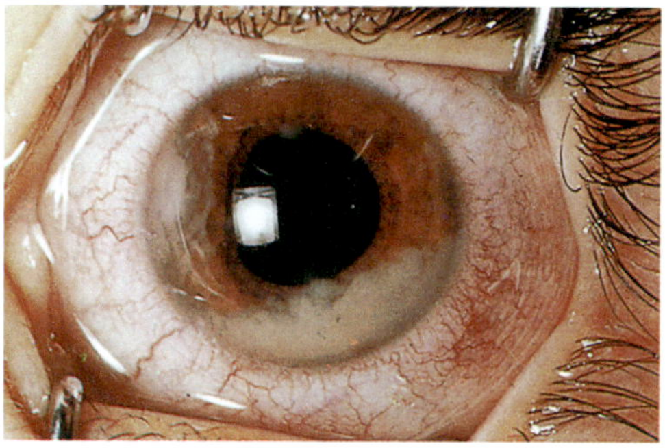

Figure 19-8 Retinoblastoma, clinical appearance. Pseudohypopyon resulting from migration of tumor cells into the anterior chamber (masquerade syndrome).

the optic nerve, orbits, and brain. MRI not only offers better soft-tissue resolution, but also avoids potentially harmful radiation exposure. Recent studies have suggested that systemic metastatic evaluation, typically bone marrow and lumbar puncture, is not indicated in children without neurologic abnormalities or evidence of extraocular extension. If optic nerve extension is suspected, lumbar puncture may be performed. Parents and siblings should be examined for evidence of untreated retinoblastoma or retinocytoma, as this would provide evidence for a hereditary predisposition to the disease. Children with retinoblastoma should have a complete history and physical examination by a pediatric oncologist.

In the United States, patients rarely present with metastases or intracranial extension at the time of diagnosis. The most frequently identified sites of metastatic involvement in children with retinoblastoma include skull bones, distal bones, brain, spinal cord, lymph nodes, and abdominal viscera. Retinoblastoma cells may escape the eye by invading the optic nerve and extending into the subarachnoid space. In addition, tumor cells may massively invade the choroid before traversing emissary canals or eroding through the sclera to enter the orbit. Extraocular extension may result in proptosis as the tumor grows in the orbit (Fig 19-9). In the anterior chamber, tumor cells may invade the trabecular meshwork, gaining access to the conjunctival lymphatics. The patient may subsequently develop palpable preauricular and cervical lymph nodes.

Differential Diagnosis

A number of lesions simulate retinoblastoma (Table 19-3). Most of these conditions can be differentiated from retinoblastoma on the basis of a comprehensive history, clinical examination, and appropriate ancillary diagnostic testing.

Persistent fetal vasculature

Persistent fetal vasculature (PFV), previously known as *persistent hyperplastic primary vitreous (PHPV),* is typically recognized within days or weeks of birth. The condition is unilateral in two-thirds of cases and is associated with microphthalmos, a shallow or flat anterior chamber, a hypoplastic iris with prominent vessels, and a retrolenticular fibrovascular mass that draws the ciliary body processes inward. On indirect ophthalmoscopy, a vascular stalk may be seen arising from the optic nerve head and attaching to the posterior lens capsule. Ultrasonography confirms the diagnosis by showing persistent hyaloid

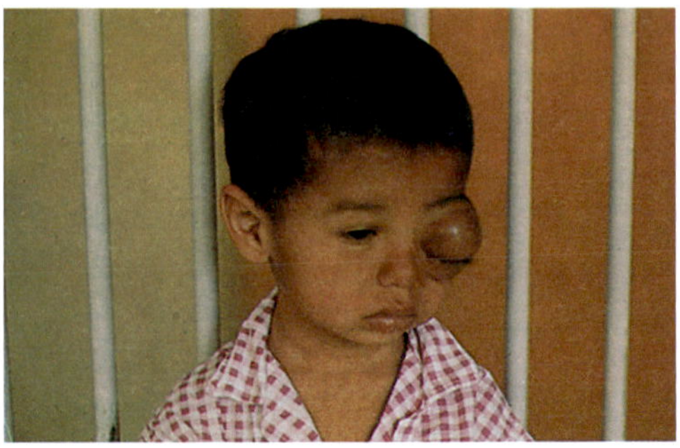

Figure 19-9 Retinoblastoma, clinical appearance. Proptosis caused by retinoblastoma with orbital invasion.

Table 19-3 Differential Diagnosis of Retinoblastoma

Clinical Diagnosis in Pseudoretinoblastoma	265 Cases*	Percent	76 Cases†	Percent
Persistent fetal vasculature	51	19	15	20
Retinopathy of prematurity	36	13	3	4
Posterior cataract	36	13	5	7
Coloboma of choroid or optic disc	30	11	7	9
Uveitis	27	10	2	3
Larval granulomatosis (Toxocara)	18	6	20	26
Congenital retinal fold	13	5		
Coats disease	10	4	12	16
Organizing vitreous hemorrhage	9	3	3	4
Retinal dysplasia	7	2		

*Modified from Howard GM, Ellsworth RM. Differential diagnosis of retinoblastoma. *Am J Ophthalmol.* 1965;60:610–618.

†From Shields JA, Stephens RT, Sarin LK. The differential diagnosis of retinoblastoma. In: Harley RD, ed. *Pediatric Ophthalmology.* 2nd ed. Philadelphia: Saunders; 1983:114.

remnants arising from the optic nerve head, usually in association with a closed funnel retinal detachment. No retinal tumor is seen, and the axial length of the eye is shortened. Calcification may be present. PFV may be managed with combined lensectomy and vitrectomy approaches in selected cases. See also Chapter 10 in this volume and BCSC Section 6, *Pediatric Ophthalmology and Strabismus.*

Coats disease

Coats disease is clinically evident within the first decade of life and is more common in boys. The lesion is typically characterized by unilateral retinal telangiectasia associated with intraretinal yellow exudation without a distinct mass (Fig 19-10). The progressive leakage of fluid may lead to an extensive retinal detachment and neovascular glaucoma. Ultrasonography documents the absence of a retinal tumor and shows the convection of cholesterol in the subretinal fluid. Fluorescein angiography shows classic telangiectatic vessels. Laser photocoagulation or cryoablation of the vascular anomalies eliminates the exudative component of the disease and may restore visual function. Subretinal fluid may be drained to facilitate these procedures. Serial evaluation and follow-up is critical for these patients.

Ocular toxocariasis

Ocular toxocariasis typically occurs in older children with a history of soil ingestion or exposure to puppies. Toxocariasis presents with posterior and peripheral granulomas, with an associated uveitis. Exudative retinal detachment, organized vitreoretinal traction, and cataracts may be present. Ultrasonography shows the vitritis, retinal detachment, granulomas, retinal traction, and the absence of calcium. See BCSC Section 9, *Intraocular Inflammation and Uveitis,* for additional discussion.

Astrocytoma

Retinal astrocytoma, or astrocytic hamartoma, generally appears as a small, smooth, white, glistening tumor located in the nerve fiber layer of the retina (Fig 19-11). It may be

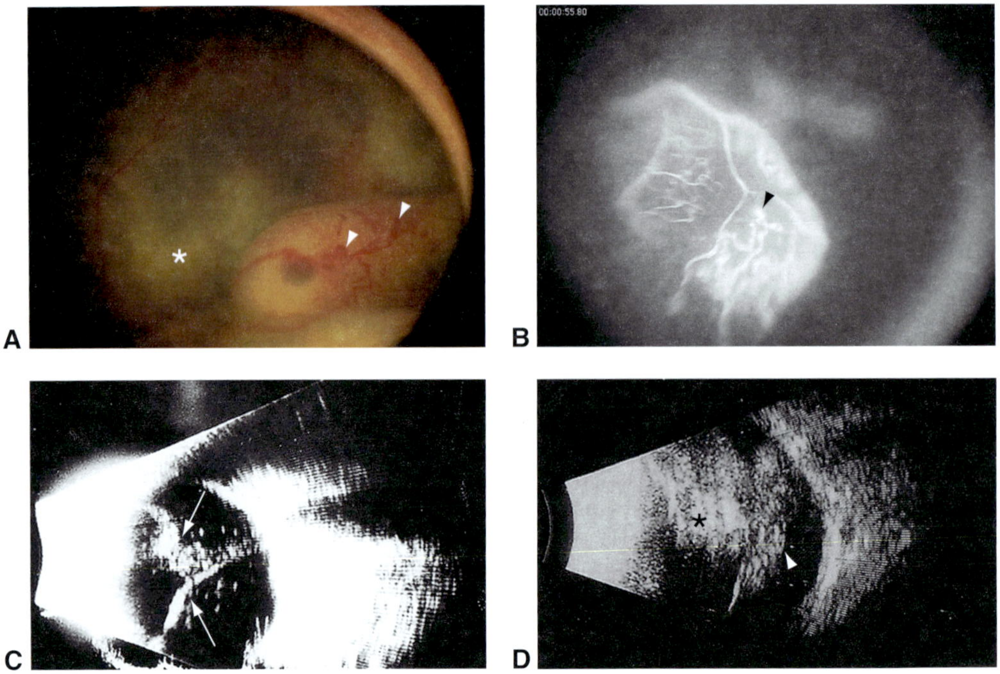

Figure 19-10 Coats disease. **A,** Clinical appearance of characteristic lightbulb aneurysms *(arrowheads)* observed in Coats disease. Note the associated exudative retinal detachment with subretinal exudate *(asterisk)*. **B,** Fluorescein angiogram showing classic telangiectatic vessels *(arrowhead)*. **C,** B-scan in Coats disease shows retinal detachment *(arrows)*. **D,** In contrast, B-scan in retinoblastoma shows total retinal detachment *(arrowhead)* and a large tumor mass *(asterisk)*. *(Parts A and B courtesy of Matthew W. Wilson, MD.)*

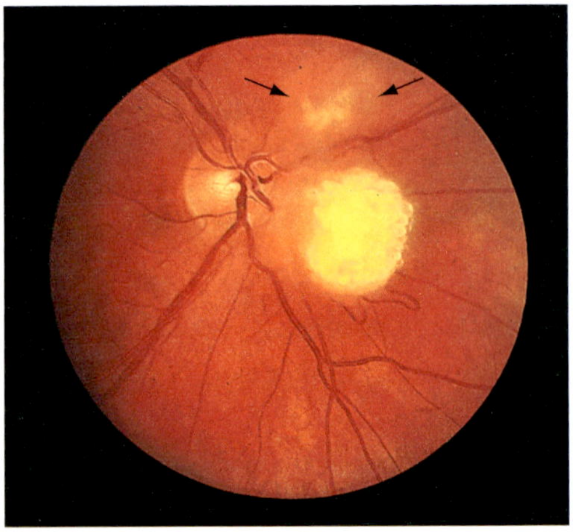

Figure 19-11 Retinal astrocytic hamartomas, clinical appearance. Note the more subtle opalescent lesion *(between arrows)* superonasal to the optic disc and the larger "mulberry" lesion inferonasal to the disc.

single or multiple, unilateral or bilateral. In some cases, it may become larger and calcified, typically having a mulberry appearance. Astrocytomas occasionally arise from the optic disc; such tumors are often referred to as *giant drusen*. Astrocytomas of the retina commonly occur in patients with tuberous sclerosis and may also be seen in patients with neurofibromatosis. Most retinal astrocytomas are not associated with a phakomatosis.

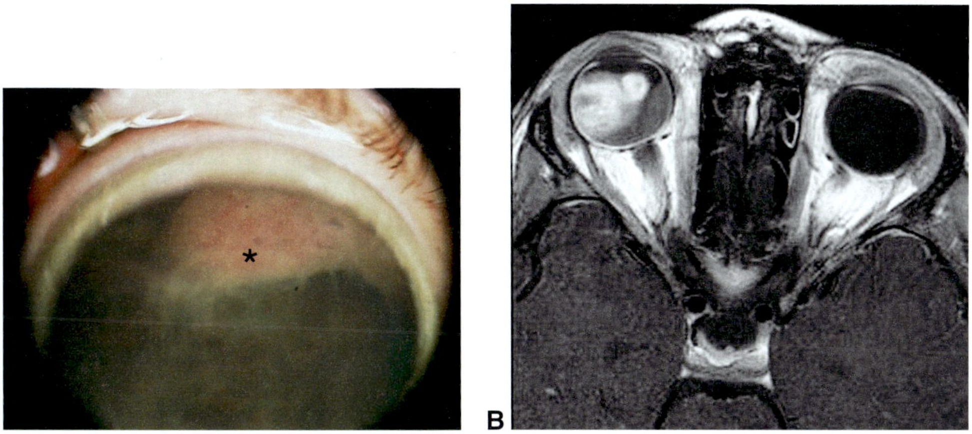

A B

Figure 19-12 Medulloepithelioma. **A,** Pigmented lesion arising in ciliary body, with amelanotic apex *(asterisk)*. **B,** T1-weighted MRI with gadolinium, showing diffuse enhancement and multiple cystic spaces. *(Courtesy of Matthew W. Wilson, MD.)*

Medulloepithelioma

Medulloepithelioma, or diktyoma, is a tumor derived from the inner layer of the optic cup (medullary epithelium) that occurs in both benign and malignant forms (see Chapter 11, Fig 11-45). This type of tumor typically becomes clinically evident in children aged 4–12 years, but it may also occur in adults. It usually appears as a variably pigmented mass arising from the ciliary body (Fig 19-12A), but it has also been documented in the retina and optic nerve. Smaller lesions may present with unexplained neovascular glaucoma with iris heterochromia. The tumor may erode through the iris root or grow along the lens zonules to enter the anterior chamber. Large cysts may be seen on the surface of the tumor or within the lesion on diagnostic imaging (Fig 19-12B). Chapter 11 discusses the histologic features of medulloepithelioma. Management usually consists of enucleation or observation. Surgical resection is specifically avoided for most of these tumors because of late complications and documented metastases associated with this treatment. Fortunately, metastasis is rare with appropriate management, even if the tumor appears frankly malignant on histologic examination. Small lesions have been successfully treated with iodine 125 plaque brachytherapy.

Classification

The Reese-Ellsworth Classification for Intraocular Tumors is the best-known method of grouping intraocular retinoblastoma (Table 19-4); it does not stage extraocular retinoblastoma. The classification takes into account the number, size, and location of tumors and the presence or absence of vitreous seeding. According to this classification, eye tumors are grouped from very favorable (group I) to very unfavorable (group V) by probability of eye preservation when treated with external-beam radiation alone. The Reese-Ellsworth classification does not provide prognostic information about patient survival or vision. The use of external-beam radiotherapy has given way to the use of primary systemic chemotherapy for the treatment of bilateral retinoblastoma. As a result, the International

Table 19-4 Reese-Ellsworth Classification of Retinoblastoma for Eye Preservation

Group	A	B
I (very favorable)	Solitary tumor 4 disc diameters (DD) at or behind equator	Multiple tumors 4 DD at or behind equator
II (favorable)	Solitary tumor 4–10 DD or behind equator	Multiple tumors 4–10 DD at or behind equator
III (doubtful)	Any lesion anterior to equator	Solitary tumor >10 DD posterior to equator
IV (unfavorable)	Multiple tumors, some larger than 10 DD	Any lesion anterior to ora serrata
V (very unfavorable)	Massive tumor occupying half or more of retina	Vitreous seeding

Classification System for Intraocular Retinoblastoma has been adopted, with the hope that it can better predict an eye's response to chemotherapy. Eyes are grouped based on the size of the tumor and the presence of subretinal fluid, as well as the extent of vitreous and subretinal seeding. Eyes with anterior chamber involvement, neovascular glaucoma, vitreous hemorrhage, and/or necrosis are grouped as being unsalvageable (Table 19-5). The American Joint Committee on Cancer (AJCC) also has a staging system for retinoblastoma that relates to both intraocular and extraocular disease; see the staging form in the appendix.

Gallie BL, Truong T, Heon E, et al. Retinoblastoma ABC classification survey. 11th International Retinoblastoma Symposium, Paris, France; 2003.

Murphree AL. Intraocular retinoblastoma: the case for a new group classification. *Ophthalmol Clin North Am.* 2005;18(1):41–53.

Reese AB. *Tumors of the Eye.* 3rd ed. Hagerstown, MD: Harper & Row; 1976:pp 90–132.

Shields CL, Mashayekhi A, Demirci H, Meadows AT, Shields JA. Practical approach to management of retinoblastoma. *Arch Ophthalmol.* 2004;122(5):729–735.

Table 19-5 International Classification System for Response to Chemotherapy

Group A	Small tumors (≤3 mm) confined to the retina; >3 mm from the fovea; >1.5 mm from the optic disc
Group B	Tumors (>3 mm) confined to the retina in any location, with clear subretinal fluid ≤6 mm from the tumor margin
Group C	Localized vitreous and/or subretinal seeding (<6 mm in total from tumor margin). If there is more than 1 site of subretinal/vitreous seeding, then the total of these sites must be <6 mm.
Group D	Diffuse vitreous and/or subretinal seeding (≥6 mm in total from tumor margin). If there is more than 1 site of subretinal/vitreous seeding, then the total of these sites must be ≥6 mm. Subretinal fluid >6 mm from tumor margin.
Group E	• No visual potential; *or* • Presence of any 1 or more of the following: ▪ tumor in the anterior segment ▪ tumor in or on the ciliary body ▪ neovascular glaucoma ▪ vitreous hemorrhage obscuring the tumor or significant hyphema ▪ phthisical or pre-phthisical eye ▪ orbital cellulitis–like presentation

Associated Conditions

Retinocytoma

Retinocytoma is clinically indistinguishable from retinoblastoma. Chapter 11 describes the histologic characteristics that distinguish retinocytoma from retinoblastoma (see Fig 11-44). The developmental biology of retinocytoma is subject to controversy. Some authorities consider retinocytoma to be retinoblastoma that has undergone differentiation, analogous to ganglioneuroma, the differentiated form of neuroblastoma. Many other authorities contend that retinocytoma is a benign counterpart of retinoblastoma.

Though histologically benign, retinocytoma carries the same genetic implications as retinoblastoma. A child harboring a retinoblastoma in one eye and a retinocytoma in the other should be considered capable of transmitting an *RB1* mutation to offspring.

Trilateral Retinoblastoma

The term *trilateral retinoblastoma* is reserved for cases of bilateral retinoblastoma associated with ectopic intracranial retinoblastoma. The ectopic focus is usually located in the pineal gland or the parasellar region and historically has been termed a *pinealoblastoma.* This tumor affects up to 5% of children with a germline *RB1* mutation. Rarely, a child may present with ectopic intracranial retinoblastoma prior to ocular involvement. More commonly, this independent malignancy presents months to years after treatment of the intraocular retinoblastoma.

Several different observations support the concept of primary intracranial pinealoblastoma. CT helped to establish that intracranial tumors in some patients dying from retinoblastoma are anatomically separate from the primary tumors in the orbit. These intracranial tumors are not associated with metastatic disease elsewhere in the body, and, unlike metastatic retinoblastoma, they often demonstrate features of differentiation such as Flexner-Wintersteiner rosettes (see Chapter 11, Fig 11-41). Embryologic, immunologic, and phylogenic evidence of photoreceptor differentiation in the pineal gland offers further support for the concept of trilateral retinoblastoma.

All patients with retinoblastoma should undergo baseline neuroimaging studies to exclude intracranial involvement. Patients with germline *RB1* gene mutations (ie, bilateral retinoblastoma, unilateral multifocal retinoblastoma, or unilateral retinoblastoma with a positive family history) should undergo serial imaging of the central nervous system (CNS). Studies suggest that serial MRI with and without contrast is most sensitive for CNS involvement and does not expose the child to radiation. Median survival of patients with retinoblastoma with CNS involvement is approximately 8 months. Recent studies report a decrease in the incidence of trilateral retinoblastoma in patients treated with systemic chemotherapy, suggesting a possible prophylactic effect.

Jubran RF, Erdreich-Epstein A, Butturini A, Murphree AL, Villablanca JG. Approaches to treatment for extraocular retinoblastoma: Children's Hospital Los Angeles experience. *J Pediatr Hematol Oncol.* 2004;26(1):31–34.

Shields CL, Meadows AT, Shields JA, Carvalho C, Smith AF. Chemoreduction for retinoblastoma may prevent intracranial neuroblastic malignancy (trilateral retinoblastoma). *Arch Ophthalmol.* 2001;119(9):1269–1272.

Treatment

When retinoblastoma is being treated, it is first and foremost important to understand that it is a malignancy. When the disease is contained within the eye, survival rates exceed 95% in the Western world. However, with extraocular spread, survival rates decrease to under 50%. Therefore, when a treatment strategy is being decided, the first goal must be preservation of life, then preservation of the eye, and, finally, preservation of vision. The modern management of intraocular retinoblastoma currently incorporates a combination of different treatment modalities, including enucleation, chemotherapy, photocoagulation, cryotherapy, external-beam radiation therapy, and plaque brachytherapy. Metastatic disease is managed using intensive chemotherapy, radiation, and bone marrow transplantation. The treatment of children with retinoblastoma requires a team approach, including an ocular oncologist, pediatric ophthalmologist, pediatric oncologist, and radiation oncologist.

Enucleation

Enucleation remains the definitive treatment for retinoblastoma, providing, in most cases, a complete surgical resection of the disease. Typically, enucleation is considered an appropriate intervention when

- the tumor involves more than 50% of the globe
- orbital or optic nerve involvement is suspected
- anterior segment involvement is present
- neovascular glaucoma is present
- there is limited visual potential in the affected eye

Enucleation techniques are aimed at minimizing the potential for inadvertent globe penetration while obtaining the greatest length of resected optic nerve that is feasible, typically longer than 10 mm. Porous integrated implants, such as hydroxyapatite or porous polyethylene, are currently used by most surgeons.

Attempts at globe-conserving therapy should be undertaken only by ophthalmologists well versed in the management of this rare childhood tumor and in conjunction with similarly experienced pediatric oncologists. Failed attempts at eye salvage may place a child at risk of metastatic disease.

Chemotherapy

A significant advance in the management of bilateral intraocular retinoblastoma in the past 2 decades has been the use of primary systemic chemotherapy. Systemic administration of chemotherapy reduces tumor volume, allowing for subsequent application of consolidative focal therapy with laser, cryotherapy, or radiotherapy (Fig 19-13). These changes have come about as a result of improvements in the treatment of both brain tumors and metastatic retinoblastoma. Current regimens incorporate varying combinations of carboplatin, vincristine, etoposide, and cyclosporine. Children receive drugs intravenously every 3–4 weeks for 4–9 cycles of chemotherapy. Meanwhile, serial EUAs are performed, during which tumor response is observed and focal therapies are administered.

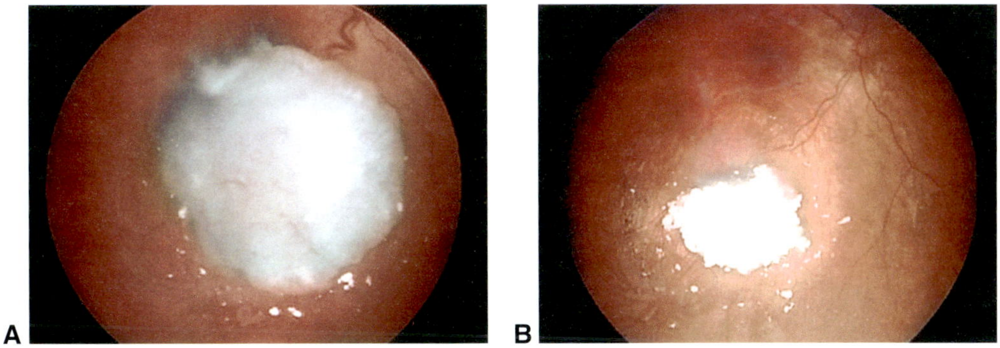

Figure 19-13 Retinoblastoma. **A,** Before chemotherapy. **B,** Reduced tumor volume after 2 cycles of chemotherapy alone.

Drug regimens, routes of administration, and dose schedules should be determined by a pediatric oncologist experienced in the treatment of children with retinoblastoma.

Local chemotherapy

Subconjunctival carboplatin with and without systemic chemotherapy has been used in the treatment of retinoblastoma. It has been abandoned by many centers because of complications such as orbital myositis, periocular fibrosis, and optic neuropathy. Local chemotherapeutic delivery to the eye with agents such as melphalan by intravitreal injection and/or selective canalization of the ophthalmic artery has been used in its place with increased success, particularly in eyes with vitreous disease.

Photocoagulation and Hyperthermia

Xenon arc and argon laser (532 nm) have traditionally been used to treat retinoblastomas smaller than 3 mm in apical height with basal dimensions less than 10 mm. Two to 3 rows of encircling retinal photocoagulation destroy the tumor's blood supply, with ensuing regression. Newer lasers allow for direct confluent treatment of the tumor surface. The diode laser (810 nm) is used to provide hyperthermia. Direct application to the surface increases the tumor's temperature to the 45°–60° Celsius range and has a direct cytotoxic effect, which can be augmented by both chemotherapy and radiation (Fig 19-14).

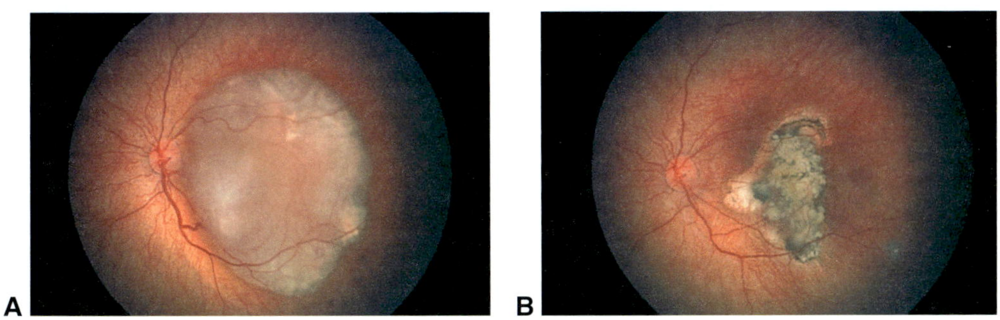

Figure 19-14 Retinoblastoma. **A,** Before treatment. **B,** Same eye 6 months later, after treatment with chemoreduction and laser therapy. *(Courtesy of Timothy G. Murray, MD.)*

Cryotherapy

Also effective for tumors in the size range of less than 10 mm in basal dimension and 3 mm in apical thickness, cryotherapy is applied under direct visualization with a triple freeze–thaw technique. Typically, laser photoablation is chosen for posteriorly located tumors and cryoablation for more anteriorly located tumors. Repetitive tumor treatments are often required for both techniques, along with close follow-up for tumor growth or treatment complications.

External-Beam Radiation Therapy

Retinoblastoma tumors are responsive to radiation. Current techniques use focused megavoltage radiation treatments, often employing lens-sparing techniques, to deliver 4000–4500 cGy over a 4–6-week treatment interval. Typically, those treated are children with bilateral disease not amenable to laser or cryotherapy. Globe salvage rates are excellent, with up to 85% of eyes being retained. Visual function is often excellent and limited only by tumor location or secondary complications.

Two major concerns have limited the application of external-beam radiotherapy using standard techniques:

1. the association of germline mutations of the *RB1* gene with a lifelong increase in the risk of second, independent primary malignancies (eg, osteosarcoma) that is exacerbated by exposure to external-beam radiotherapy
2. the potential for radiation-related sequelae, which include midface hypoplasia, radiation-induced cataract, and radiation optic neuropathy and retinopathy

Evidence suggests that combined-modality therapy that uses lower-dose external-beam radiotherapy coupled with chemotherapy may allow for increased globe conservation with decreased radiation morbidity. In addition, the use of systemic chemotherapy may delay the need for external-beam radiotherapy, allowing for greater orbital development and significantly decreasing the risk of second malignancies once the child is older than 1 year.

Plaque Radiotherapy (Brachytherapy)

Radioactive plaque therapy may be used both as salvage therapy for eyes in which globe-conserving therapies have failed to destroy all viable tumor and as a primary treatment for some children with relatively small to medium-sized tumors. This technique is generally applicable for tumors less than 16 mm in basal diameter and 8 mm in apical thickness. The most commonly used isotopes are iodine 125 and ruthenium 106. Intraoperative localization with ultrasound enhances local tumor control for plaque brachytherapy. A greater likelihood of radiation optic neuropathy or retinopathy may be associated with this radiotherapy modality compared with external-beam radiotherapy. Limiting the radiation dose to periocular structures may lower the incidence of radiation-induced second malignancies.

Targeted Therapy

New frontiers in the treatment of retinoblastoma include the use of gene therapy and small-molecule inhibition. Adenoviral-mediated transfection of tumor cells with thymidine kinase renders the tumor susceptible to systemically administered ganciclovir. Phase 1 clinical trials have been completed, documenting both safety and efficacy. Although this targeted therapy is currently reserved as salvage therapy for eyes failing all conventional modalities of treatment, there is hope that it may become a mainstream treatment. The use of small-molecule inhibitors in aberrant cellular pathways has shown promise in preclinical models.

Spontaneous Regression

Retinoblastoma is one of the more common malignant tumors to undergo complete and spontaneous necrosis (although this is rarely recognized with active disease). Spontaneous regression is recognized clinically after involutional changes such as phthisis have occurred. The incidence of spontaneous regression is unknown, as no child with active retinoblastoma is observed with the hope of spontaneous involution. Although the mechanism by which spontaneous regression occurs is not understood, its histologic appearance is diagnostic. The vitreous cavities of these phthisical eyes are filled with islands of calcified cells embedded in a mass of fibroconnective tissue. Close inspection of the peripheral portion of these calcified islands reveals the ghosted contours of fossilized tumor cells. The process is often accompanied by exuberant proliferation of retinal pigment and ciliary epithelia.

Prognosis

Children with intraocular retinoblastoma who have access to modern medical care have a very good prognosis for survival, with overall survival rates of over 95% for children in developed countries. The most important risk factor associated with death is extraocular extension of tumor, either directly through the sclera or, more commonly, by invasion of the optic nerve, especially to the surgically resected margin (see Chapter 11, Fig 11-43). The importance of choroidal invasion is unclear. Although a multivariate analysis of a large case series has shown that choroidal invasion is not predictive of metastases, the significance of this pathologic finding remains the subject of debate. A current multicenter study is investigating this further. Some evidence suggests, however, that bilateral tumors may increase the risk of death because of their association with primary intracranial tumors (see the discussion of trilateral retinoblastoma earlier in this chapter).

Children who survive bilateral retinoblastoma have an increased incidence of nonocular malignancies later in life. The mean latency for second tumor development is approximately 9 years from management of the primary retinoblastoma. The *RB1* mutation is associated with approximately a 25% incidence of second tumor development within 50 years in patients treated without exposure to radiation therapy. External-beam

Table 19-6 Nonretinoblastoma Malignancies in Retinoblastoma Survivors

Tumors Arising in the Field of Radiation of the Eye		Tumors Arising Outside the Field of Radiation of the Eye	
Pathologic Type	**Percent**	**Pathologic Type**	**Percent**
Osteosarcoma	40	Osteosarcoma	36
Fibrosarcoma	10	Melanoma	12
Soft-tissue sarcoma	8	Pinealoma	9
Anaplastic and unclassifiable	8	Ewing sarcoma	6
Squamous cell carcinoma	5	Papillary thyroid carcinoma	6
Rhabdomyosarcoma	5	Assorted other	30
Assorted other	24		

Modified with permission from Abramson DH, Ellsworth RM, Kitchin FD, el al. Second nonocular tumors in retinoblastoma survivors. Are they radiation-induced? *Ophthalmology.* 1984;91:1351–1355.

radiation therapy decreases the latency period, in turn increasing the incidence of second tumors in the first 30 years of life, as well as increasing the proportion of tumors in the head and neck. The most common type of second cancer in these patients is osteogenic sarcoma. Other relatively common second malignancies include pinealomas, brain tumors, cutaneous melanomas, soft-tissue sarcomas, and primitive unclassifiable tumors (Table 19-6). Estimates suggest that up to 20% of patients who have bilateral retinoblastoma will develop an apparently unrelated neoplasm within 20 years and that up to 40% will develop a third malignancy within 30 years. The prognosis for survival in retinoblastoma patients who later develop sarcomas is less than 50%.

CHAPTER 20

Ocular Involvement in Systemic Malignancies

Secondary Tumors of the Eye

Metastatic Carcinoma

Since the first description in 1872 of a metastatic tumor in the eye of a patient with carcinoma, a large body of literature has indicated that the most common type of intraocular or orbital tumor in adults is metastatic. There are several comprehensive studies of ocular metastatic tumors: some have reported the incidence of tumor metastases in a consecutive series in autopsies, some have dealt with tumor incidence in patients with generalized malignancy, and others have used a clinicopathologic approach. As long-term survival from systemic primary malignancy continues to increase, the ophthalmologist will be confronted with a growing incidence of intraocular and orbital metastatic disease requiring prompt recognition and appropriate diagnostic and therapeutic management.

Metastases to the eye are being diagnosed with increasing frequency for various reasons:

- increasing incidence of certain tumor types that metastasize to the eye (eg, breast, lung)
- prolonged survival of patients with certain cancer types (eg, breast cancer)
- increasing awareness among medical oncologists and ophthalmologists of the pattern of metastatic disease

Primary tumor sites

The vast majority of metastatic solid tumors to the eye are carcinomas from various organs. Cutaneous melanoma rarely metastasizes to the eye. Table 20-1 shows the most common primary tumors that metastasize to the choroid.

Mechanisms of metastasis to the eye

The mechanism of intraocular metastasis depends on hematogenous dissemination of tumor cells. The anatomy of the arterial blood supply to the eye dictates the predilection of tumor cell deposits within the eye. The posterior choroid, with its rich vascular supply, is the most favored site of intraocular metastases, and it is affected 10–20 times more frequently than is the iris or ciliary body. The retina and optic disc, supplied by the single

Table 20-1 Primary Sites of Choroidal Metastasis

Males (*N* = 137)	Females (*N* = 287)
Lung (40%)	Breast (70%)
Unknown (30%)	Lung (10%)
Gastrointestinal (10%)	Unknown (10%)
Kidney (5%)	Others (<5%)
Prostate (5%)	Gastrointestinal (<5%)
Skin (<5%)	Skin (1%)
Others (<5%)	Kidney (<1%)
Breast (1%)	

Modified from Shields CL, Shields JA, Gross NE, et al. Survey of 520 eyes with uveal metastases. *Ophthalmology.* 1997;104:1265–1276.

central retinal artery, are rarely the sole site of involvement. Bilateral ocular involvement has been reported in approximately 25% of cases, and multifocal deposits are frequently seen within the involved eye. Many patients with ocular metastases also have concurrent central nervous system (CNS) metastases.

Clinical evaluation

The clinical features of intraocular metastases depend on the site of involvement. Metastases to the iris and ciliary body usually appear as white or gray-white gelatinous nodules (Figs 20-1, 20-2, 20-3). The clinical features of anterior uveal metastases may include

- iridocyclitis
- secondary glaucoma
- rubeosis iridis

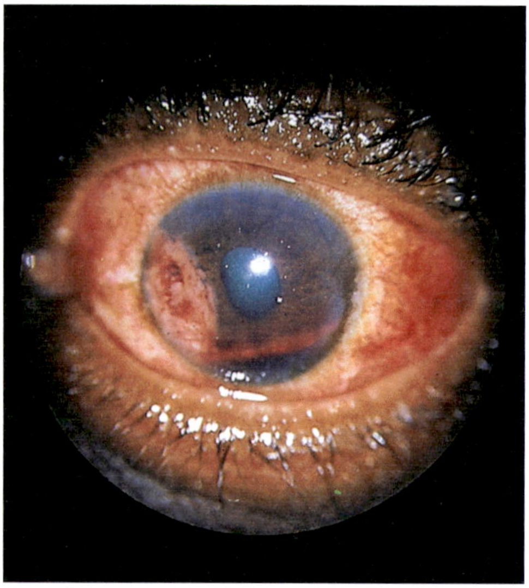

Figure 20-1 Metastasis to the iris associated with hyphema.

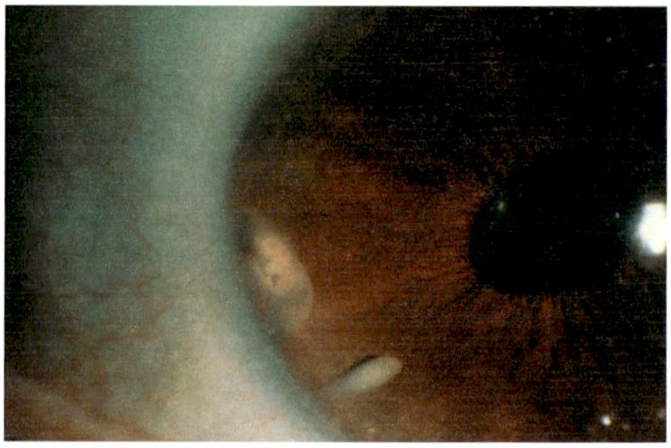

Figure 20-2 Metastasis from breast carcinoma to the iris. *(Courtesy of Timothy G. Murray, MD.)*

- hyphema
- irregular pupil

Anterior segment tumors are best evaluated with slit-lamp biomicroscopy coupled with gonioscopy. High-resolution ultrasound imaging may quantify tumor size and anatomical relationships.

Patients with a tumor in the posterior pole commonly complain of loss of vision. Pain and photopsia may be concurrent symptoms. Indirect binocular ophthalmoscopy may reveal a nonrhegmatogenous (ie, exudative) retinal detachment associated with a placoid amelanotic tumor mass (Figs 20-4, 20-5, 20-6). Multiple or bilateral lesions may be present in approximately 25% of cases, highlighting the importance of close evaluation of the fellow eye. These lesions are usually relatively flat and ill defined, often gray-yellow or yellow-white, with secondary alterations at the level of the retinal pigment epithelium (RPE) presenting as clumps of brown pigment ("leopard spotting"; Fig 20-7).

The mushroom configuration frequently seen in primary choroidal melanoma from breakthrough of the Bruch membrane is rarely present in uveal metastases. The retina overlying the metastasis may appear opaque and become detached. Rapid tumor growth

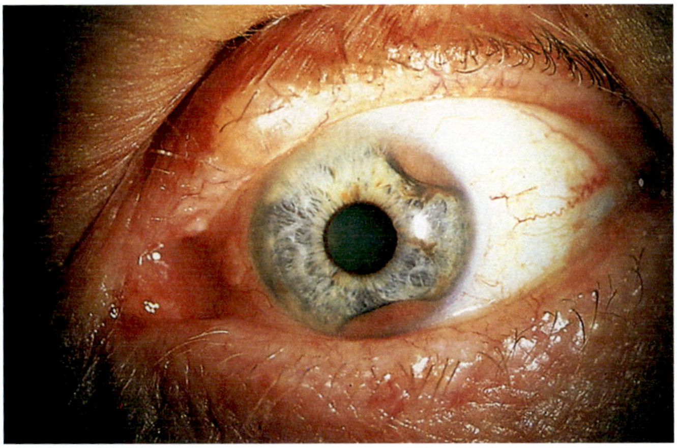

Figure 20-3 Metastatic cutaneous melanoma to the iris. Note both lesions at periphery.

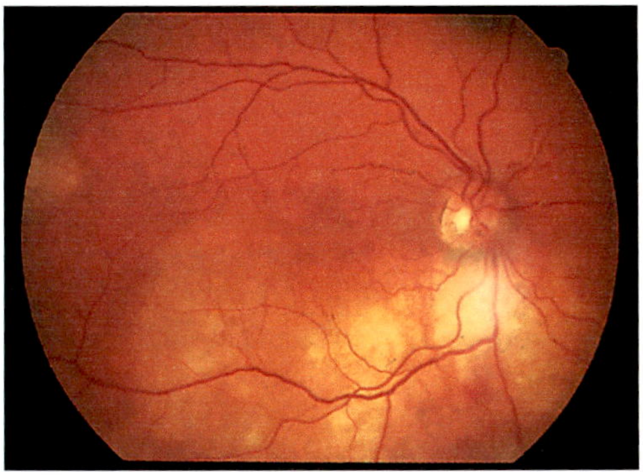

Figure 20-4 Multiple metastatic lesions to the choroid. Note the pale yellow color and relative flatness.

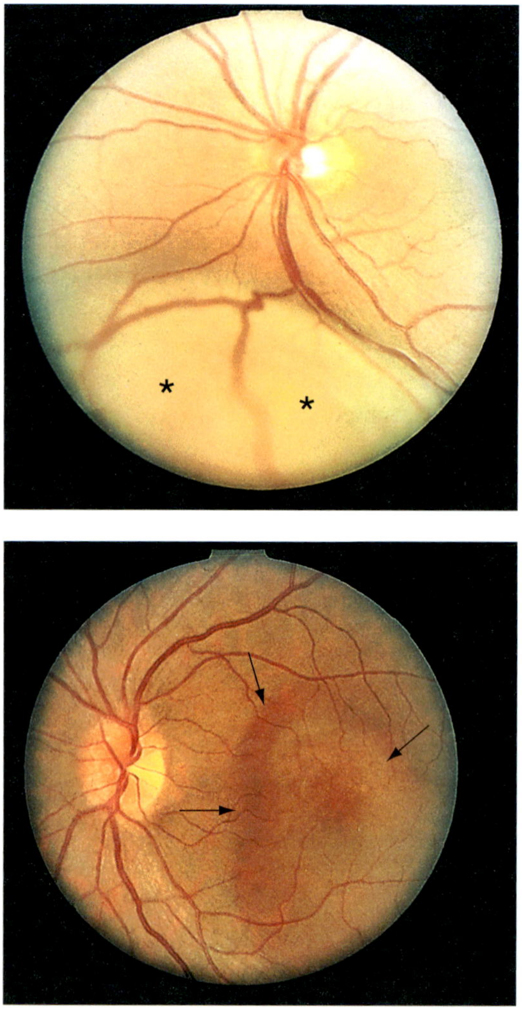

Figure 20-5 A, Metastatic lesion to the choroid inferiorly, associated with bullous retinal detachment *(asterisks).* **B,** Subtle metastatic lesion to the choroid *(arrows),* near the fovea, associated with serous effusion.

with necrosis and uveitis are occasionally observed. Dilated epibulbar vessels may be seen in the quadrant overlying the metastasis. For a differential diagnosis of choroidal metastasis, see Table 20-2.

Ancillary tests

Although *fluorescein angiography* may be helpful in defining the margins of a metastatic tumor, it is typically less useful in differentiating a metastasis from a primary intraocular neoplasm. The double circulation pattern and prominent early choroidal filling often seen in choroidal melanomas are rarely found in metastatic tumors.

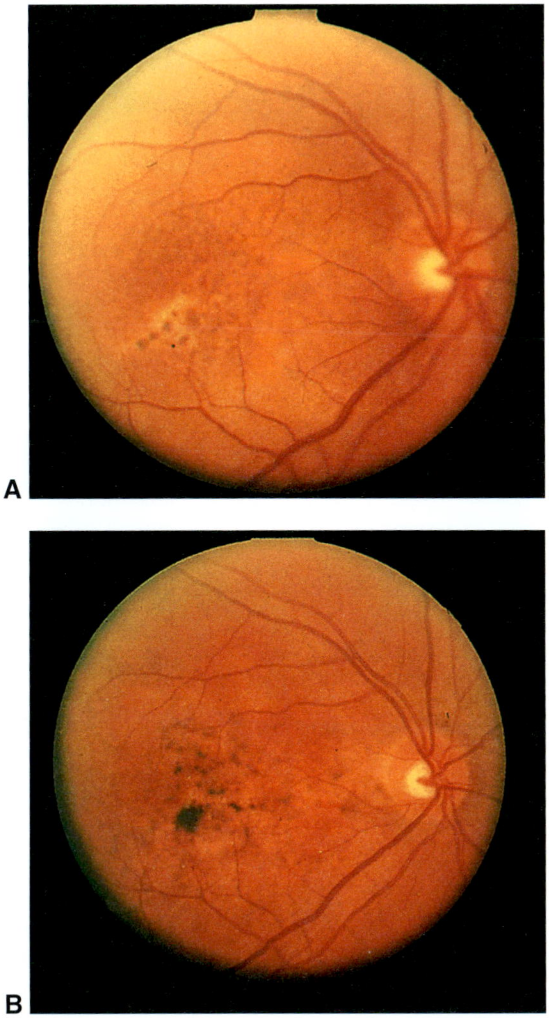

Figure 20-6 **A,** Metastatic carcinoma to the choroid. Vision was reduced to finger counting because of macular involvement. Note irregular pigmentation on surface. **B,** Same eye, 1 month after radiation therapy. Visual acuity has improved to 20/20. Note increased pigmentation, characteristic of irradiation effects.

Ultrasonography is diagnostically valuable in patients with a metastatic tumor. B-scan shows an echogenic choroidal mass with an ill-defined, sometimes lobulated, outline. Overlying secondary retinal detachment is commonly detected in these cases. A-scan demonstrates moderate to high internal reflectivity.

Fine-needle aspiration biopsy may be helpful in rare cases when the diagnosis cannot be established by noninvasive procedures. Although metastatic tumors may recapitulate the histology of the primary tumor, they are often less differentiated. Special histochemical and immunohistochemical stains assist in the diagnosis of metastatic tumors.

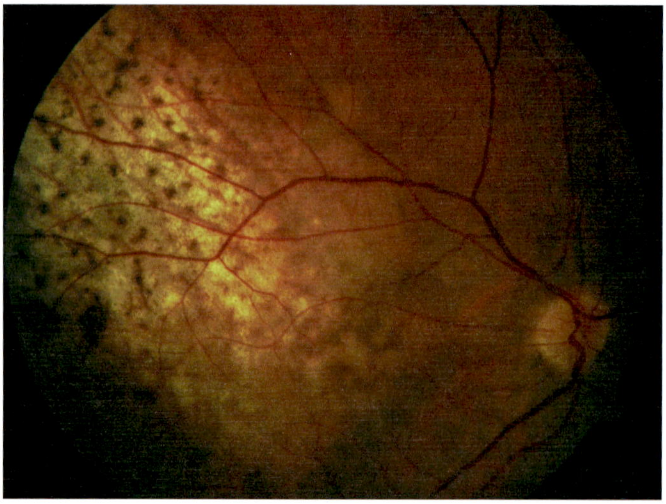

Figure 20-7 Breast metastases, clinical appearance. Note the amelanotic infiltrative choroidal mass with secondary overlying retinal pigment epithelial changes accounting for the characteristic "leopard spots." *(Courtesy of Matthew W. Wilson, MD.)*

Table 20-2 Differential Diagnosis of Choroidal Metastasis

Amelanotic nevus	Vogt-Koyanagi-Harada syndrome
Amelanotic melanoma	Central serous retinopathy
Choroidal hemangioma	Infectious lesions
Choroidal osteoma	Organized subretinal hemorrhage
Choroidal detachment	Extensive neovascular membranes
Posterior scleritis	Rhegmatogenous retinal detachment

Metastases to the optic nerve may produce disc edema, decreased visual acuity, and visual field defects. Because the metastases may involve the parenchyma or the optic nerve sheath, MRI as well as ultrasonography may be valuable in detecting the presence and location of the lesion(s).

Metastases to the retina, which are very rare, appear as white, noncohesive lesions, often distributed in a perivascular location suggestive of cotton-wool spots (Fig 20-8). Because of secondary vitreous seeding of tumor cells, these metastases sometimes resemble retinitis more than they do a true tumor. Vitreous aspirates for cytologic studies may confirm the diagnosis.

Other diagnostic factors

One of the most important diagnostic factors in the evaluation of suspected metastatic tumors is a history of systemic malignancy. More than 90% of patients with uveal metastasis from carcinoma of the breast, for example, have a history of treatment prior to the development of ocular involvement. In the remaining 10% of patients, the primary tumor can usually be diagnosed by breast examination at the time the suspicious ocular lesion is detected. For other patients, however, often there is no prior history of malignancy. This is especially true of patients with ocular metastasis from the lung. A complete systemic

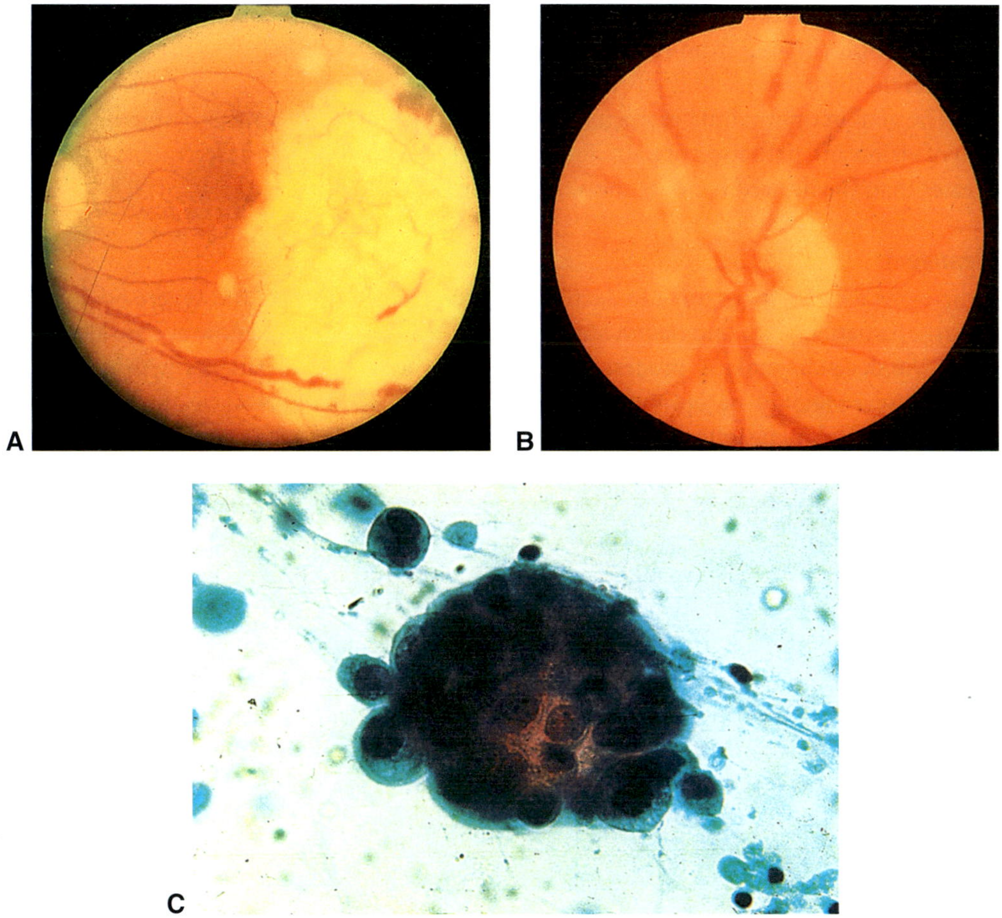

Figure 20-8 A, Metastatic lung carcinoma to the retina, involving the macula. Vision was reduced to finger counting. B, Same eye, showing characteristic perivascular distribution of metastases. C, Vitreous aspirate from same eye, showing an aggregate of tumor cells, characteristic of adenocarcinoma of the lung.

evaluation, a family history, and a history of smoking may alert the ophthalmologist to the suspected site of an occult primary tumor. Any patient with an amelanotic fundus mass suspected of being a metastatic focus should have a thorough systemic evaluation, including imaging of the breast, chest, abdomen, and pelvis. PET-CT scanning may help direct a more targeted evaluation.

Prognosis

The diagnosis of tumor metastatic to the uvea implies a poor prognosis, because widespread dissemination of the primary tumor has usually occurred. In one report, the survival time following the diagnosis of metastasis to the uvea ranged from 1 to 67 months, depending on the primary cancer type. Metastatic carcinoid is associated with long survival times. Patients with breast carcinoma metastatic to the uvea survive an average of 9–13 months after the metastasis is recognized, but cases with long-term survival have now been reported. Shorter survival time is typically seen in patients with lung carcinoma and carcinomas arising from the gastrointestinal or genitourinary tracts, in which metastases herald the presence of the primary tumor.

The goal in ophthalmic management of ocular metastases is preservation or restoration of vision and palliation of pain. Radical surgical procedures and treatments with risks greater than the desired benefits should be avoided.

Treatment

Indications for treatment include decreased vision, pain, diplopia, and severe ocular proptosis. The patient's age and health status and the condition of the fellow eye are also critical in the decision-making process. The treatment modality in patients with metastatic ocular disease should be individually tailored. When ocular metastases are concurrent with widespread metastatic disease, systemic chemotherapy alone or in combination with local therapy is reasonable. In patients manifesting metastases in the eye alone, local therapy modalities may be sufficient, allowing conservation of visual function with minimal systemic morbidity.

Chemotherapy or hormonal therapy for sensitive tumors (eg, breast cancer) may induce a prompt response. In such patients, no additional ocular treatment may be indicated. However, when vision is endangered by choroidal metastases in spite of chemotherapy, additional modalities of local therapy such as external-beam radiation, brachytherapy, laser photocoagulation, or transpupillary thermotherapy may be necessary. Radiotherapy is frequently associated with rapid improvement of the patient's symptoms, along with rapid resolution of exudative retinal detachment and, often, direct reduction in tumor size. Possible adverse effects of the radiation include cataract, radiation retinopathy, and radiation optic neuropathy. Rarely, enucleation is performed because of severe, unrelenting pain.

Amer R, Pe'er J, Chowers I, Anteby I. Treatment options in the management of choroidal metastases. *Ophthalmologica.* 2004;218(6):372–377.

Ferry AP, Font RL. Carcinoma metastatic to the eye and orbit. I. A clinicopathologic study of 227 cases. *Arch Ophthalmol.* 1974;92(4):276–286.

Shields CL, Shields JA, Gross NE, Schwartz GP, Lally SE. Survey of 520 eyes with uveal metastases. *Ophthalmology.* 1997;104(8):1265–1276.

Shields JA, Shields CL, Brotman HK, Carvalho C, Perez N, Eagle RC Jr. Cancer metastatic to the orbit: the 2000 Robert M. Curts lecture. *Ophthal Plast Reconstr Surg.* 2001;17(5):346–354.

Direct Intraocular Extension

Direct extension of extraocular tumors into the eye is rare. Intraocular extension occurs most commonly with conjunctival squamous cell carcinoma and less frequently with conjunctival melanoma and basal cell carcinoma of the eyelid. The sclera is usually an effective barrier against intraocular invasion. Only a small minority of carcinomas of the conjunctiva ever successfully penetrate the globe, but those that do are often variants of squamous cell carcinoma: mucoepidermoid carcinoma or spindle cell variant. These more aggressive neoplasms usually recur several times after local excision before they invade the eye.

Lymphomatous Tumors

Intraocular lymphomas may arise in different parts of the eye, expressing various clinical manifestations. *Primary intraocular lymphoma* (also known as *large cell lymphoma, vitreoretinal lymphoma,* or *retinal lymphoma*), is the most common and most aggressive type of lymphoma involving the eye and is usually associated with primary central nervous system lymphoma (PCNSL). In these cases, the vitreous and retina are involved. Less frequently, the eye can be involved in *systemic/visceral/nodal lymphoma.* In these cases, the uveal tract is more commonly involved, usually in a pattern of metastatic disease. In advanced cases, the intraocular findings of the 2 types may overlap. In recent decades, the incidence of PCNSL has increased significantly in both immunocompetent and immunocompromised persons.

Primary Intraocular Lymphoma

Clinical evaluation

Ocular signs and symptoms may occur before CNS findings. In such cases, the disease may masquerade as a nonspecific uveitis. The onset of bilateral posterior uveitis in patients older than 50 years is suggestive of large cell lymphoma, as is "chronic" uveitis in patients in their fifth to seventh decades. Although 30% of patients present with unilateral involvement, delayed involvement of the second eye occurs in approximately 85% of patients.

Diffuse vitreous cells may be associated with deep subretinal yellow-white infiltrates (Fig 20-9). Often, fine details of the retina are obscured by the density of the vitritis ("headlight in the fog"). Retinal vasculitis and/or vascular occlusion may be observed. The RPE may reveal characteristic clumping overlying the subretinal/sub-RPE infiltrates (see Fig 10-14 and the discussion of histologic findings in Chapter 10). Anterior chamber reaction may be minimal.

Photographic and fluorescein angiographic studies document baseline clinical findings but are rarely helpful in defining a differential diagnosis. Ultrasonographic

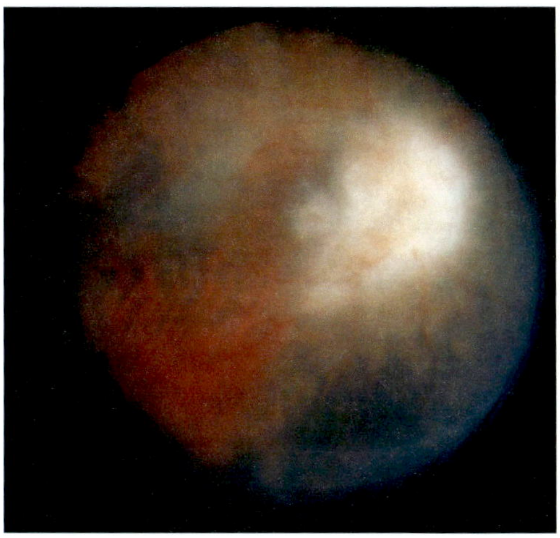

Figure 20-9 Fundus picture of a patient with vitreoretinal lymphoma. Note the vitreous haze, optic disc involvement, and peripapillary subretinal infiltrates. *(Courtesy of Jacob Pe'er, MD.)*

examination may reveal discrete nodular or placoid infiltration of the subretinal space, associated retinal detachment, and vitreous syneresis with increased reflectivity. Clinical history and neurologic evaluation may reveal neurologic deficits in up to 10% of patients, and 60% of patients show concomitant CNS involvement at the time of presentation. If the diagnosis is suspected, neurologic consultation coupled with CT or MRI studies and lumbar puncture should be coordinated with diagnostic vitrectomy.

Pathologic studies

Diagnostic confirmation of ocular involvement requires sampling of the vitreous and, when appropriate, the subretinal space. Coordinated planning with the ophthalmic pathologist prior to surgery regarding sample handling is important. The ophthalmic pathologist should be skilled in the handling of small-volume intraocular specimens and experienced in the evaluation of vitreous samples.

The best approach to pathologic evaluation of the specimen remains controversial. Diagnostic pars plana vitrectomy is indicated to obtain an undiluted or diluted vitreous specimen. If a subretinal nodule is accessible in a region of the retina unlikely to compromise visual function, subretinal aspiration of the lesion can be performed. A single-vitrectomy biopsy may not be adequate, and a second biopsy may be required. Evaluation of the vitreous and subretinal specimen may be performed using cytopathology (see Chapter 10, Fig 10-15), including immunohistochemical studies for subclassification of the cells, flow cytometry, and polymerase chain reaction/fluorescence in situ hybridization (PCR/FISH) analysis for gene rearrangements and the ratio of interleukin-10 (IL-10) to IL-6 (see Chapters 3, 4, and 10).

Preferably, a pathologist familiar with the diagnosis of intraocular large cell lymphoma should evaluate the specimen. If an adequate specimen is obtained, multiple pathologic approaches may be employed. Cytologic evaluation is essential in establishing the diagnosis, with flow cytometry, PCR, and cytokine levels (IL-10/IL-6) serving as ancillary studies. Specimens that reveal malignant lymphocytic cells establish the diagnosis (Fig 20-10), and evaluation of cell surface markers may allow for subclassification of the tumor.

Treatment

Because the blood–ocular barriers may limit penetration of chemotherapeutic agents into the eye, irradiation of the affected eye using fractionated external-beam radiation has remained popular in some centers for treatment of intraocular lymphoma. However, although radiotherapy may induce an ocular remission, the tumor invariably recurs, and further irradiation places the patient at high risk for irreversible vision loss caused by radiation retinopathy. Radiotherapy to the eye is often given with systemic or intrathecal chemotherapy. Some centers use systemic chemotherapy alone, mainly high-dose methotrexate, for the treatment of vitreoretinal lymphoma. However, studies have shown that drug penetration into the retina and vitreous is limited with systemic administration, and recurrence is common. Because of concern about the disadvantages of ocular irradiation and systemic chemotherapy, several groups use intraocular chemotherapy, injecting methotrexate into the vitreous, with very good responses and low recurrence rates. Recently, intravitreal injections of rituximab have been used experimentally. Parallel to the treatment of the intraocular disease, the CNS and/or systemic lymphoma should be treated by a medical oncologist.

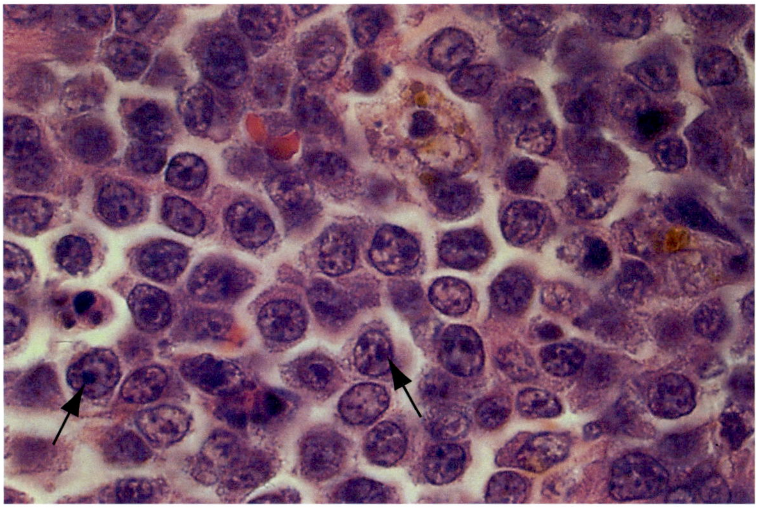

Figure 20-10 Large cell lymphoma, cytology. Note the unusual nuclei and prominent nucleoli *(arrows)* of these neoplastic lymphoid cells obtained by fine-needle aspiration biopsy.

Prognosis

The prognosis for patients with large cell lymphoma is poor, although advances in early diagnosis have produced a cohort of long-term survivors. Serial follow-up with consultative management by an experienced medical oncologist is critical in the management of this disease. Patients with PCNSL should be observed carefully by an ophthalmologist for possible ocular involvement, even after remission of the CNS disease.

Chan CC, Wallace DJ. Intraocular lymphoma: update on diagnosis and management. *Cancer Control.* 2004;11(5):285–295.

Coupland SE, Damato B. Understanding intraocular lymphomas. *Clin Exp Ophthalmol.* 2008; 36(6):564–578.

Frenkel S, Hendler K, Siegal T, Shalom E, Pe'er J. Intravitreal methotrexate for treating vitreoretinal lymphoma. Ten years of experience. *Br J Ophthalmol.* 2008;92(3):383–388.

Uveal Lymphoid Infiltration

Uveal lymphoid infiltration, formerly known as *reactive lymphoid hyperplasia,* typically presents in patients in the sixth decade of life; it can occur at any uveal site. Similar lymphoid proliferation can occur in the conjunctiva and orbit (see also Chapter 5 for conjunctival involvement, Chapter 12 for uveal involvement, and Chapter 14 for orbital involvement).

Clinical evaluation

Patients typically notice painless, progressive vision loss. Ophthalmoscopically, a diffuse or, rarely, nodular amelanotic thickening of the choroid is noted. Exudative retinal detachment and secondary glaucoma may be present in up to 85% of eyes. Frequently, delay between the onset of symptoms and diagnostic intervention is significant.

This rare disorder is characterized pathologically by localized or diffuse infiltration of the uveal tract by lymphoid cells. The etiology is unknown. Clinically, this condition can simulate posterior uveal melanoma, metastatic carcinoma to the uvea, sympathetic ophthalmia, Vogt-Koyanagi-Harada syndrome, and posterior scleritis. Proptosis of the affected eye occurs in up to 15% of patients who develop simultaneous orbital infiltration with benign lymphoid cells. Ultrasonographic testing reveals a diffuse, homogeneous choroidal infiltrate with associated secondary retinal detachment. Extraocular extension or orbital involvement may be best demonstrated with ultrasonography.

Pathologic studies

Biopsy confirmation should be targeted to the most accessible tissue. If extraocular involvement is present, biopsy of the involved conjunctiva or orbit may be considered. Fine-needle aspiration biopsy or pars plana vitrectomy with biopsy may be indicated for isolated uveal involvement. Coordination with the ophthalmic pathologist is crucial to achieve the greatest likelihood of appropriate confirmation and cell marker studies.

Treatment

Historically, eyes with this type of lymphoid infiltration were generally managed by enucleation because of presumed malignancy. Current management emphasizes globe-conserving therapy aimed at preservation of vision. High-dose oral steroids may induce tumor regression and decrease exudative retinal detachment. Early intervention with low-dose ocular and orbital fractionated external-beam radiotherapy may definitively manage the disease.

Prognosis

The prognosis for survival is excellent for patients with uveal lymphoid infiltration, with the rare exception of patients with systemic lymphoma. Preservation of visual function appears related to primary tumor location and secondary sequelae, including exudative retinal detachment or glaucoma. Early intervention appears to enhance the likelihood of vision preservation.

Ocular Manifestations of Leukemia

Ocular involvement with leukemia is common, occurring in as many as 80% of the eyes of patients examined at autopsy. Clinical studies have documented ophthalmic findings in as many as 40% of patients at diagnosis. Patients may be asymptomatic, or they may complain of blurred or decreased vision. Clinically, the retina is the most commonly affected intraocular structure. Leukemic retinopathy is characterized by intraretinal and subhyaloidal hemorrhages, hard exudates, cotton-wool spots, and white-centered retinal hemorrhages (pseudo–Roth spots)—all of which are usually the result of associated anemia, hyperviscosity, and/or thrombocytopenia (Fig 20-11). Leukemic infiltrates appear as yellow deposits in the retina and the subretinal space. Perivascular leukemic infiltrates produce gray-white streaks in the retina. Vitreous involvement by leukemia is rare and most often results from direct extension via retinal hemorrhage. If necessary, a diagnostic vitrectomy can be performed to establish a diagnosis.

Although, clinically, the retina is the most commonly affected ocular structure, histologic studies have shown that the uvea is more commonly affected than the retina. The

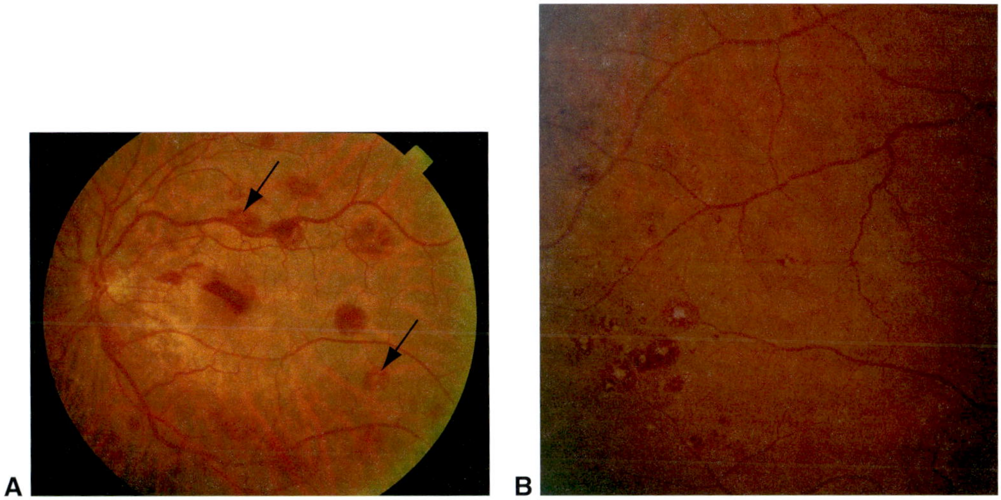

Figure 20-11 Retinal involvement in leukemia. **A,** Leukemic retinopathy. Clinical photograph shows scattered intraretinal hemorrhages, some of which have white centers *(arrows)*. **B,** White-centered hemorrhages. *(Part A courtesy of Robert H. Rosa, Jr, MD; part B courtesy of Jacob Pe'er, MD.)*

uveal tract may serve as a "sanctuary site," predisposing the eye to be the structure in which recurrent disease first manifests clinically. Choroidal infiltrates may be difficult to detect with indirect ophthalmoscopy; they may be better detected on ultrasonography as diffuse thickening of the choroid. Serous retinal detachments may overlie these infiltrates. Leukemic involvement of the iris manifests as a diffuse thickening with loss of the iris crypts, and, in some cases, small nodules may be seen at the margin of the pupil (see Chapter 17, Fig 17-4D). Leukemic cells may invade the anterior chamber, forming a pseudohypopyon. Infiltration of the angle by these cells can give rise to secondary glaucoma.

A patient with leukemic infiltration of the optic nerve (Fig 20-12) may present with severe vision loss and optic nerve edema. One or both eyes may be affected. This is an ophthalmic emergency and requires immediate treatment to preserve as much vision as

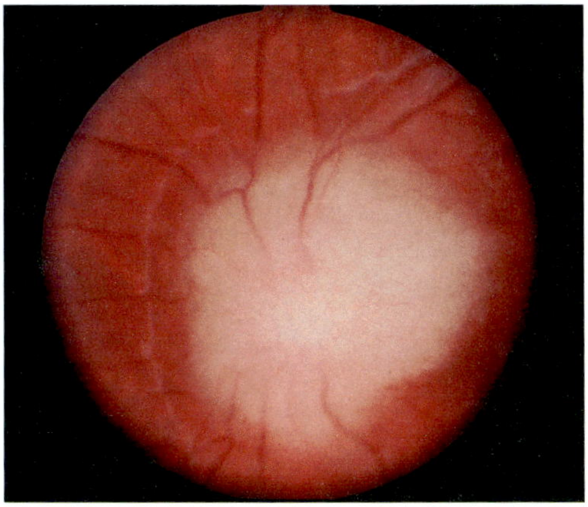

Figure 20-12 Leukemic infiltration of optic nerve. *(Courtesy of Robert H. Rosa, Jr, MD.)*

possible. Systemic and intrathecal combination chemotherapy is needed with or without radiation.

Leukemic infiltrates may also involve the orbital soft tissue, with resultant proptosis. These tumors, which are more common with myelogenous leukemias, are referred to as *granulocytic sarcomas* or *chloromas.* They have a predilection for the lateral and medial walls of the orbit.

Treatment of leukemic involvement of the eye generally consists of low-dose radiation therapy to the eye and systemic chemotherapy. The prognosis for vision depends on the type of leukemia and the extent of ocular involvement.

APPENDIX

American Joint Committee on Cancer (AJCC) Staging Forms, 2010

[The material in this appendix is used with permission from Edge SB, Byrd DR, Compton CC, Fritz AG, Greene FL, Trotti A, eds. Ophthalmic Sites. In: *AJCC Staging Manual.* 7th ed. New York, NY: Springer; 2010:part X, pp 521–589.]

Carcinoma of the Eyelid Staging Form			
Clinical *Extent of disease before any treatment*	**Stage Category Definitions**		**Pathologic** *Extent of disease through completion of definitive surgery*
❏ y clinical—staging completed after neoadjuvant therapy but before subsequent surgery	**Tumor Size:** ________	**Laterality:** ☐ left ☐ right ☐ bilateral	❏ y pathologic—staging completed after neoadjuvant therapy AND subsequent surgery
	Primary Tumor (T)		
❏ **TX**	Primary tumor cannot be assessed.		❏ **TX**
❏ **T0**	No evidence of primary tumor.		❏ **T0**
❏ **Tis**	Carcinoma *in situ.*		❏ **Tis**
❏ **T1**	Tumor 5 mm or less in greatest dimension. Not invading the tarsal plate or eyelid margin.		❏ **T1**
❏ **T2a**	Tumor more than 5 mm, but not more than 10 mm in greatest dimension. Or, any tumor that invades the tarsal plate or eyelid margin.		❏ **T2a**
❏ **T2b**	Tumor more than 10 mm, but not more than 20 mm in greatest dimension. Or, involves full thickness eyelid.		❏ **T2b**
❏ **T3a**	Tumor more than 20 mm in greatest dimension. Or, any tumor that invades adjacent ocular, or orbital structures. Any T with perineural tumor invasion.		❏ **T3a**
❏ **T3b**	Tumor complete resection requires enucleation, exenteration or bone resection.		❏ **T3b**
❏ **T4**	Tumor is not resectable due to extensive invasion of ocular, orbital, craniofacial structures or brain.		❏ **T4**

(Continued)

Carcinoma of the Eyelid Staging Form *(continued)*

Clinical *Extent of disease before any treatment*	**Stage Category Definitions**	**Pathologic** *Extent of disease through completion of definitive surgery*
	Regional Lymph Nodes (N)	
❑ **NX**	Regional lymph nodes cannot be assessed.	❑ **NX**
❑ **N0**	No regional lymph node metastasis, based upon clinical evaluation or imaging.	
	No regional lymph node metastasis, based upon lymph node biopsy.	❑ **N0**
❑ **N1**	Regional lymph node metastasis.	❑ **N1**
	Distant Metastasis (M)	
❑ **M0**	No distant metastasis (no pathologic M0; use clinical M to complete stage group).	
❑ **M1**	Distant metastasis.	❑ **M1**

Anatomic Stage • Prognostic Groups

Clinical				**Pathologic**			
Group	**T**	**N**	**M**	**Group**	**T**	**N**	**M**
❑ 0	Tis	N0	M0	❑ 0	Tis	N0	M0
❑ IA	T1	N0	M0	❑ IA	T1	N0	M0
❑ IB	T2a	N0	M0	❑ IB	T2a	N0	M0
❑ IC	T2b	N0	M0	❑ IC	T2b	N0	M0
❑ II	T3a	N0	M0	❑ II	T3a	N0	M0
❑ IIIA	T3b	N0	M0	❑ IIIA	T3b	N0	M0
❑ IIIB	Any T	N1	M0	❑ IIIB	Any T	N1	M0
❑ IIIC	T4	Any N	M0	❑ IIIC	T4	Any N	M0
❑ IV	Any T	Any N	M1	❑ IV	Any T	Any N	M1
❑ Stage unknown				❑ Stage unknown			

Prognostic Factors (Site-Specific Factors)

Required for Staging: None

Clinically Significant:

Sentinel Lymph Node Biopsy (SLNB) results ________________

Regional nodes identified on clinical or radiographic examination ________

Perineural invasion ________________

Tumor necrosis ________________

Pagetoid spread ________________

More than 3 Mohs micrographic surgical layers required ________

Immunosuppression—patient has HIV ________________

Immunosuppression—history of solid organ transplant or leukemia ________

Prior radiation to the tumor field ________________

Excluding skin cancer, patient has history of two or more carcinomas ________

Patient has Muir-Torre syndrome ________________

Patient has xeroderma pigmentosa ________________

For Eyelid Cutaneous Squamous Cell Carcinoma only:

Required for Staging:

Tumor thickness (in mm) ________________

Clark's Level ________________

Presence/absence of perineural invasion ________________

Primary site location on ear or non-glabrous lip ________________

Histologic grade ________________

Size of largest lymph node metastasis ________________

General Notes:

For identification of special cases of TNM or pTNM classifications, the "m" suffix and "y," "r," and "a" prefixes are used. Although they do not affect the stage grouping, they indicate cases needing separate analysis.

m suffix indicates the presence of multiple primary tumors in a single site and is recorded in parentheses: pT(m)NM.

y prefix indicates those cases in which classification is performed during or following initial multimodality therapy. The cTNM or pTNM category is identified by a "y" prefix. The ycTNM or ypTNM categorizes the extent of tumor actually present at the time of that examination.

Carcinoma of the Eyelid Staging Form *(continued)*

Histologic Grade (G) *(also known as overall grade)*

Grading system	***Grade***
❑ 2 grade system	❑ Grade I or 1
❑ 3 grade system	❑ Grade II or 2
❑ 4 grade system	❑ Grade III or 3
❑ No 2, 3, or 4 grade system is available	❑ Grade IV or 4

Additional Descriptors

Lymphatic Vessel Invasion (L) and Venous Invasion (V) have been combined into Lymph-Vascular Invasion (LVI) for collection by cancer registrars. The College of American Pathologists' (CAP) Checklist should be used as the primary source. Other sources may be used in the absence of a Checklist. Priority is given to positive results.

- ❑ Lymph-Vascular Invasion Not Present (absent)/Not Identified
- ❑ Lymph-Vascular Invasion Present/Identified
- ❑ Not Applicable
- ❑ Unknown/Indeterminate

Residual Tumor (R)

The absence or presence of residual tumor after treatment. In some cases treated with surgery and/or with neoadjuvant therapy there will be residual tumor at the primary site after treatment because of incomplete resection or local and regional disease that extends beyond the limit of ability of resection.

- ❑ RX Presence of residual tumor cannot be assessed
- ❑ R0 No residual tumor
- ❑ R1 Microscopic residual tumor
- ❑ R2 Macroscopic residual tumor

General Notes *(continued)*:

The "y" categorization is not an estimate of tumor prior to multimodality therapy.

r prefix indicates a recurrent tumor when staged after a disease-free interval, and is identified by the "r" prefix: rTNM.

a prefix designates the stage determined at autopsy: aTNM.

surgical margins is data field recorded by registrars describing the surgical margins of the resected primary site specimen as determined only by the pathology report.

neoadjuvant treatment is radiation therapy or systemic therapy (consisting of chemotherapy, hormone therapy, or immunotherapy) administered prior to a definitive surgical procedure. If the surgical procedure is not performed, the administered therapy no longer meets the definition of neoadjuvant therapy.

Histologic Grade (G)

Grade is reported in registry systems by the grade value. A two-grade, three-grade, or four-grade system may be used. If a grading system is not specified, generally the following system is used:

GX Grade cannot be assessed
G1 Well differentiated
G2 Moderately differentiated
G3 Poorly differentiated
G4 Undifferentiated

Histopathologic Type

The primary eyelid carcinoma tumors include the following group and list of histologies:

Basal cell carcinoma
Squamous cell carcinoma
Mucoepidermoid carcinoma
Sebaceous carcinoma
Primary eccrine adenocarcinoma
Primary apocrine adenocarcinoma
Adenoid cystic carcinoma
Merkel cell carcinoma

Carcinoma of the Conjunctiva Staging Form

Clinical *Extent of disease before any treatment*	**Stage Category Definitions**		**Pathologic** *Extent of disease through completion of definitive surgery*
❑ y clinical—staging completed after neoadjuvant therapy but before subsequent surgery	**Tumor Size:** ________	**Laterality:** ☐ left ☐ right ☐ bilateral	❑ y pathologic—staging completed after neoadjuvant therapy AND subsequent surgery
	Primary Tumor (T)		
❑ **TX**	Primary tumor cannot be assessed		❑ **TX**
❑ **T0**	No evidence of primary tumor		❑ **T0**
❑ **Tis**	Carcinoma *in situ*		❑ **Tis**
❑ **T1**	Tumor 5 mm or less in greatest dimension		❑ **T1**
❑ **T2**	Tumor more than 5 mm in greatest dimension, without invasion of adjacent structures		❑ **T2**
❑ **T3**	Tumor invades adjacent structures (excluding the orbit)		❑ **T3**
❑ **T4**	Tumor invades the orbit with or without further extension		❑ **T4**
❑ **T4a**	Tumor invades orbital soft tissues, without bone invasion		❑ **T4a**
❑ **T4b**	Tumor invades bone		❑ **T4b**
❑ **T4c**	Tumor invades adjacent paranasal sinuses		❑ **T4c**
❑ **T4d**	Tumor invades brain		❑ **T4d**
	Regional Lymph Nodes (N)		
❑ **NX**	Regional lymph nodes cannot be assessed		❑ **NX**
❑ **N0**	No regional lymph node metastasis		❑ **N0**
❑ **N1**	Regional lymph node metastasis		❑ **N1**
	Distant Metastasis (M)		
❑ **M0**	No distant metastasis (no pathologic M0; use clinical M to complete stage group)		
❑ **M1**	Distant metastasis		❑ **M1**

Anatomic Stage • Prognostic Groups

Clinical	**Pathologic**
No stage grouping is presently recommended	No stage grouping is presently recommended

Prognostic Factors (Site-Specific Factors)

Required for Staging: None

Clinically Significant: Ki-67 growth fraction ________________

Histologic Grade (G) *(also known as overall grade)*

Grading system	***Grade***
❑ 2 grade system	❑ Grade I or 1
❑ 3 grade system	❑ Grade II or 2
❑ 4 grade system	❑ Grade III or 3
❑ No 2, 3, or 4 grade system is available	❑ Grade IV or 4

General Notes:

For identification of special cases of TNM or pTNM classifications, the "m" suffix and "y," "r," and "a" prefixes are used. Although they do not affect the stage grouping, they indicate cases needing separate analysis.

m suffix indicates the presence of multiple primary tumors in a single site and is recorded in parentheses: pT(m)NM.

Carcinoma of the Conjunctiva Staging Form *(continued)*

Additional Descriptors

Lymphatic Vessel Invasion (L) and Venous Invasion (V) have been combined into Lymph-Vascular Invasion (LVI) for collection by cancer registrars. The College of American Pathologists' (CAP) Checklist should be used as the primary source. Other sources may be used in the absence of a Checklist. Priority is given to positive results.

- ❑ Lymph-Vascular Invasion Not Present (absent)/Not Identified
- ❑ Lymph-Vascular Invasion Present/Identified
- ❑ Not Applicable
- ❑ Unknown/Indeterminate

Residual Tumor (R)

The absence or presence of residual tumor after treatment. In some cases treated with surgery and/or with neoadjuvant therapy there will be residual tumor at the primary site after treatment because of incomplete resection or local and regional disease that extends beyond the limit of ability of resection.

- ❑ RX Presence of residual tumor cannot be assessed
- ❑ R0 No residual tumor
- ❑ R1 Microscopic residual tumor
- ❑ R2 Macroscopic residual tumor

General Notes *(continued)*:

y prefix indicates those cases in which classification is performed during or following initial multimodality therapy. The cTNM or pTNM category is identified by a "y" prefix. The ycTNM or ypTNM categorizes the extent of tumor actually present at the time of that examination. The "y" categorization is not an estimate of tumor prior to multimodality therapy.

r prefix indicates a recurrent tumor when staged after a disease-free interval, and is identified by the "r" prefix: rTNM.

a prefix designates the stage determined at autopsy: aTNM.

surgical margins is data field recorded by registrars describing the surgical margins of the resected primary site specimen as determined only by the pathology report.

neoadjuvant treatment is radiation therapy or systemic therapy (consisting of chemotherapy, hormone therapy, or immunotherapy) administered prior to a definitive surgical procedure. If the surgical procedure is not performed, the administered therapy no longer meets the definition of neoadjuvant therapy.

Histopathologic Type

The classification applies only to carcinoma of the conjunctiva.

Conjunctival intraepithelial neoplasia (CIN) including in situ squamous cell carcinoma
Squamous cell carcinoma
Mucoepidermoid carcinoma
Spindle cell carcinoma
Sebaceous gland carcinoma including pagetoid (conjunctival) spread
Basal cell carcinoma

Histologic Grade (G)

Grade is reported in registry systems by the grade value. A two-grade, three-grade, or four-grade system may be used. If a grading system is not specified, generally the following system is used:

GX Grade cannot be assessed
G1 Well differentiated
G2 Moderately differentiated
G3 Poorly differentiated
G4 Undifferentiated

Malignant Melanoma of the Conjunctiva Staging Form			
Clinical *Extent of disease before any treatment*	**Stage Category Definitions**		**Pathologic** *Extent of disease through completion of definitive surgery*
❑ y clinical—staging completed after neoadjuvant therapy but before subsequent surgery	**Tumor Size:** ______	**Laterality:** ☐ left ☐ right ☐ bilateral	❑ y pathologic—staging completed after neoadjuvant therapy AND subsequent surgery
	Primary Tumor (T) Quadrants are defined by clock hour, starting at the limbus (eg, 6, 9, 12, 3) extending from the central cornea to and beyond the eyelid margins. This will bisect the caruncle.		
❑ **TX**	Primary tumor cannot be assessed		❑ **TX**
❑ **T0**	No evidence of primary tumor		❑ **T0**
❑ **Tis**	Melanoma confined to the conjunctival epithelium		❑ **Tis**
❑ **T1**	Malignant conjunctival melanoma of the bulbar conjunctiva		
❑ **T1a**	Less than or equal to 1 quadrant*		
pT1a	Melanoma of the bulbar conjunctiva not more than 0.5 mm in thickness with invasion of the substantia propria		❑ **pT1a**
❑ **T1b**	More than 1 but less than or equal to 2 quadrants		
pT1b	Melanoma of the bulbar conjunctiva more than 0.5 mm but not more than 1.5 mm in thickness with invasion of the substantia propria		❑ **pT1b**
❑ **T1c**	More than 2 but less than or equal to 3 quadrants		
pT1c	Melanoma of the bulbar conjunctiva greater than 1.5 mm in thickness with invasion of the substantia propria		❑ **pT1c**
❑ **T1d**	Greater than 3 quadrants		
❑ **T2**	Malignant conjunctival melanoma of the non-bulbar (palpebral, forniceal, caruncular)		
❑ **T2a**	Non-caruncular, less than or equal to 1 quadrant		
pT2a	Melanoma of the palpebral, forniceal or caruncular conjunctiva not more than 0.5 mm in thickness with invasion of the substantia propria		❑ **pT2a**
❑ **T2b**	Non-caruncular, greater than 1 quadrant		
pT2b	Melanoma more than 0.5 but not greater than 1.5 mm in thickness with invasion of the substantia propria		❑ **pT2b**
❑ **T2c**	Any caruncular, less than or equal to 1 quadrant		
pT2c	Melanoma of the palpebral, forniceal or caruncular conjunctiva greater than 1.5 mm in thickness with invasion of the substantia propria		❑ **pT2c**
❑ **T2d**	Any caruncular, greater than 1 quadrant		

Malignant Melanoma of the Conjunctiva Staging Form *(continued)*

Clinical *Extent of disease before any treatment*	**Stage Category Definitions**	**Pathologic** *Extent of disease through completion of definitive surgery*
❑ **T3**	Any malignant conjunctival melanoma with local invasion	
pT3	Melanoma invades the eye, eyelid, nasolacrimal system, sinuses or orbit	❑ **pT3**
❑ **T3a**	Globe	
❑ **T3b**	Eyelid	
❑ **T3c**	Orbit	
❑ **T3d**	Sinus	
❑ **T4**	Tumor invades the central nervous system	
pT4	Melanoma invades the central nervous system	❑ **pT4**
	*pT(is) Melanoma *in situ* (includes the term primary acquired melanosis) with atypia replacing greater than 75% of the normal epithelial thickness, with cytologic features of epithelioid cells, including abundant cytoplasm, vesicular nuclei or prominent nucleoli, and/or presence of intraepithelial nests of atypical cells.	
	Regional Lymph Nodes (N)	
	Clinical	
❑ **NX**	Regional lymph nodes cannot be assessed	❑ **NX**
❑ **N0a (biopsy)**	No regional lymph node metastasis, biopsy performed	❑ **N0**
❑ **N0b (no biopsy)**	No regional lymph node metastasis, biopsy not performed	
❑ **N1**	Regional lymph node metastasis	❑ **N1**
	Distant Metastasis (M)	
❑ **M0**	No distant metastasis (no pathologic M0; use clinical M to complete stage group)	
❑ **M1**	Distant metastasis	❑ **M1**

Anatomic Stage • Prognostic Grouping

Clinical	**Pathologic**
No stage grouping is presently recommended	No stage grouping is presently recommended

Prognostic Factors (Site-Specific Factors)

Required for Staging: None

Clinically Significant: Measured thickness (depth) ____________

Histologic Grade (G) *(also known as overall grade)*

Grading system	***Grade***
❑ 2 grade system	❑ Grade I or 1
❑ 3 grade system	❑ Grade II or 2
❑ 4 grade system	❑ Grade III or 3
❑ No 2, 3, or 4 grade system is available	❑ Grade IV or 4

General Notes:

For identification of special cases of TNM or pTNM classifications, the "m" suffix and "y," "r," and "a" prefixes are used. Although they do not affect the stage grouping, they indicate cases needing separate analysis.

m suffix indicates the presence of multiple primary tumors in a single site and is recorded in parentheses: pT(m)NM.

(Continued)

Malignant Melanoma of the Conjunctiva Staging Form *(continued)*	
Additional Descriptors ***Lymphatic Vessel Invasion (L) and Venous Invasion (V)*** have been combined into Lymph-Vascular Invasion (LVI) for collection by cancer registrars. The College of American Pathologists' (CAP) Checklist should be used as the primary source. Other sources may be used in the absence of a Checklist. Priority is given to positive results. ❑ Lymph-Vascular Invasion Not Present (absent)/Not Identified ❑ Lymph-Vascular Invasion Present/Identified ❑ Not Applicable ❑ Unknown/Indeterminate ***Residual Tumor (R)*** The absence or presence of residual tumor after treatment. In some cases treated with surgery and/or with neoadjuvant therapy there will be residual tumor at the primary site after treatment because of incomplete resection or local and regional disease that extends beyond the limit of ability of resection. ❑ RX Presence of residual tumor cannot be assessed ❑ R0 No residual tumor ❑ R1 Microscopic residual tumor ❑ R2 Macroscopic residual tumor	**General Notes** *(continued):* **y prefix** indicates those cases in which classification is performed during or following initial multimodality therapy. The cTNM or pTNM category is identified by a "y" prefix. The ycTNM or ypTNM categorizes the extent of tumor actually present at the time of that examination. The "y" categorization is not an estimate of tumor prior to multimodality therapy. **r prefix** indicates a recurrent tumor when staged after a disease-free interval, and is identified by the "r" prefix: rTNM. **a prefix** designates the stage determined at autopsy: aTNM. **surgical margins** is data field recorded by registrars describing the surgical margins of the resected primary site specimen as determined only by the pathology report. **neoadjuvant treatment** is radiation therapy or systemic therapy (consisting of chemotherapy, hormone therapy, or immunotherapy) administered prior to a definitive surgical procedure. If the surgical procedure is not performed, the administered therapy no longer meets the definition of neoadjuvant therapy.

Histopathologic Type

This categorization applies only to melanoma of the conjunctiva.

Histologic Grade (G)

Histologic grade represents the origin of the primary tumor.

- GX Origin cannot be assessed
- G0 Primary acquired melanosis without cellular atypia
- G1 Conjunctival nevus
- G2 Primary acquired melanosis with cellular atypia (epithelial disease only)
- G3 Primary acquired melanosis with epithelial cellular atypia and invasive melanoma
- G4 De novo malignant melanoma

Malignant Melanoma of the Uvea Staging Form			
Clinical *Extent of disease before any treatment*	**Stage Category Definitions**		**Pathologic** *Extent of disease through completion of definitive surgery*
❑ y clinical—staging completed after neoadjuvant therapy but before subsequent surgery	**Tumor Size:** ________	**Laterality:** ☐ left ☐ right ☐ bilateral	❑ y pathologic—staging completed after neoadjuvant therapy AND subsequent surgery
	Primary Tumor (T)		
	All Uveal Melanomas		
❑ **TX**	Primary tumor cannot be assessed		❑ **TX**
❑ **T0**	No evidence of primary tumor		❑ **T0**
	Iris*		
❑ **T1**	Tumor limited to the iris		❑ **T1**
❑ **T1a**	Tumor limited to the iris not more than 3 clock hours in size		❑ **T1a**
❑ **T1b**	Tumor limited to the iris more than 3 clock hours in size		❑ **T1b**
❑ **T1c**	Tumor limited to the iris with secondary glaucoma		❑ **T1c**
❑ **T2**	Tumor confluent with or extending into the ciliary body, choroid or both		❑ **T2**
❑ **T2a**	Tumor confluent with or extending into the ciliary body, choroid or both, with secondary glaucoma		❑ **T2a**
❑ **T3**	Tumor confluent with or extending into the ciliary body, choroid or both, with scleral extension		❑ **T3**
❑ **T3a**	Tumor confluent with or extending into the ciliary body, choroid or both, with scleral extension and secondary glaucoma		❑ **T3a**
❑ **T4**	Tumor with extrascleral extension		❑ **T4**
❑ **T4a**	Tumor with extrascleral extension less than or equal to 5 mm in diameter		❑ **T4a**
❑ **T4b**	Tumor with extrascleral extension more than 5 mm in diameter		❑ **T4b**
	*Iris melanomas originate from, and are predominantly located in, this region of the uvea. If less than half of the tumor volume is located within the iris, the tumor may have originated in the ciliary body and consideration should be given to classifying it accordingly.		
	Ciliary Body and Choroid *(see Figure below)*		
	Primary ciliary body and choroidal melanomas are classified according to the four tumor size categories below:		
❑ **T1**	Tumor size category 1		❑ **T1**
❑ **T1a**	Tumor size category 1 without ciliary body involvement and extraocular extension		❑ **T1a**

(Continued)

Malignant Melanoma of the Uvea Staging Form *(continued)*		
Clinical *Extent of disease before any treatment*	**Stage Category Definitions**	**Pathologic** *Extent of disease through completion of definitive surgery*
❑ **T1b**	Tumor size category 1 with ciliary body involvement	❑ **T1b**
❑ **T1c**	Tumor size category 1 without ciliary body involvement but with extraocular extension less than or equal to 5 mm in diameter	❑ **T1c**
❑ **T1d**	Tumor size category 1 with ciliary body involvement and extraocular extension less than or equal to 5 mm in diameter	❑ **T1d**
❑ **T2**	Tumor size category 2	❑ **T2**
❑ **T2a**	Tumor size category 2 without ciliary body involvement and extraocular extension	❑ **T2a**
❑ **T2b**	Tumor size category 2 with ciliary body involvement	❑ **T2b**
❑ **T2c**	Tumor size category 2 without ciliary body involvement but with extraocular extension less than or equal to 5 mm in diameter	❑ **T2c**
❑ **T2d**	Tumor size category 2 with ciliary body involvement and extraocular extension less than or equal to 5 mm in diameter	❑ **T2d**
❑ **T3**	Tumor size category 3	❑ **T3**
❑ **T3a**	Tumor size category 3 without ciliary body involvement and extraocular extension	❑ **T3a**
❑ **T3b**	Tumor size category 3 with ciliary body involvement	❑ **T3b**
❑ **T3c**	Tumor size category 3 without ciliary body involvement but with extraocular extension less than or equal to 5 mm in diameter	❑ **T3c**
❑ **T3d**	Tumor size category 3 with ciliary body involvement and extraocular extension less than or equal to 5 mm in diameter	❑ **T3d**
❑ **T4**	Tumor size category 4	❑ **T4**
❑ **T4a**	Tumor size category 4 without ciliary body involvement and extraocular extension	❑ **T4a**
❑ **T4b**	Tumor size category 4 with ciliary body involvement	❑ **T4b**
❑ **T4c**	Tumor size category 4 without ciliary body involvement but with extraocular extension less than or equal to 5 mm in diameter	❑ **T4c**
❑ **T4d**	Tumor size category 4 with ciliary body involvement and extraocular extension less than or equal to 5 mm in diameter	❑ **T4d**
❑ **T4e**	Any size tumor category with extraocular extension more than 5 mm in diameter	❑ **T4e**
	*__Clinical:__ In clinical practice, the largest tumor basal diameter may be estimated in optic disc diameters (dd, average: 1 dd = 1.5 mm). Tumor	

Malignant Melanoma of the Uvea Staging Form *(continued)*

Clinical *Extent of disease before any treatment*	**Stage Category Definitions**	**Pathologic** *Extent of disease through completion of definitive surgery*
	thickness may be estimated in diopters (average: 2.5 diopters = 1 mm). However, techniques such as ultrasonography and fundus photography are used to provide more accurate measurements. Ciliary body involvement can be evaluated by the slit-lamp, ophthalmoscopy, gonioscopy and transillumination. However, high frequency ultrasonography (ultrasound biomicroscopy) is used for more accurate assessment. Extension through the sclera is evaluated visually before and during surgery, and with ultrasonography, computed tomography or magnetic resonance imaging. †**Pathologic:** When histopathologic measurements are recorded after fixation, tumor diameter and thickness may be underestimated because of tissue shrinkage.	
	Regional Lymph Nodes (N)	
❑ **NX**	Regional lymph nodes cannot be assessed	❑ **NX**
❑ **N0**	No regional lymph node metastasis	❑ **N0**
❑ **N1**	Regional lymph node metastasis	❑ **N1**
	Distant Metastasis (M)	
❑ **M0**	No distant metastasis (no pathologic M0; use clinical M to complete stage group)	
❑ **M1**	Distant metastasis	❑ **M1**
❑ **M1a**	Largest diameter of the largest metastasis ≤3 cm	❑ **M1a**
❑ **M1b**	Largest diameter of the largest metastasis 3.1–8.0 cm	❑ **M1b**
❑ **M1c**	Largest diameter of the largest metastasis 8.1 cm or more	❑ **M1c**

Thickness (mm)	≤3.0	3.1–6.0	6.1–9.0	9.1–12.0	12.1–15.0	15.1–18.0	>18.0
>15.0					4	4	4
12.1–15.0				3	3	4	4
9.1–12.0		3	3	3	3	3	4
6.1–9.0	2	2	2	2	3	3	4
3.1–6.0	1	1	1	2	2	3	4
≤3.0	1	1	1	1	2	2	4

Largest basal diameter (mm)

Classification for ciliary body and choroid uveal melanoma based on thickness and diameter.

(Continued)

Malignant Melanoma of the Uvea Staging Form *(continued)*

Anatomic Stage • Prognostic Grouping

Clinical

Group	T	N	M
❑ I	T1a	N0	M0
❑ IIA	T1b–d	N0	M0
	T2a	N0	M0
❑ IIB	T2b	N0	M0
	T3a	N0	M0
❑ IIIA	T2c–d	N0	M0
	T3b–c	N0	M0
	T4a	N0	M0
❑ IIIB	T3d	N0	M0
	T4b–c	N0	M0
❑ IIIC	T4d–e	N0	M0
❑ IV	Any T	N1	M0
	Any T	Any N	M1a–c
❑ Stage unknown			

Pathologic

Group	T	N	M
❑ I	T1a	N0	M0
❑ IIA	T1b–d	N0	M0
	T2a	N0	M0
❑ IIB	T2b	N0	M0
	T3a	N0	M0
❑ IIIA	T2c–d	N0	M0
	T3b–c	N0	M0
	T4a	N0	M0
❑ IIIB	T3d	N0	M0
	T4b–c	N0	M0
❑ IIIC	T4d–e	N0	M0
❑ IV	Any T	N1	M0
	Any T	Any N	M1a–c
❑ Stage unknown			

Prognostic Factors (Site-Specific Factors)

Required for Staging: Tumor height and largest diameter

Clinically Significant:

Measured thickness (depth) ____________

Chromosomal alterations ____________

Gene expression profile ____________

Positron emission tomography/computed tomography ____________

Confocal indocyanine green angiography ____________

Mitotic count per 40 high power fields (HPF) ____________

Mean diameter of the ten largest nucleoli (MLN) ____________

Presence of extravascular matrix patterns ____________

Microvascular density (MVD) ____________

Insulin-like growth factor 1 receptor (IGF1-R) ____________

Tumor-infiltrating lymphocytes ____________

Tumor-infiltrating macrophages ____________

HLA Class I expression ____________

Histologic Grade (G) *(also known as overall grade)*

Grading system	***Grade***
❑ 2 grade system	❑ Grade I or 1
❑ 3 grade system	❑ Grade II or 2
❑ 4 grade system	❑ Grade III or 3
❑ No 2, 3, or 4 grade system is available	❑ Grade IV or 4

Additional Descriptors

Lymphatic Vessel Invasion (L) and Venous Invasion (V) have been combined into Lymph-Vascular Invasion (LVI) for collection by cancer registrars. The College of American Pathologists' (CAP) Checklist should be used as the primary source. Other sources may be used in the absence of a Checklist. Priority is given to positive results.

- ❑ Lymph-Vascular Invasion Not Present (absent)/Not Identified
- ❑ Lymph-Vascular Invasion Present/Identified
- ❑ Not Applicable
- ❑ Unknown/Indeterminate

General Notes:

For identification of special cases of TNM or pTNM classifications, the "m" suffix and "y," "r," and "a" prefixes are used. Although they do not affect the stage grouping, they indicate cases needing separate analysis.

m suffix indicates the presence of multiple primary tumors in a single site and is recorded in parentheses: pT(m)NM.

y prefix indicates those cases in which classification is performed during or following initial multimodality therapy. The cTNM or pTNM category is identified by a "y" prefix. The ycTNM or ypTNM categorizes the extent of tumor actually present at the time of that examination. The "y" categorization is not an estimate of tumor prior to multimodality therapy.

r prefix indicates a recurrent tumor when staged after a disease-free interval, and is identified by the "r" prefix: rTNM.

a prefix designates the stage determined at autopsy: aTNM.

surgical margins is data field recorded by registrars describing the surgical margins of the resected primary site specimen as determined only by the pathology report.

Malignant Melanoma of the Uvea Staging Form *(continued)*	
Residual Tumor (R) The absence or presence of residual tumor after treatment. In some cases treated with surgery and/or with neoadjuvant therapy there will be residual tumor at the primary site after treatment because of incomplete resection or local and regional disease that extends beyond the limit of ability of resection. ❏ RX Presence of residual tumor cannot be assessed ❏ R0 No residual tumor ❏ R1 Microscopic residual tumor ❏ R2 Macroscopic residual tumor	**General Notes** *(continued):* **neoadjuvant treatment** is radiation therapy or systemic therapy (consisting of chemotherapy, hormone therapy, or immunotherapy) administered prior to a definitive surgical procedure. If the surgical procedure is not performed, the administered therapy no longer meets the definition of neoadjuvant therapy.

Histopathologic Type

The histopathologic types are as follows:

Spindle cell melanoma (greater than 90% spindle cells)
Mixed cell melanoma (>10% epithelioid cells and <90% spindle cells)
Epithelioid cell melanoma (greater than 90% epithelioid cells)

Histologic Grade (G)*

GX Grade cannot be assessed
G1 Spindle cell melanoma
G2 Mixed cell melanoma
G3 Epithelioid cell melanoma

**Note:* Because of general lack of agreement regarding which proportion of epithelioid cells classifies a tumor as mixed and epithelioid in type, some ophthalmic pathologists currently combine grades 2 and 3 (nonspindle, epithelioid cells detected) and contrast them with grade 1 (spindle, no epithelioid cells detected).

Retinoblastoma Staging Form			
Clinical *Extent of disease before any treatment*	**Stage Category Definitions**		**Pathologic** *Extent of disease through completion of definitive surgery*
❏ y clinical—staging completed after neoadjuvant therapy but before subsequent surgery	**Tumor Size:** ________	**Laterality:** ☐ left ☐ right ☐ bilateral	❏ y pathologic—staging completed after neoadjuvant therapy AND subsequent surgery
	Primary Tumor (T)		
❏ **TX**	Primary tumor cannot be assessed.		❏ **pTX**
❏ **T0**	No evidence of primary tumor.		❏ **pT0**
❏ **T1**	Tumors no more than ⅔ the volume of the eye with no vitreous or subretinal seeding.		
pT1	Tumor confined to eye with no optic nerve or choroidal invasion.		❏ **pT1**
❏ **T1a**	No tumor in either eye is greater than 3 mm in largest dimension or located closer than 1.5 mm to the optic nerve or fovea.		
❏ **T1b**	At least one tumor is greater than 3 mm in largest dimension or located closer than 1.5 mm to the optic nerve or fovea. No retinal detachment or subretinal fluid beyond 5 mm from the base of the tumor.		
❏ **T1c**	At least one tumor is greater than 3 mm in largest dimension or located closer than 1.5 mm to the optic nerve or fovea. With retinal detachment or subretinal fluid beyond 5 mm from the base of the tumor.		
❏ **T2**	Tumors no more than ⅔ the volume of the eye with vitreous or subretinal seeding. Can have retinal detachment.		
pT2	Tumor with minimal optic nerve and/or choroidal invasion.		❏ **pT2**
❏ **T2a**	Focal vitreous and/or subretinal seeding of fine aggregates of tumor cells is present, but no large clumps or "snowballs" of tumor cells.		
pT2a	Tumor superficially invades optic nerve head but does not extend past lamina cribrosa *or* tumor exhibits focal choroidal invasion.		❏ **pT2a**
❏ **T2b**	Massive vitreous and/or subretinal seeding is present, defined as diffuse clumps or "snowballs" of tumor cells.		
pT2b	Tumor superficially invades optic nerve head but does not extend past lamina cribrosa *and* exhibits focal choroidal invasion.		❏ **pT2b**
❏ **T3**	Severe intraocular disease.		
pT3	Tumor with significant optic nerve and/or choroidal invasion.		❏ **pT3**
❏ **T3a**	Tumor fills more than ⅔ of the eye.		
pT3a	Tumor invades optic nerve past lamina cribrosa but not to surgical resection line *or* tumor exhibits massive choroidal invasion.		❏ **pT3a**

Retinoblastoma Staging Form *(continued)*

Clinical *Extent of disease before any treatment*	**Stage Category Definitions**	**Pathologic** *Extent of disease through completion of definitive surgery*
❑ **T3b**	One or more complications present, which may include tumor-associated neovascular or angle closure glaucoma, tumor extension into the anterior segment, hyphema, vitreous hemorrhage, or orbital cellulitis.	
pT3b	Tumor invades optic nerve past lamina cribrosa but not to surgical resection line *and* exhibits massive choroidal invasion.	❑ **pT3b**
❑ **T4**	Extraocular disease detected by imaging studies.	
pT4	Tumor invades optic nerve to resection line or exhibits extraocular extension elsewhere.	❑ **pT4**
❑ **T4a**	Invasion of optic nerve.	
pT4a	Tumor invades optic nerve to resection line but no extraocular extension identified.	❑ **pT4a**
❑ **T4b**	Invasion into the orbit.	
pT4b	Tumor invades optic nerve to resection line and extraocular extension identified.	❑ **pT4b**
❑ **T4c**	Intracranial extension not past chiasm.	
❑ **T4d**	Intracranial extension past chiasm.	
	Regional Lymph Nodes (N)	
	Clinical	
❑ **NX**	Regional lymph nodes cannot be assessed.	❑ **NX**
❑ **N0**	No regional lymph node involvement.	❑ **N0**
❑ **N1**	Regional lymph node involvement (preauricular, cervical, submandibular).	❑ **N1**
❑ **N2**	Distant lymph node involvement.	❑ **N2**
	Distant Metastasis (M)	
	Clinical	
❑ **M0**	No distant metastasis (no pathologic M0; use clinical M to complete stage group).	
❑ **M1**	Systemic metastasis.	
❑ **M1a**	Single lesion to sites other than CNS.	
❑ **M1b**	Multiple lesions to sites other than CNS.	
❑ **M1c**	Prechiasmatic CNS lesion(s).	
❑ **M1d**	Postchiasmatic CNS lesion(s).	
❑ **M1e**	Leptomeningeal and/or CSF involvement.	
	Pathologic	
	Metastasis to sites other than CNS.	❑ **M1**
	Single lesion.	❑ **M1a**
	Multiple lesions.	❑ **M1b**
	CNS metastasis.	❑ **M1c**
	Discrete mass(es) without leptomeningeal and/or CSF involvement.	❑ **M1d**
	Leptomeningeal and/or CSF involvement.	❑ **M1e**

Anatomic Stage • Prognostic Groups

Clinical	**Pathologic**
No stage grouping is presently recommended	No stage grouping is presently recommended

(Continued)

Retinoblastoma Staging Form *(continued)*

Prognostic Factors (Site-Specific Factors)

Required for Staging: None

Clinically Significant:

Extension evaluated at enucleation ______

RB gene mutation ______

Positive family history of retinoblastoma ______

Primary globe-sparing treatment failure ______

Greatest linear extent of choroid involved by choroidal tumor invasion ______

Histologic Grade (G) *(also known as overall grade)*

Grading system	***Grade***
❑ 2 grade system	❑ Grade I or 1
❑ 3 grade system	❑ Grade II or 2
❑ 4 grade system	❑ Grade III or 3
❑ No 2, 3, or 4 grade system is available	❑ Grade IV or 4

Additional Descriptors

Lymphatic Vessel Invasion (L) and Venous Invasion (V) have been combined into Lymph-Vascular Invasion (LVI) for collection by cancer registrars. The College of American Pathologists' (CAP) Checklist should be used as the primary source. Other sources may be used in the absence of a Checklist. Priority is given to positive results.

❑ Lymph-Vascular Invasion Not Present (absent)/Not Identified
❑ Lymph-Vascular Invasion Present/Identified
❑ Not Applicable
❑ Unknown/Indeterminate

Residual Tumor (R)

The absence or presence of residual tumor after treatment. In some cases treated with surgery and/or with neoadjuvant therapy there will be residual tumor at the primary site after treatment because of incomplete resection or local and regional disease that extends beyond the limit of ability of resection.

❑ RX Presence of residual tumor cannot be assessed
❑ R0 No residual tumor
❑ R1 Microscopic residual tumor
❑ R2 Macroscopic residual tumor

General Notes:

For identification of special cases of TNM or pTNM classifications, the "m" suffix and "y," "r," and "a" prefixes are used. Although they do not affect the stage grouping, they indicate cases needing separate analysis.

m suffix indicates the presence of multiple primary tumors in a single site and is recorded in parentheses: pT(m)NM.

y prefix indicates those cases in which classification is performed during or following initial multimodality therapy. The cTNM or pTNM category is identified by a "y" prefix. The ycTNM or ypTNM categorizes the extent of tumor actually present at the time of that examination. The "y" categorization is not an estimate of tumor prior to multimodality therapy.

r prefix indicates a recurrent tumor when staged after a disease-free interval, and is identified by the "r" prefix: rTNM.

a prefix designates the stage determined at autopsy: aTNM.

surgical margins is data field recorded by registrars describing the surgical margins of the resected primary site specimen as determined only by the pathology report.

neoadjuvant treatment is radiation therapy or systemic therapy (consisting of chemotherapy, hormone therapy, or immunotherapy) administered prior to a definitive surgical procedure. If the surgical procedure is not performed, the administered therapy no longer meets the definition of neoadjuvant therapy.

Histologic Grade (G)

Grade is reported in registry systems by the grade value. A two-grade, three-grade, or four-grade system may be used. If a grading system is not specified, generally the following system is used:

GX Grade cannot be assessed
G1 Well differentiated
G2 Moderately differentiated
G3 Poorly differentiated
G4 Undifferentiated

Histopathologic Type

This classification applies only to retinoblastoma.

Carcinoma of the Lacrimal Gland Staging Form

Clinical *Extent of disease before any treatment*	**Stage Category Definitions**		**Pathologic** *Extent of disease through completion of definitive surgery*
❑ y clinical—staging completed after neoadjuvant therapy but before subsequent surgery	**Tumor Size:** ________	**Laterality:** ☐ left ☐ right ☐ bilateral	❑ y pathologic—staging completed after neoadjuvant therapy AND subsequent surgery
	Primary Tumor (T)		
❑ **TX**	Primary tumor cannot be assessed		❑ **TX**
❑ **T0**	No evidence of primary tumor		❑ **T0**
❑ **T1**	Tumor 2 cm or less in greatest dimension, with or without extraglandular extension into the orbital soft tissue		❑ **T1**
❑ **T2**	Tumor more than 2 cm but not more than 4 cm in greatest dimension*		❑ **T2**
❑ **T3**	Tumor more than 4 cm in greatest dimension*		❑ **T3**
❑ **T4**	Tumor invades periosteum or orbital bone or adjacent structures		❑ **T4**
❑ **T4a**	Tumor invades periosteum		❑ **T4a**
❑ **T4b**	Tumor invades orbital bone		❑ **T4b**
❑ **T4c**	Tumor invades adjacent structures (brain, sinus, pterygoid fossa, temporal fossa)		❑ **T4c**
	*As the maximum size of the lacrimal gland is 2 cm, T2 and greater tumors will usually extend into the orbital soft tissue.		
	Regional Lymph Nodes (N)		
❑ **NX**	Regional lymph nodes cannot be assessed		❑ **NX**
❑ **N0**	No regional lymph node metastasis		❑ **N0**
❑ **N1**	Regional lymph node metastasis		❑ **N1**
	Distant Metastasis (M)		
❑ **M0**	No distant metastasis (no pathologic M0; use clinical M to complete stage group)		
❑ **M1**	Distant metastasis		❑ **M1**

Anatomic Stage • Prognostic Groups

Clinical	**Pathologic**
No stage grouping is presently recommended	No stage grouping is presently recommended

Prognostic Factors (Site-Specific Factors)	**General Notes:**
Required for Staging: None **Clinically Significant:** Ki-67 growth fraction ________ Nuclear NM23 staining ________	For identification of special cases of TNM or pTNM classifications, the "m" suffix and "y," "r," and "a" prefixes are used. Although they do not affect the stage grouping, they indicate cases needing separate analysis.

(Continued)

Carcinoma of the Lacrimal Gland Staging Form *(continued)*

Histologic Grade (G) *(also known as overall grade)*

Grading system	***Grade***
❑ 2 grade system	❑ Grade I or 1
❑ 3 grade system	❑ Grade II or 2
❑ 4 grade system	❑ Grade III or 3
❑ No 2, 3, or 4 grade system is available	❑ Grade IV or 4

Additional Descriptors

Lymphatic Vessel Invasion (L) and Venous Invasion (V) have been combined into Lymph-Vascular Invasion (LVI) for collection by cancer registrars. The College of American Pathologists' (CAP) Checklist should be used as the primary source. Other sources may be used in the absence of a Checklist. Priority is given to positive results.

❑ Lymph-Vascular Invasion Not Present (absent)/Not Identified
❑ Lymph-Vascular Invasion Present/Identified
❑ Not Applicable
❑ Unknown/Indeterminate

Residual Tumor (R)

The absence or presence of residual tumor after treatment. In some cases treated with surgery and/or with neoadjuvant therapy there will be residual tumor at the primary site after treatment because of incomplete resection or local and regional disease that extends beyond the limit of ability of resection.

❑ RX Presence of residual tumor cannot be assessed
❑ R0 No residual tumor
❑ R1 Microscopic residual tumor
❑ R2 Macroscopic residual tumor

General Notes *(continued)*:

m suffix indicates the presence of multiple primary tumors in a single site and is recorded in parentheses: pT(m)NM.

y prefix indicates those cases in which classification is performed during or following initial multimodality therapy. The cTNM or pTNM category is identified by a "y" prefix. The ycTNM or ypTNM categorizes the extent of tumor actually present at the time of that examination. The "y" categorization is not an estimate of tumor prior to multimodality therapy.

r prefix indicates a recurrent tumor when staged after a disease-free interval, and is identified by the "r" prefix: rTNM.

a prefix designates the stage determined at autopsy: aTNM.

surgical margins is data field recorded by registrars describing the surgical margins of the resected primary site specimen as determined only by the pathology report.

neoadjuvant treatment is radiation therapy or systemic therapy (consisting of chemotherapy, hormone therapy, or immunotherapy) administered prior to a definitive surgical procedure. If the surgical procedure is not performed, the administered therapy no longer meets the definition of neoadjuvant therapy.

Histologic Grade (G)

In most cases, the histology defines the grade of malignancy in lacrimal gland carcinomas as in salivary gland carcinomas.

GX Grade cannot be assessed
G1 Well differentiated
G2 Moderately differentiated: includes adenoid cystic carcinoma without basaloid (solid) pattern
G3 Poorly differentiated: includes adenoid cystic carcinoma with basaloid (solid) pattern
G4 Undifferentiated

Histopathologic Type

The major malignant primary epithelial tumors include the following:

Low Grade

Carcinoma ex pleomorphic adenoma [where the carcinoma is noninvasive or minimally invasive as defined by the WHO classification (extension <1.5 mm beyond the capsule—into surrounding tissue)]
Polymorphous low-grade carcinoma
Mucoepidermoid carcinoma, grades 1 and 2
Epithelial-myoepithelial carcinoma

Cystadenocarcinoma and papillary cystadenocarcinoma
Acinic cell carcinoma
Basal cell adenocarcinoma
Mucinous adenocarcinoma

High Grade

Carcinoma ex pleomorphic adenoma (malignant mixed tumor) that includes adenocarcinoma and adenoid cystic carcinoma arising in a pleomorphic adenoma [where the carcinoma is invasive as defined by the WHO classification (extension >1.5 mm beyond the capsule—into surrounding tissue)]
Adenoid cystic carcinoma, not otherwise specified
Adenocarcinoma, not otherwise specified
Mucoepidermoid carcinoma, grade 3
Ductal adenocarcinoma
Squamous cell carcinoma
Sebaceous adenocarcinoma
Myoepithelial carcinoma
Lymphoepithelial carcinoma

Other Rare and Unclassifiable Carcinomas

Sarcoma of the Orbit Staging Form

Clinical *Extent of disease before any treatment*	**Stage Category Definitions**		**Pathologic** *Extent of disease through completion of definitive surgery*
❑ y clinical—staging completed after neoadjuvant therapy but before subsequent surgery	**Tumor Size:** ______	**Laterality:** ☐ left ☐ right ☐ bilateral	❑ y pathologic—staging completed after neoadjuvant therapy AND subsequent surgery

Clinical	Primary Tumor (T)	Pathologic
❑ **TX**	Primary tumor cannot be assessed	❑ **TX**
❑ **T0**	No evidence of primary tumor	❑ **T0**
❑ **T1**	Tumor 15 mm or less in greatest dimension	❑ **T1**
❑ **T2**	Tumor more than 15 mm in greatest dimension without invasion of globe or bony wall	❑ **T2**
❑ **T3**	Tumor of any size with invasion of orbital tissues and/or bony walls	❑ **T3**
❑ **T4**	Tumor invasion of globe or periorbital structure, such as eyelids, temporal fossa, nasal cavity and paranasal sinuses, and/or central nervous system	❑ **T4**

Clinical	Regional Lymph Nodes (N)	Pathologic
❑ **NX**	Regional lymph nodes cannot be assessed	❑ **NX**
❑ **N0**	No regional lymph node metastasis	❑ **N0**
❑ **N1**	Regional lymph node metastasis	❑ **N1**

Clinical	Distant Metastasis (M)	Pathologic
❑ **M0**	No distant metastasis (no pathologic M0; use clinical M to complete stage group)	
❑ **M1**	Distant metastasis	❑ **M1**

Anatomic Stage • Prognostic Groups

Clinical	**Pathologic**
No stage grouping is presently recommended	No stage grouping is presently recommended

Prognostic Factors (Site-Specific Factors)

Required for Staging: None
Clinically Significant: None

Histologic Grade (G) *(also known as overall grade)*

Grading system	***Grade***
❑ 2 grade system	❑ Grade I or 1
❑ 3 grade system	❑ Grade II or 2
❑ 4 grade system	❑ Grade III or 3
❑ No 2, 3, or 4 grade system is available	❑ Grade IV or 4

General Notes:
For identification of special cases of TNM or pTNM classifications, the "m" suffix and "y," "r," and "a" prefixes are used. Although they do not affect the stage grouping, they indicate cases needing separate analysis.

m suffix indicates the presence of multiple primary tumors in a single site and is recorded in parentheses: pT(m)NM.

Sarcoma of the Orbit Staging Form *(continued)*

Additional Descriptors

Lymphatic Vessel Invasion (L) and Venous Invasion (V) have been combined into Lymph-Vascular Invasion (LVI) for collection by cancer registrars. The College of American Pathologists' (CAP) Checklist should be used as the primary source. Other sources may be used in the absence of a Checklist. Priority is given to positive results.

- ❑ Lymph-Vascular Invasion Not Present (absent)/Not Identified
- ❑ Lymph-Vascular Invasion Present/Identified
- ❑ Not Applicable
- ❑ Unknown/Indeterminate

Residual Tumor (R)

The absence or presence of residual tumor after treatment. In some cases treated with surgery and/or with neoadjuvant therapy there will be residual tumor at the primary site after treatment because of incomplete resection or local and regional disease that extends beyond the limit of ability of resection.

- ❑ RX Presence of residual tumor cannot be assessed
- ❑ R0 No residual tumor
- ❑ R1 Microscopic residual tumor
- ❑ R2 Macroscopic residual tumor

General Notes *(continued)*:

y prefix indicates those cases in which classification is performed during or following initial multimodality therapy. The cTNM or pTNM category is identified by a "y" prefix. The ycTNM or ypTNM categorizes the extent of tumor actually present at the time of that examination. The "y" categorization is not an estimate of tumor prior to multimodality therapy.

r prefix indicates a recurrent tumor when staged after a disease-free interval, and is identified by the "r" prefix: rTNM.

a prefix designates the stage determined at autopsy: aTNM.

surgical margins is data field recorded by registrars describing the surgical margins of the resected primary site specimen as determined only by the pathology report.

neoadjuvant treatment is radiation therapy or systemic therapy (consisting of chemotherapy, hormone therapy, or immunotherapy) administered prior to a definitive surgical procedure. If the surgical procedure is not performed, the administered therapy no longer meets the definition of neoadjuvant therapy.

Histologic Grade (G)

Grade is reported in registry systems by the grade value. A two-grade, three-grade, or four-grade system may be used. If a grading system is not specified, generally the following system is used:

GX Grade cannot be assessed
G1 Well differentiated
G2 Moderately differentiated
G3 Poorly differentiated
G4 Undifferentiated

Histopathologic Type

Malignancies of the orbit primarily include a broad spectrum of malignant soft tissue tumors.

Ocular Adnexal Lymphoma Staging Form			
Clinical *Extent of disease before any treatment*	**Stage Category Definitions**		**Pathologic** *Extent of disease through completion of definitive surgery*
❑ y clinical—staging completed after neoadjuvant therapy but before subsequent surgery	**Tumor Size:** ________	**Laterality:** ☐ left ☐ right ☐ bilateral	❑ y pathologic—staging completed after neoadjuvant therapy AND subsequent surgery
	Primary Tumor (T)		
❑ **TX**	Lymphoma extent not specified		❑ **TX**
❑ **T0**	No evidence of lymphoma		❑ **T0**
❑ **T1**	Lymphoma involving the conjunctiva alone without orbital involvement		❑ **T1**
❑ **T1a**	Bulbar conjunctiva only		❑ **T1a**
❑ **T1b**	Palpebral conjunctiva +/– fornix +/– caruncle		❑ **T1b**
❑ **T1c**	Extensive conjunctival involvement		❑ **T1c**
❑ **T2**	Lymphoma with orbital involvement +/– any conjunctival involvement		❑ **T2**
❑ **T2a**	Anterior orbital involvement (+/– conjunctival involvement)		❑ **T2a**
❑ **T2b**	Anterior orbital involvement (+/– conjunctival involvement + lacrimal involvement)		❑ **T2b**
❑ **T2c**	Posterior orbital involvement (+/– conjunctival involvement +/– anterior involvement and +/– any extraocular muscle involvement)		❑ **T2c**
❑ **T2d**	Nasolacrimal drainage system involvement (+/– conjunctival involvement but not including nasopharynx)		❑ **T2d**
❑ **T3**	Lymphoma with pre-septal eyelid involvement (defined above) +/– orbital involvement +/– any conjunctival involvement		❑ **T3**
❑ **T4**	Orbital adnexal lymphoma extending beyond orbit to adjacent structures such as bone and brain		❑ **T4**
❑ **T4a**	Involvement of nasopharynx		❑ **T4a**
❑ **T4b**	Osseous involvement (including periosteum)		❑ **T4b**
❑ **T4c**	Involvement of maxillofacial, ethmoidal and/or frontal sinuses		❑ **T4c**
❑ **T4d**	Intracranial spread		❑ **T4d**
	Regional Lymph Nodes (N)		
❑ **NX**	Regional lymph nodes cannot be assessed		❑ **NX**
❑ **N0**	No evidence of lymph node involvement		❑ **N0**
❑ **N1**	Involvement of ipsilateral regional lymph nodes*		❑ **N1**
❑ **N2**	Involvement of contra lateral or bilateral regional lymph nodes*		❑ **N2**
❑ **N3**	Involvement of peripheral lymph nodes not draining ocular adnexal region		❑ **N3**
❑ **N4**	Involvement of central lymph nodes		❑ **N4**
	*The regional lymph nodes included preauricular (parotid), submandibular, and cervical.		

Ocular Adnexal Lymphoma Staging Form *(continued)*

Clinical *Extent of disease before any treatment*	**Stage Category Definitions**	**Pathologic** *Extent of disease through completion of definitive surgery*
	Distant Metastasis (M)	
❑ **M0**	No evidence of involvement of other extranodal sites (no pathologic M0; use clinical M to complete stage group)	
❑ **M1a**	Noncontiguous involvement of tissues or organs external to the ocular adnexa (eg, parotid glands, submandibular gland, lung, liver, spleen, kidney, breast, etc)	❑ **M1a**
❑ **M1b**	Lymphomatous involvement of the bone marrow	❑ **M1b**
❑ **M1c**	Both M1a and M1b involvement	❑ **M1c**

Anatomic Stage • Prognostic Groups

Clinical	**Pathologic**
No stage grouping is presently recommended	No stage grouping is presently recommended

Prognostic Factors (Site-Specific Factors)

Required for Staging: None
Clinically Significant:
Tumor cell growth fraction (Ki-67, MIB-1) ______________
Serum lactate dehydrogenase (LDH) at diagnosis ______________
History of rheumatoid arthritis ______________
History of Sjögren's syndrome ______________
History of connective tissue disease ______________
History of recurrent dry eye syndrome (sicca syndrome) ______________
Any evidence of a viral infection (eg Hepatitis C or HIV) ______________
Any evidence of a bacterial infection (eg *Helicobacter pylori*) ______________
Any evidence of an infection caused by other micro-organisms (eg *Chlamydia psittaci*) ______________

Histologic Grade (G) *(also known as overall grade)*

Grading system	***Grade***
❑ 2 grade system	❑ Grade I or 1
❑ 3 grade system	❑ Grade II or 2
❑ 4 grade system	❑ Grade III or 3
❑ No 2, 3, or 4 grade system is available	❑ Grade IV or 4

Additional Descriptors
Lymphatic Vessel Invasion (L) and Venous Invasion (V) have been combined into Lymph-Vascular Invasion (LVI) for collection by cancer registrars. The College of American Pathologists' (CAP) Checklist should be used as the primary source. Other sources may be used in the absence of a Checklist. Priority is given to positive results.

❑ Lymph-Vascular Invasion Not Present (absent)/Not Identified
❑ Lymph-Vascular Invasion Present/Identified
❑ Not Applicable
❑ Unknown/Indeterminate

General Notes:
For identification of special cases of TNM or pTNM classifications, the "m" suffix and "y," "r," and "a" prefixes are used. Although they do not affect the stage grouping, they indicate cases needing separate analysis.

m suffix indicates the presence of multiple primary tumors in a single site and is recorded in parentheses: pT(m)NM.

y prefix indicates those cases in which classification is performed during or following initial multimodality therapy. The cTNM or pTNM category is identified by a "y" prefix. The ycTNM or ypTNM categorizes the extent of tumor actually present at the time of that examination. The "y" categorization is not an estimate of tumor prior to multimodality therapy.

r prefix indicates a recurrent tumor when staged after a disease-free interval, and is identified by the "r" prefix: rTNM.

a prefix designates the stage determined at autopsy: aTNM.

surgical margins is data field recorded by registrars describing the surgical margins of the resected primary site specimen as determined only by the pathology report.

(Continued)

Ocular Adnexal Lymphoma Staging Form *(continued)*	
Residual Tumor (R) The absence or presence of residual tumor after treatment. In some cases treated with surgery and/or with neoadjuvant therapy there will be residual tumor at the primary site after treatment because of incomplete resection or local and regional disease that extends beyond the limit of ability of resection. ❑ RX Presence of residual tumor cannot be assessed ❑ R0 No residual tumor ❑ R1 Microscopic residual tumor ❑ R2 Macroscopic residual tumor	**General Notes** *(continued)*: **neoadjuvant treatment** is radiation therapy or systemic therapy (consisting of chemotherapy, hormone therapy, or immunotherapy) administered prior to a definitive surgical procedure. If the surgical procedure is not performed, the administered therapy no longer meets the definition of neoadjuvant therapy.

Histologic Grade (G)

Grades are given only to *follicular lymphomas* as described by the 2002 WHO classification for malignant lymphomas as follows:

G1 1–5 centroblasts per 10 high power field
G2 Between 5 and 15 centroblasts per 10 high power fields
G3a More than 15 centroblasts per 10 high power fields but with admixed centrocytes
G3b More than 15 centroblasts per 10 high power fields but without centrocytes

Histopathologic Type

The lymphomas arising as *primary tumors* in the ocular adnexa are subtyped according to the WHO Lymphoma classification. The main ocular adnexal lymphoma subtypes include the following:

Extranodal marginal zone B-cell lymphoma (MALT lymphoma)
Diffuse large B-cell lymphoma
Follicular lymphoma
Mantle cell lymphoma
Lymphoplasmacytic lymphoma
Plasmacytoma
Burkitt lymphoma
Peripheral T-cell lymphoma, unspecified
Mycosis fungoides
Extranodal NK/T-cell lymphoma, nasal type
Anaplastic large cell lymphoma

Jaffe ES, Harris NL, Stein H, Vardiman JW. *World Health Organization Classification of Tumours: Tumours of Haematopoietic and Lymphoid Tissues. Pathology and Genetics.* Lyon, France: IARC; 2001.

Basic Texts

Ophthalmic Pathology and Intraocular Tumors

Albert DM, Jakobiec FA, eds. *Atlas of Clinical Ophthalmology.* Philadelphia: Saunders; 1996.

Albert DM, Miller JW, eds. *Albert & Jakobiec's Principles & Practice of Ophthalmology.* 3rd ed. Philadelphia: Saunders; 2008.

Apple DJ, Rabb MF. *Ocular Pathology: Clinical Applications and Self-Assessment.* 5th ed. St Louis: Mosby; 1998.

Bornfeld N, Gragoudas ES, Höpping W, et al, eds. *Tumors of the Eye.* New York: Kugler; 1991.

Char DH. *Clinical Ocular Oncology.* 2nd ed. Philadelphia: Lippincott Williams & Wilkins; 1998.

Cohen IK, Diegelmann RF, Lindblad WJ, eds. *Wound Healing: Biochemical and Clinical Aspects.* Philadelphia: Saunders; 1992.

Dutton JJ. *Atlas of Clinical and Surgical Orbital Anatomy.* Philadelphia: Saunders; 1994.

Garner A, Klintworth GK, eds. *Pathobiology of Ocular Disease: A Dynamic Approach.* 2nd ed. New York: Informa Healthcare; 1994.

Isenberg SJ, ed. *The Eye in Infancy.* 2nd ed. St Louis: Mosby; 1994.

Margo CE, Grossniklaus HE. *Ocular Histopathology: A Guide to Differential Diagnosis.* Philadelphia: Saunders; 1991.

McLean IW, Burnier MN, Zimmerman LE, Jakobiec FA. *Tumors of the Eye and Ocular Adnexa.* Washington: Armed Forces Institute of Pathology; 1994.

Nauman GOH, Apple DJ. *Pathology of the Eye.* New York: Springer-Verlag; 1986.

Sanborn GE, Gonder JR, Shields JA. *Atlas of Intraocular Tumors.* Philadelphia: Saunders; 1994.

Sassani JW, ed. *Ophthalmic Pathology With Clinical Correlations.* Philadelphia: Lippincott Williams & Wilkins; 1997.

Shields JA, Shields CL. *Atlas of Eyelid and Conjunctival Tumors.* Philadelphia: Lippincott Williams & Wilkins; 1999.

Shields JA, Shields CL. *Atlas of Intraocular Tumors.* Philadelphia: Lippincott Williams & Wilkins; 1999.

Spencer WH, ed. *Ophthalmic Pathology: An Atlas and Textbook.* 4th ed. Philadelphia: Saunders; 1996.

Yanoff M, Fine BS. *Ocular Pathology.* 5th ed. St Louis: Mosby; 2002.

Related Academy Materials

The Academy is dedicated to providing a wealth of high-quality clinical education resources for ophthalmologists.

Print Publications and Electronic Products

For a complete listing of Academy products related to topics covered in this BCSC Section, visit our online store at http://store.aao.org/clinical-education/topic/comprehensive-ophthalmology.html. Or call Customer Service at 866.561.8558 (toll free, US only) or +1 415.561.8540, Monday through Friday, between 8:00 AM and 5:00 PM (PST).

Online Resources

Visit the Ophthalmic News and Education (ONE®) Network at www.aao.org/one to find relevant videos, online courses, journal articles, practice guidelines, self-assessment quizzes, images and more. The ONE Network is a free Academy-member benefit.

Access free, trusted articles and content with the Academy's collaborative online encyclopedia, EyeWiki, at www.aao.org/eyewiki.

Requesting Continuing Medical Education Credit

The American Academy of Ophthalmology is accredited by the Accreditation Council for Continuing Medical Education to provide continuing medical education for physicians.

The American Academy of Ophthalmology designates this enduring material for a maximum of 10 *AMA PRA Category 1 Credits*™. Physicians should claim only the credit commensurate with the extent of their participation in the activity.

The American Medical Association requires that all learners participating in activities involving enduring materials complete a formal assessment before claiming continuing medical education (CME) credit. To assess your achievement in this activity and ensure that a specified level of knowledge has been reached, a posttest for this Section of the Basic and Clinical Science Course is provided. A minimum score of 80% must be obtained to pass the test and claim CME credit.

To take the posttest and request CME credit online:

1. Go to www.aao.org/cme and log in.
2. Click on "Claim CME Credit and View My CME Transcript" and then "Report AAO Credits."
3. Select the appropriate Academy activity. You will be directed to the posttest.
4. Once you have passed the test with a score of 80% or higher, you will be directed to your transcript. *If you are not an Academy member, you will be able to print out a certificate of participation once you have passed the test.*

Originally released June 2011; reviewed for currency September 2, 2014. **CME expiration date: June 1, 2016.** *AMA PRA Category 1 Credits*™ may be claimed only once during this period.

For assistance, contact the Academy's Customer Service department at 866-561-8558 (US only) or 415-561-8540 between 8:00 AM and 5:00 PM (PST), Monday through Friday, or send an e-mail to customer_service@aao.org.

Study Questions

Please note that these questions are *not* part of your CME reporting process. They are provided here for self-assessment and identification of personal professional practice gaps. The required CME posttest is available online (see "Requesting CME Credit").

Following the questions are a blank answer sheet and answers with discussions. Although a concerted effort has been made to avoid ambiguity and redundancy in these questions, the authors recognize that differences of opinion may occur regarding the "best" answer. The discussions are provided to demonstrate the rationale used to derive the answer. They may also be helpful in confirming that your approach to the problem was correct or, if necessary, in fixing the principle in your memory. The Section 4 faculty would like to thank the Self-Assessment Committee for working with them to provide these study questions and discussions.

1. What is a lesion composed of normal, mature tissue in an abnormal location?
   a. hamartoma
   b. choristoma
   c. hemangioma
   d. granuloma

2. Which of the following cells would most likely be observed on histologic examination of a specimen of a bacterial corneal ulcer?
   a. eosinophils
   b. basophils
   c. epithelioid histiocytes
   d. neutrophils

3. Which of the following choices is a general histologic sign of malignancy?
   a. nuclear/cellular pleomorphism
   b. dyskeratosis
   c. dysplasia
   d. calcification

4. When glaucoma occurs in association with angle recession, it is most commonly because of which of the following?
   a. damage to the trabecular meshwork
   b. associated lens subluxation
   c. iridodialysis
   d. a tear in the ciliary body muscle

5. If a conjunctival biopsy is being performed for suspicion of ocular cicatricial pemphigoid, then half of the specimen should be submitted in formalin for routine histology and the other half should be submitted in what medium for immunofluorescence studies?
   a. Michel medium
   b. glutaraldehyde
   c. saline
   d. absolute alcohol

6. What is the first step in preparing a specimen for electron microscopy?
   a. glutaraldehyde fixation
   b. thick sections
   c. thin sections
   d. osmification process

7. Frozen sections are appropriate for which one of the following?
   a. to surgically control the margins of a neoplasm
   b. to interpret a conjunctival lesion
   c. to interpret a cutaneous lesion
   d. to make a formal diagnosis

8. What is the best way to diagnose orbital hemangiopericytoma?
   a. radiologic imaging
   b. ultrasound testing
   c. fine-needle aspiration or open orbital biopsy
   d. clinical symptoms and examination

9. A 40-year-old man has a painless, palpable mass in the right superolateral orbit that displaces the globe down and inward. A CT scan shows a heterogeneous mass in the region of the lacrimal gland with adjacent bone remodeling. Which biopsy approach is correct?
   a. total primary excision through a lateral orbitotomy
   b. incisional biopsy through a lateral orbitotomy
   c. incisional biopsy through a medial orbitotomy
   d. total primary excision through a medial orbitotomy

10. What method can identify infectious agents, neoplastic cells, or degenerative conditions and distinguish lesions of neuroectodermal origin from neuroendocrine lesions?
    a. Gram stain
    b. chromatography
    c. routine histologic examination
    d. immunohistochemistry

11. Which of the following corneal stromal dystrophies is characterized by both hyaline and amyloid deposits?
    a. granular
    b. lattice
    c. Avellino
    d. macular

12. Which of the following forms of infectious keratitis displays double-walled cysts in the corneal stroma on histology?
    a. pseudomonal ulcer
    b. herpetic keratitis
    c. *Acanthamoeba* keratitis
    d. *Fusarium* keratitis

13. A 55-year-old diabetic black female has unilateral elevated intraocular pressure associated with long-standing intraocular hemorrhage. The pertinent slit-lamp finding consists of golden brown cells in the anterior chamber. What is the most likely etiology of her elevated intraocular pressure?
    a. aqueous fluid overproduction
    b. artifactual readings due to corneal edema
    c. outflow obstruction due to red blood cell membrane rigidity
    d. traumatic pupillary block

14. What disease may be diagnosed by finding Heinz bodies on red blood cell membranes in an anterior chamber aspirate?
    a. lymphoma
    b. siderosis
    c. pseudoexfoliation
    d. ghost cell glaucoma

15. A 35-year-old woman, recently diagnosed with rheumatoid arthritis, presents with a violaceous scleral nodule. The biopsy will most likely reveal which of the following?
    a. palisading arrangement of histiocytes/giant cells around necrotic/necrobiotic collagen fibers
    b. sparse inflammatory infiltrate composed of lymphocytes and plasma cells
    c. colonies of gram-negative bacteria associated with acute necrotizing inflammation
    d. circumscribed proliferation of spindle cells in chronically inflamed, richly vascular, and myxoid stroma

16. The pathophysiology of posterior subcapsular cataract may best be described by which of the following?
    a. posterior migration of lens epithelial cells
    b. disorganization of posterior lens fibers
    c. infiltration of the posterior lens by inflammatory cells
    d. retention of lens fiber nuclei

17. What is the histopathologic appearance of the anterior chamber angle in a case of phacolytic glaucoma?
    a. infiltration by hemosiderin-laden macrophages
    b. lack of significant inflammatory cell infiltrate
    c. infiltration by neutrophils
    d. infiltration by protein-laden macrophages

18. Of the following, which anatomic boundary is not a component of the vitreous?
    a. hyaloid face
    b. internal limiting membrane
    c. hyaloideocapsular ligament
    d. vitreous base

19. Which of the following vitreous degenerations is *not* age related?
    a. vitreous syneresis
    b. macular hole
    c. posterior vitreous detachment
    d. asteroid hyalosis

20. Pathologic examination of cystoid macular edema reveals cysts in which retinal layer?
    a. outer plexiform
    b. Bruch membrane
    c. internal limiting membrane
    d. retinal pigment epithelium

21. A 6-week-old child is brought by his parents because of a 1-cm reddish mass on the left upper eyelid, which prevents the eye from opening fully. It has grown rapidly since birth. MRI shows an enhancing vascular lesion. Which entity is most likely?
    a. plexiform neurofibroma
    b. acute dacryocystitis
    c. capillary hemangioma
    d. benign mixed tumor of the lacrimal gland

22. Histopathologically, the uveitis seen in Vogt-Koyanagi-Harada syndrome most closely resembles the uveitis seen in which one of the following diseases?
   a. juvenile idiopathic arthritis
   b. intraocular lymphoma
   c. pars planitis
   d. sympathetic ophthalmia

23. An asymptomatic, dome-shaped, orange mass is noted in the midperipheral fundus of a 30-year-old woman. An overlying exudative retinal detachment is present. A-scan ultrasonography shows high internal reflectivity. Which entity is most likely?
   a. posterior scleritis
   b. central serous retinopathy
   c. amelanotic choroidal melanoma
   d. circumscribed choroidal hemangioma

24. Which pathologic finding would differentiate between a ruptured dermoid and ruptured epidermoid cyst?
   a. hair follicles
   b. lamellated keratin
   c. mixed inflammation
   d. squamous epithelium

25. What is the most common type of intraocular tumor?
   a. melanoma
   b. retinoblastoma
   c. lymphoma
   d. metastatic neoplasm

26. A 25-year-old white male with a history of conjunctivitis presents with a flesh-colored mass with a central umbilication on the upper eyelid. Examination of the pathologic specimen reveals invasive lobular acanthosis, a central umbilication, and eosinophilic and basophilic intracytoplasmic inclusions. What is the most likely diagnosis?
   a. squamous papilloma
   b. xanthelasma
   c. basal cell carcinoma
   d. Molluscum contagiosum

27. A 22-year-old female presents with a painless, nontender, flesh-colored, hyperkeratotic eyelid mass. Pathologic examination shows acanthotic epithelium surrounding a fibrovascular core. What is the most likely etiology?
    a. bacterial
    b. inflammation
    c. sun exposure
    d. viral

28. Squamous cell carcinoma in situ is defined as a pathologic anatomic limitation by which one of the following?
    a. superficial epithelium
    b. stromal keratocytes
    c. basal epithelium
    d. basement membrane

29. With which of the following is aniridia most commonly associated?
    a. retinal pigment epithelial hyperplasia
    b. optic nerve coloboma
    c. glaucoma
    d. optically empty vitreous

30. What physiologic changes are associated with acquired optic atrophy?
    a. increased myelin with thinning of the pial septa
    b. shrinkage of the nerve diameter with widening of the subarachnoid space
    c. uniform changes across the nerve without variation
    d. increased myelin and shrinking of the subarachnoid space

31. What is optic nerve glioma most frequently associated with?
    a. Sturge-Weber syndrome
    b. neurofibromatosis type 1
    c. Peters anomaly
    d. neurofibromatosis type 2

32. Which of the following is *not* a clinical risk factor for metastatic disease in patients with uveal melanoma?
    a. large tumor size
    b. ciliary body involvement
    c. young age
    d. extraocular extension

33. Which of the following is the most important risk factor for the development of uveal melanoma?
    a. dysplastic nevus syndrome
    b. light-colored complexion
    c. ocular melanocytosis
    d. ultraviolet light exposure

34. At the time a choroidal melanoma is diagnosed, which test is recommended to help rule out metastasis?
    a. serum glucose
    b. brain MRI
    c. bone marrow biopsy
    d. abdominal imaging

35. With which of the following organs must the ophthalmologist be most concerned about in a patient with retinal capillary hemangioblastoma?
    a. brain and kidney
    b. liver and lung
    c. bowel and skin
    d. organs of the immune system and central nervous system

36. What association distinguishes von Hippel–Lindau syndrome from von Hippel disease?
    a. intracranial calcifications, ash-leaf spots, retinal astrocytomas
    b. café-au-lait spots, Lisch nodules, optic pathway gliomas
    c. pheochromocytomas, cerebellar hemangioblastomas, renal cell carcinomas
    d. limbal dermoids, upper eyelid colobomas, preauricular tags

37. Which of the following is the most important histopathologic risk factor for mortality in the enucleated globe from a patient with retinoblastoma?
    a. the presence of anterior segment involvement
    b. the extent of retinal detachment
    c. the extent of optic nerve and choroidal invasion
    d. the size of the tumor

38. Which of the following clinical characteristics is typical of Coats disease?
    a. unilateral
    b. associated with HLA-B27
    c. found in female patients
    d. bilateral

39. Intraocular calcification in the eye of a child is most diagnostic of what disease?
    a. retinoblastoma
    b. toxocariasis
    c. persistent fetal vasculature
    d. Coats disease

40. What is the most common secondary tumor in retinoblastoma patients?
    a. fibrosarcoma
    b. melanoma
    c. pinealoblastoma
    d. osteosarcoma

41. When a parent has bilateral retinoblastoma, which risk factors apply to the affected parent's children?
    a. 85% risk of developing retinoblastoma
    b. risk of bilateral disease in all affected children
    c. risk of developing retinoblastoma in males only
    d. 45% risk of developing retinoblastoma

42. What is the primary treatment for a 2-year-old child with unilateral retinoblastoma classified as International Classification Group E?
    a. systemic chemotherapy alone
    b. intra-arterial chemotherapy
    c. enucleation
    d. radiation alone

43. What is the treatment of choice for metastatic carcinoma to the eye?
    a. chemotherapy
    b. external-beam radiation
    c. brachytherapy
    d. individually tailored in each case

44. What is the most common finding in ocular involvement in leukemia?
    a. retinal hemorrhages
    b. aqueous cells
    c. retinal perivascular sheathing
    d. vitreous cells

45. What tumor frequently occurs in conjunction with central nervous system involvement?
    a. basal cell carcinoma of the eyelid
    b. primary intraocular lymphoma
    c. retinoblastoma
    d. ciliary body melanoma

46. Leukemic retinopathy may cause hemorrhages in which level(s) of the retina?
    a. preretinal (subhyaloidal) and intraretinal
    b. subretinal
    c. choroidal
    d. Leukemic retinopathy does not cause retinal hemorrhages.

Answer Sheet for Section 4 Study Questions

Question	Answer	Question	Answer
1	a b c d	24	a b c d
2	a b c d	25	a b c d
3	a b c d	26	a b c d
4	a b c d	27	a b c d
5	a b c d	28	a b c d
6	a b c d	29	a b c d
7	a b c d	30	a b c d
8	a b c d	31	a b c d
9	a b c d	32	a b c d
10	a b c d	33	a b c d
11	a b c d	34	a b c d
12	a b c d	35	a b c d
13	a b c d	36	a b c d
14	a b c d	37	a b c d
15	a b c d	38	a b c d
16	a b c d	39	a b c d
17	a b c d	40	a b c d
18	a b c d	41	a b c d
19	a b c d	42	a b c d
20	a b c d	43	a b c d
21	a b c d	44	a b c d
22	a b c d	45	a b c d
23	a b c d	46	a b c d

Answers

1. **b.** A choristoma is normal, mature tissue in an abnormal location. A limbal dermoid is an example of a choristoma—skin that is present at the abnormal location of the limbus but otherwise normal and mature. The term *hamartoma* describes an exaggerated hypertrophy and hyperplasia (abnormal amount) of mature tissue at a normal location. An example of a hamartoma is a cavernous hemangioma, an encapsulated mass of mature venous channels in the orbit. A granuloma is an aggregate of epithelioid histiocytes within tissue in the setting of chronic granulomatous inflammation.
2. **d.** Neutrophils, or polymorphonuclear leukocytes (PMNs), are identified by their multisegmented nuclei and intracytoplasmic granules, and they predominate in the acute inflammatory response in bacterial infections. Eosinophils have bilobed nuclei and prominent eosinophilic intracytoplasmic granules and are commonly observed in allergic reactions. Basophils contain basophilic intracytoplasmic granules, circulate in the bloodstream, and play a role in parasitic infections and allergic responses. Epithelioid histiocytes have abundant eosinophilic cytoplasm and sharp cell borders and are histologic markers of granulomatous inflammation.
3. **a.** Malignant tumor cells are characterized histologically by cellular and nuclear pleomorphism (ie, cells and nuclei of different sizes and shapes). Premature individual cell keratinization, or dyskeratosis, may be seen in both benign and malignant epithelial lesions. Dysplasia (abnormal epithelial maturation) is a premalignant change. Calcification may be seen in benign and malignant lesions.
4. **a.** Traumatic recession of the anterior chamber angle is due to a tear in the ciliary body, between the longitudinal and circular muscles, with posterior displacement of the iris root. Concurrent damage to the trabecular meshwork may lead to glaucoma. Lens subluxation and iridodialysis may be observed in addition to angle recession after blunt ocular trauma; however, the glaucoma that occurs in association with angle recession is most commonly caused by damage to the trabecular meshwork.
5. **a.** Michel (pronounced mee-SHELL) transport medium is used to transport specimens for immunofluorescence studies. In ocular cicatricial pemphigoid, immunofluorescence studies demonstrate IgG, IgM, and/or IgA immunoglobulins, and/or complement (C3) positivity in the epithelial basement membrane zone. Michel medium is not a fixative. It should be stored refrigerated (not frozen) until use. Specimens may be kept in Michel medium for up to 5 days at room temperature. Glutaraldehyde is the preferred fixative for electron microscopy. Normal saline solution (0.9% sodium chloride) and absolute ethyl alcohol may be employed to transport tissue within 24 hours for RNA studies.
6. **a.** Glutaraldehyde (2.5% solution in phosphate buffered saline) fixation is the first step in preparing a specimen for electron microscopy. The tissue is then washed in buffered solution and postfixed in osmium tetroxide (osmification process). Representative pieces of tissue are processed in graded alcohol baths for dehydration and embedded in epoxy resin. Thick sections (1 µm in thickness) are cut to examine the tissue under light microscopy and identify regions of greatest interest for ultrathin sectioning. The ultrathin sections (50 nm in thickness) are cut with diamond or glass knives attached to an ultramicrotome and then mounted on a 3-mm-diameter copper grid. The mounted sections are then stained with uranyl acetate (or lead citrate) to impart contrast to the tissue for electron microscopy.

7. **a.** A frozen section is indicated when the results of the study will affect management of the patient in the operating room. Two common indications for frozen section are to determine whether resection margins are free of tumor and to determine whether the surgeon has obtained a representative biopsy specimen in the case of metastases. Interpretation or diagnosis of a lesion requires permanent sections. Permanent sections are always preferred and are the standard for formal diagnosis based on pathologic findings.

8. **c.** Hemangiopericytoma is a solid tumor, and radiologic imaging and ultrasonography would therefore provide only nonspecific features that are of poor diagnostic value. Hemangiopericytoma is a primary orbital tumor, and the clinical symptoms will be the same as the symptoms for any orbital tumor. One can expect proptosis, pain, and diplopia as presenting features. The diagnosis requires positive immunohistochemical staining for CD34. The staining can be done on fine-needle or open orbital biopsy specimen.

9. **a.** Pleomorphic adenoma (benign mixed tumor) is the most common epithelial tumor of the lacrimal gland. The tumor is pseudoencapsulated and grows by expansion. Progressive growth into the bone of the lacrimal fossa may cause excavation and stimulate new bone (cortication) formation in the area. Total primary excision through a lateral orbitotomy is the correct approach because when part of a tumor is left behind, tumor recurrence and, in rare instances, malignant transformation are possible. A lateral orbitotomy provides the best surgical exposure and allows for complete removal of the tumor.

10. **d.** Immunohistochemistry takes advantage of the property that a given cell can express specific antigens. In immunohistochemistry, a primary antibody binds to a specific antigen on the surface of or within a cell. The antibody is linked to a chromogen, whose colored end-product is visualized under a microscope to determine the cell type. Hundreds of antibodies specific for cellular products or surface antigens are available, and immunohistochemistry is the only method capable of distinguishing lesions of neuroendocrine origin from those of neuroectodermal origin. *Chromatography* is the collective term for a set of laboratory techniques used to separate colored chemical mixtures and is not routinely used in pathologic examination of tissues. A Gram stain can identify the morphology of an infectious bacterium and the bacterium's affinity for a specific histological stain, thus distinguishing between gram-positive and gram-negative bacteria. This information can be used in the selection of an antibiotic. Routine histologic examination cannot distinguish neuroendocrine from neuroectodermal lesions because their pathologic appearance is very similar.

11. **c.** Avellino dystrophy, or combined granular-lattice dystrophy, displays features of both granular dystrophy (type 1) and lattice dystrophy (type 1). Histologically, hyaline deposits (highlighted by the Masson trichrome stain) and amyloid deposits (highlighted by the Congo red stain) are present within the corneal stroma, which is characteristic of granular dystrophy and lattice dystrophy, respectively. Macular dystrophy exhibits mucopolysaccharide deposits (highlighted by the alcian blue and colloidal iron stains).

12. **c.** *Acanthamoeba* protozoa have a double-walled cyst morphology, and these cysts are difficult to eradicate from the corneal stroma. Less commonly, trophozoite forms may also be identified. Epithelial cells infected with herpes virus may display intranuclear inclusions, but these are rarely seen histologically because corneal grafting is not generally performed during the acute phase of infection. *Pseudomonas* is a gram-negative bacterium and is rod shaped (bacillus).

13. **c.** Long-standing intraocular hemorrhage leads to degenerative changes in erythrocytes, which lose intracellular hemoglobin and, clinically, appear golden brown or "khaki col-

ored." These rigid, spherical ghost cells may obstruct the trabecular meshwork, leading to ghost cell glaucoma.

14. **d.** Ghost cells are hemolyzed erythrocytes that have lost most of their intracellular hemoglobin. Heinz bodies are the remaining denatured, precipitated hemoglobin particles within the ghost cells.
15. **a.** The clinical presentation is suggestive of nodular scleritis, related to rheumatoid arthritis. Choice *a* describes the histology of a rheumatoid nodule.
16. **a.** Under normal conditions, the lens epithelial cells terminate at the lens equator. When the equatorial lens epithelial cells migrate onto the posterior lens capsule, they swell (referred to as *bladder cells of Wedl*), resulting in posterior subcapsular cataract formation.
17. **d.** In phacolytic glaucoma, denatured lens protein in a hypermature cataract leaks through microscopic openings in an intact lens capsule. This lens protein is then phagocytosed by macrophages, which are present in the anterior chamber angle.
18. **b.** The internal limiting membrane is the innermost layer of the neurosensory retina and, though attached to the vitreous, is not considered a component of the vitreous. The hyaloid face is the outer surface of the vitreous cortex. The hyaloideocapsular ligament forms the anterior border of the vitreous, which is attached to the lens capsule. The vitreous base is a firm circumferential attachment of the vitreous straddling the ora serrata.
19. **d.** The development of asteroid hyalosis is not known to be a consequence of age. Vitreous syneresis, macular hole, and posterior vitreous detachment can be considered age related, as the incidence of these conditions increases with age.
20. **a.** Nerve fiber layers in the outer plexiform layer (nerve fiber layer of Henle) run obliquely, allowing for the accumulation of fluid in the macula, which appears as cysts when there is abnormal permeability of the blood–retina barrier.
21. **c.** Capillary hemangioma is the most common neoplasm of the eyelid in childhood and has a bright red appearance clinically. Plexiform neurofibromas typically affect the upper eyelid, are not particularly vascular, and do not typically cause discoloration of the eyelid. Acute dacryocystitis can occur in children, but it would affect the medial canthal region of the lower eyelid. Benign mixed tumor of the lacrimal gland is rare in children. It may cause a mass in the upper outer eyelid, typically without discoloration. If the eyelid is everted, the mass may be appreciated through the conjunctiva.
22. **d.** The inflammation seen in Vogt-Koyanagi-Harada (VKH) syndrome is very similar to that seen in sympathetic ophthalmia. Both demonstrate the presence of lymphocytes and epithelioid histiocytes (granulomatous inflammation) in the posterior uveal tract. VKH involves the choriocapillaris more often than does sympathetic ophthalmia. Juvenile idiopathic arthritis typically involves the anterior uveal tract and does not demonstrate granulomatous inflammation. Pars planitis involves the peripheral retina, vitreous, and choroid. Typically, the inflammation is not granulomatous.
23. **d.** Circumscribed choroidal hemangioma typically has a red or orange appearance clinically, and it is characteristically highly reflective on ultrasonography. Posterior scleritis may be very difficult to appreciate on fundus examination but may have an associated exudative retinal detachment. On B-scan echography, the sclera will appear thickened, and a "T sign" may be seen around the optic nerve. Central serous retinopathy will have a localized exudative retinal detachment, typically without significant findings in the choroid. Amelanotic melanomas usually appear cream colored clinically and have low to medium internal reflectivity on A-scan echography.

24. **a.** The correct answer is the presence of hair follicles. An epidermoid cyst is lined with keratinized stratified squamous epithelium similar to epidermis but does not have skin adnexal structures such as hair follicles or glands. A dermoid cyst is lined with epidermal epithelium and has adnexal structures. Both types of cysts will generate a mixed inflammatory response if they rupture.
25. **d.** The most common type of intraocular tumor overall is a metastatic neoplasm. The second most common type in adults is uveal melanoma. Retinoblastoma is uncommon overall, and lymphomas are rare.
26. **d.** Molluscum contagiosum is characterized by marked focal acanthosis of the epidermis with a central umbilication. Viral inclusions are present in most of the superficial epithelial cells. Squamous papilloma has an upward rather than downward growth pattern histologically. Xanthelasma consists of aggregates of foamy macrophages in the dermis. Basal cell carcinoma has an invasive (downward) growth pattern, with multiple islands of blue cells with the characteristic peripheral palisading border of tumor cells. Basal cell carcinoma is more common on the lower eyelid.
27. **d.** The correct answer is viral. A papilloma, typical of infection of the skin with human papillomavirus, is defined as acanthotic epithelium with a fibrovascular core. Bacterial infections typically cause an abscess or cellulitis. Inflammatory lesions are typically erythematous. Sun exposure may cause hyperpigmentation, wrinkling, or actinic keratosis (ie, a flat, red, scaly lesion).
28. **d.** Squamous cell carcinoma in situ implies that the neoplasm is confined to the epithelium and does not break through the basement membrane and extend into the underlying stroma.
29. **c.** Aniridia is most commonly associated with glaucoma. Foveal hypoplasia, cataract, and corneal pannus may also be present.
30. **b.** In acquired optic atrophy, there is loss of axonal fibers, which results in a decrease in the optic nerve diameter with corresponding widening of the intermeningeal (subarachnoid) space. Additional changes include gliosis and thickening of the fibrovascular pial septa.
31. **b.** Optic nerve glioma is most frequently associated with neurofibromatosis type 1.
32. **c.** Old age was found to be a risk factor for metastatic uveal melanoma. The other choices are also well-established risk factors.
33. **b.** The risk of developing uveal melanoma is closely related to a person's complexion. Uveal melanoma appears mostly in whites, mainly in those of European origin, and is rare in other races.
34. **d.** The liver is by far the most frequent site of metastasis from uveal melanoma, and metastasis to other organs, such as the lungs, skin, and bones, is rarely found without liver involvement.
35. **a.** The presence of a retinal capillary hemangioblastoma (previously known as *retinal capillary hemangioma*) suggests the possibility of von Hippel–Lindau (VHL) syndrome resulting from a mutation of the *VHL* gene on chromosome 3. Patients with VHL syndrome are at risk for cerebellar hemangioblastomas, pheochromocytomas, and renal cell carcinomas. Genetic screening of such patients should be considered.
36. **c.** von Hippel disease is limited to a solitary finding, retinal capillary hemangioblastoma. VHL syndrome is associated with cerebellar hemangioblastomas. Patients with this syndrome are also at risk of developing pheochromocytomas and renal cell carcinomas.

37. **c.** Invasion of the optic nerve increases the risk of central nervous system metastasis either by direct access in or along the nerve or by seeding of the subarachnoid space. Massive, deep invasion of the choroid increases the risk of hematogenous spread (metastases).

38. **a.** Coats disease is a unilateral retinal vasculopathy occurring most commonly in boys younger than 10 years. Some studies have linked Coats disease to mutations in the Norrie disease gene *(NDP)*. There is no association with HLA-B27.

39. **a.** Intraocular calcifications are the hallmark of retinoblastoma and signify retinoblastoma until proven otherwise. In rare instances, intraocular calcifications may be seen in toxocariasis, persistent fetal vasculature, and Coats disease. In these cases, calcifications are usually focal and discrete, occurring within granulomas (toxocariasis) or a retrolental membrane (persistent fetal vasculature) or at the level of the retinal pigment epithelium (Coats disease).

40. **d.** Osteosarcomas represent 40% of tumors arising within the field of radiation and 36% outside the field of radiation in patients previously treated for retinoblastoma.

41. **d.** A parent with retinoblastoma, in theory, has a somatic mutation of at least 1 allele of the retinoblastoma gene *(RB1)*. Thus, there is a 50% chance that the parent will pass the mutated allele to each of his or her children. There is a 90% chance of penetrance if the abnormal allele is inherited. Therefore, the child's risk of developing retinoblastoma is the sum of 0.50×0.90, which is 0.45, or 45%.

42. **c.** A 2-year-old child with unilateral retinoblastoma at diagnosis is unlikely to develop disease in the other eye. Any tumors that form would most likely be peripheral to the macula and, with close surveillance, amenable to local treatment with laser or cryotherapy alone. Eyes classified as International Group E have the most advanced intraocular disease with limited visual potential. Tumors may invade the anterior chamber and ciliary body, and there may be associated neovascular glaucoma. Such eyes are unlikely to respond to conservative treatment measures.

43. **d.** Treatment of a patient with a metastasis to the eye should be individually tailored after consultation with the patient's oncologist. When the patient has other systemic metastases, systemic chemotherapy—which may also affect the ocular metastasis—may be considered. When there are multiple ocular metastases and chemotherapy is not planned, external-beam radiation may be considered. When the ocular metastasis is solitary and no other systemic metastases are known, brachytherapy may be the treatment of choice.

44. **a.** Retinal hemorrhages, typically white-centered hemorrhages, are the most common ocular manifestation of leukemia. Patients with leukemia and retinal hemorrhages typically have anemia and thrombocytopenia. The other findings are much less common.

45. **b.** Primary intraocular lymphoma (also known as *large cell lymphoma, vitreoretinal lymphoma,* or *retinal lymphoma*), occurs in 15%–25% of patients with primary central nervous system lymphoma (PCNSL). On the other hand, more than half of patients with primary intraocular lymphoma have or will develop PCNSL.

46. **a.** Leukemic retinopathy is characterized by intraretinal and preretinal (subhyaloidal) hemorrhages. The hemorrhages most often result from associated anemia or thrombocytopenia. Retinal hemorrhages may have white centers, so-called pseudo–Roth spots. Additional findings may include hard exudates, cotton-wool spots, and perivascular infiltrates.

Index

(*f* = figure; *t* = table)